# Classic Works
# in Medical Ethics

*Core Philosophical Readings*

# Classic Works
# in Medical Ethics
## Core Philosophical Readings

*EDITED BY*
### Gregory E. Pence
*Department of Philosophy*
*School of Medicine*
*University of Alabama at Birmingham*

Boston, Massachusetts   Burr Ridge, Illinois   Dubuque, Iowa
Madison, Wisconsin   New York, New York
San Francisco, California   St. Louis, Missouri

# McGraw-Hill

*A Division of The* **McGraw·Hill** *Companies*

CLASSIC WORKS IN MEDICAL ETHICS: CORE PHILOSOPHICAL READINGS

7 8 9 0 QWF/QWF 0 9 8

ISBN 978-0-07-038115-5
MHID 0-07-038115-1

Editorial director: *Philip Butcher*
Sponsoring editor: *Sarah Moyers*
Marketing manager: *Daniel M. Loch*
Project manager: *Robert A. Preskill*
Production supervisor: *Heather D. Burbridge*
Designer: *Michael Warrell*
Compositor: *Shepherd Incorporated*
Typeface: *10/12 Palatino*
Printer: *Quebecor Printing Book Group/Fairfield*

**Library of Congress Cataloging-in-Publication Data**

Classic works in medical ethics : core philosophical readings /
  edited by Gregory E. Pence.
    p.  cm.
   ISBN 0–07–038115–1
   1. Medical ethics.    I. Pence, Gregory E.
  R724.C524  1998
  174'.2--dc21
                                              97–1300

http://www.mhcollege.com

# About the Author

GREGORY E. PENCE is a professor in the Department of Philosophy and School of Medicine at the University of Alabama at Birmingham. For over two decades, he served on the Institutional Review Board on human experimentation. He is a past chair of the board for Birmingham AIDS Outreach. He has published in *Bioethics, Journal of the American Medical Association, American Philosophical Quarterly, Canadian Journal of Philosophy,* the *New York Times, Newsweek,* and *The Wall Street Journal.* He has twice won teaching awards, and he has given many talks on bioethics in places that include China and Israel.

# Contents

Part Six
# IMPERILED NEWBORNS

Part Seven
# EXPERIMENTATION AND ANIMALS

Part Eight
# JUST ALLOCATION OF SCARCE MEDICAL RESOURCES

Part Nine
# INVOLUNTARY PSYCHIATRIC TREATMENT

## Part Ten
## GENETIC INFORMATION AND GENETIC THERAPY

## Part Eleven
## JUSTICE, MEDICAL FINANCE, AND MEDICAL CARE

## Part Twelve
## AIDS

# *Preface*

Some professors teaching Medical Ethics want to ensure that students get a basic grounding in the core writings of the field. After thirty years, Medical Ethics has matured to where such a collection of core writings is now possible. Indeed, there is a growing danger that some of the classic articles will cease to be known because they are no longer included in "issue-of-the-year" anthologies.

This book offers:

1. Classic well-written articles that have stood the test of time and that have something to teach.
2. Articles with good philosophical analysis dealing with important topics and making significant contributions to understanding of issues.
3. An introductory essay discussing ethical theories and medical ethics.

This anthology includes no long, boring selections from government commissions or technical pieces from scientific journals. Most articles emphasize cogent philosophical analysis applied to classic problems in medical ethics. Many selections illustrate how and why philosophers contributed to the progress of medical ethics.

These articles cluster around several broad philosophical questions that have emerged over the past decades of Medical Ethics:

1. How active can ethical physicians be in *terminating* the lives of dying patients?
2. How active can ethical physicians be in *assisting* human life to begin outside the womb?
3. How active can ethical physicians be in *terminating* the beginnings of human life at embryonic, fetal, and newborn stages?
4. How should the circle of *personhood* be expanded and/or contracted to include and/or exclude certain types of beings, such as higher animals, fetuses, impaired newborns, and comatose patients?

5. How should *individual rights* be balanced against the *greater social good?*
6. Does anyone act so badly as not to deserve certain kinds of medical treatments?
7. By which *standard* should medicine justly *allocate* scarce medical resources where not everyone can get the resource and live?

Articles were selected in various ways by: (1) determining which articles have been reprinted the most and the longest in all the anthologies in medical ethics, (2) scanning the World Wide Web for syllabi in medical ethics to see what articles are actually used and assigned, (3) reviewing syllabi in Medical Ethics on file at the Kennedy Institute of Ethics Library, (4) perusing packets of articles on specific topics used to teach medical ethics by intensive seminars or Bioethics Centers around the United States, and (5) the advice of philosopher-reviewers who teach Medical Ethics to undergraduates.

Ultimately, selection of an article depended on the editor's reading of the article and affirmative answers to the questions: Is this a good piece of philosophical analysis? Does it discuss an important subject? Was it important to the field? Can undergraduate students profit from reading it? If a "yes" answer could be made to all four questions, the article was included.

I am especially indebted to Mark Waymack, the late David James, Mark Yarborough, and James Rachels for advice in editing this book. Phil Butcher, Alexis Walker, and Sarah Moyers were great at McGraw-Hill.

# Ethical Theories and Medical Ethics

## Gregory E. Pence

## THE GREEKS AND THE VIRTUES

The teachings of the major ancient Greek philosophers—Socrates, Plato, and Aristotle—as well as the general culture of fifth-century (B.C.E.) Athens—advocated virtue ethics, the ethical theory that emphasizes acquiring good traits of character. Virtue theory applied to medicine emphasizes creating physicians with such traits.

Our English word "ethics" derives from the Greek *ethos*, meaning "disposition" or "character." *Ethos* was an inseparable part of the Greek phrase *ethike aretai* (literally "skills of character"). The Greek word *arete* means at once "excellence," "good," and "skill." Our modern "ethics" builds on, but differs from, *ethike aretai* because two millennia of later theories of ethics built other meanings onto the original concept.

From at least as early as the time of Homer (sometime from eighth- to sixth-century B.C.E.), presocratic Greek ethics emphasized *ethike arete* in performing a role well. That is to say, the scope of ethical inquiry was limited to the roles one fulfilled. If one wanted to know about ethics, one asked about the traits of a good soldier, physician, mother, or ruler. For example, one would ask, "What is the goal of being a soldier?" Answer: "To defend one's country." Then one asks, "What excellences are needed to defend one's country?" Answer: physical strength, courage, skill in using weapons, organization in fighting in groups, temperance, and cunning.

Such ethics were teleological. In other words, they assumed that things developed towards a natural goal. In Greek medicine, if we want to know what makes a good physician, we need to know the purpose of medicine. That purpose is to heal the sick. What virtues are needed to do so? Answer: compassion, knowledge of healing, and skill in human relations.

1

Role-defined ethics remain powerful today and are the bases on which more universal principles build. For example, medical students first try to master the excellences of the traditional role of physicians before attempting to live by principles beyond that role.

Socrates, Plato, and Aristotle, in a combined move of ethical genius, attempted to transcend role-defined ethics and to argue that there were distinctive *ethika aretai* of a good person. What are they? In their view, they were the cardinal (primary) virtues of courage, temperance, wisdom, and justice (in dealing with people). These are the distinctive excellences necessary to function best in human society.

The implications of this view for medical ethics is that moral inquiry must not only ask, "What virtues should a good physician possess?" but also, "What virtues should a good person possess who happens to be a physician?" The narrow question is, "What should a good physician do?" The broader question is, "What should a *good person* do?"

Not all physicians in ancient times agreed about the role of a good physician, and here looms one of the great divides in medical ethics. Hippocrates and his brethren adopted not only a patient-centered ethics but also a sanctity-of-all-life worldview, holding that physicians should neither perform abortions nor assist in euthanasia of any kind. But most ancient Greek physicians took a *naturalistic* approach that was a precursor to the scientific worldview. In other words, they advocated forming conclusions based on what one could see and feel. These physicians did not practice medicine based on assumptions about gods and goddesses or about an afterlife, so they were more oriented to helping patients in the here-and-now. Accordingly, they often helped terminally ill patients to die. Most such Greek physicians adopted a quality-of-life view, believing that it was futile to maintain a life of pain and suffering that had little chance of amelioration. It is unclear whether their aid was role-defined, or whether it stemmed from compassion. In either case, the majority of naturalistic physicians used their factual knowledge and technical skills for very different evaluative ends than their Hippocratic counterparts.

## CHRISTIAN ETHICS, CHRISTIAN VIRTUES

By the fourth century C.E., Christianity had added its theological virtues of faith, hope, and charity to the list of human virtues. The paradigmatic virtue of compassion (charity) that many today associate with a good physician comes in part from Christianity's emphasis on helping others. The etymological root of "compassion" means "to suffer with," as Jesus of Nazareth is held by Christians to have suffered with, and for, humans on the cross.

Here we have two differences of emphasis that later came to be fused. Where naturalistic physicians emphasized technical competence in curing disease, religious physicians emphasized compassion in *being with* patients. When the limits of technical competence had been reached—as they were often reached very soon during these centuries—compassion became the supreme virtue. Both traditions contributed to today's definition of good physicians: every patient wants a physician who is both knowledgeable and merciful.

Virtue ethics in medicine also underlies the apprentice system of medical education, in which young medical students gradually assume more responsibility by assisting older physicians in treating patients. The attending physician teaches the resident, who teaches the intern, who teaches the third year student. What is taught, theoretically, is not only how to perform a procedure but also how to be compassionate, wise, courageous, and patient-centered.

What would virtue ethics say about a particular issue in medical ethics? The general answer is that with every new case, the physician-in-training should imitate the reasoning and empathy of good physicians. Thus confronted with a 14-year-old patient who refuses to eat after being partially paralyzed after an auto accident, most experienced physicians are likely to say, "Let's work with him until he's of legal age, then he can decide for himself. By that time, he'll probably find a reason to live."

It should be emphasized that Socratic virtues also celebrated an elitist, anti-democratic ethics that scorned the ordinary person and his worth. The Greeks believed themselves superior to all the peoples they had conquered. Aristotle's student, Alexander the Great, attempted to instill Greek values, culture, and language on everyone, and he had no tolerance for the cultures of other, "inferior" peoples. The Greek ethics that Alexander inherited was perfectionistic, aristocratic, and meritocratic. In this sense, the quality-of-life attitude of ancient Greek physicians was elitist and perfectionistic, whereas the sanctity-of-life ethic of Hippocratic physicians was much less so.

In contrast to Greek elitism, the three great religions of the West emphasize duties to the poor and sick: the rabbinic ethics of Bar Hillel stress acts that help one's fellow man; Jesus says that as you treat the poor, so you treat Him; and Mohammed made the *zakat,* the tax on property for the poor, one of the pillars of Islam. So for a Jew, Christian, or Moslem, a good physician is first a Jew, Christian, or Moslem, and second a physician.

As such, a good Christian physician must care for the poor as part of his duties as a physician. To put this point in more religious terms, the physician's license, knowledge, and wisdom is not a proprietary right to make money but an instrument of a higher calling from God. In the movie, *Chariots of Fire,* the Presbyterian Olympic runner says, "I run not for me but to glorify the Lord" and for this reason refuses to compete on the sabbath. Similarly, to use a medical degree only to make money is to abase a degree given in trust for a higher cause.

One area in which the contrast between religious and nonreligious ethics in medicine becomes salient is in thinking about genetics. Greek ethics advocated eugenics ("good birth"). Plato advocated mystery-shrouded mating festivals where those men judged to be "most perfect" would impregnate similar females. For Plato, breeding would be arranged to perfect humanity, not by choice or for love. Just as the Greeks improved the stock of their animals by selective breeding, so Plato wanted to improve humans. Just as the young Greek gentleman should try to perfect his body and life as a work of art, so human society should try to perfect itself by creating better children.

In contrast, the three western religious traditions have preached for centuries that the goal of human life has been either to create a God-based society on earth or to save the most souls for the afterlife. Accordingly, western religions have resisted attempts to tamper with the genes of humans, asserting that humans were created in the image of God and denying that humans should try to perfect themselves through genetics. (In modern times, however, some liberal believers have argued that eliminating genetic disease is not sinful.)

Applying virtue ethics to medical ethics has several limitations. One is that it has little to say about how to make particular, ethical decisions, aside from the injunction to imitate good physicians. Another limitation is that as ethics becomes more role-defined, the less it meets universal standards. Finally, both religious and nonreligious theories of the virtues tend to emphasize the status quo over fundamental, social change. One outcome is that physicians adopting a traditional role tend to be paternalistic, treating patients as children and overruling their decisions.

## NATURAL LAW THEORY

It has become a truism that when the Romans conquered Greece (in the second century B.C.E.), they themselves were conquered by many aspects of Greek culture. The Stoic philosophers of Roman times elevated one aspect of the Greek world view to a higher level. Rules for human beings, the Stoics argued, were so embedded in the texture of the world that they were "law" for humans. These came to be known as "natural laws." They were apprehended by unaided reason, in other words, without Scripture or divine revelation.

Behind the notion of a natural law, of course, is that of a hidden law-giver. In the eleventh century, Thomas Aquinas synthesized many aspects of Aristotelianism with what had become orthodox teachings of the Christian church. Aquinas made explicit the connection between God and the natural laws of the world: a rational god made the world work rationally and gave humans reason to discover his rational, natural laws. Studying ethical theory was a rational process of discovery about the world that revealed rules about how humans should act. Correct *descriptions* of the world would yield correct *prescriptions* about how to act. To act rationally was to act morally, which in turn was to act in accordance with natural law.

One thing that these rules commanded was to go against one's natural feelings. St. Augustine taught in the fourth century C.E. that human nature was contaminated by sin and, as such, human feelings were mired in lust, sloth, avarice, and the other deadly sins. In stunning contrast to modern times, Aquinas held that thinking about ethics was emphatically *not* about examining one's feelings. Instead, it was a matter of following rules laid down by God and his agents, the clergy and theologians of the Church.

An example of natural law theory in medical ethics concerns homosexuality. Aquinas believed that God made two sexes for procreation and that it was natural and rational for a man and woman to mate to have children. On the other hand, for two people of the same gender to have sex (or form a lifelong union) was contrary to natural law, and hence, immoral.

One problem with natural law theory is seen in the above example in that what is considered "against natural law" may vary over the centuries. Many rational people today do not consider homosexuality to be unnatural, especially because it has been practiced since the beginning of human history and because some great cultures, such as the ancient Greeks, celebrated it as ideal.

As another example of problems of natural law theory, consider sex in marriage. Augustine held that the *only* permissible justification for sexual relations between a man and wife was to produce children. Modern Catholic teaching is very different, and regards loving sexual relations between man and wife as natural and good, even when there is no desire to have children. Indeed, the Catholic Church today holds *in vitro* fertilization to be immoral precisely *because* no act of loving sex is involved between man and woman.

Natural law theory bequeathed to medical ethics the famous *doctrine of double effect*. This doctrine held that if an action had two effects, one good and the other evil, the evil was morally permitted: (1) if the action was good in itself or not evil, (2) if the good followed as immediately from the cause as did the evil effect, (3) if only the good effect was intended, and (4) if there was as important a reason for performing the action as for allowing the evil effect. For example, exceptions could be made to the rule banning abortions in cases of an ectopic pregnancy (an embryo growing in a fallopian tube) and a cancerous uterus (where uterus and fetus had to be removed together). In both cases, this doctrine allowed abortions if the direct intention was to save the life of the mother. Similarly, the doctrine of double effect would not allow physicians to assist in executions, since it would not allow a direct intention to assist in the taking of a life, although it might allow a physician to be present to ease the suffering of a prisoner in the event of a botched execution.

Also derived from the natural law tradition is the *principle of totality,* which covers what kinds of changes may be made to the human body: changes are permitted only to ensure the proper functioning of the total body. The underlying idea is that one's body is not something that one owns, but that one holds in trust for God: "The body is the temple of the Lord." So a gangrenous leg may be amputated or a cancerous breast removed, because the fundamental health of the body is at risk from these threats. According to this principle, we are given our bodies as they are for a reason and we should not change our bodies for frivolous reasons. Thus the principle of totality rules out all forms of sterilization to prevent pregnancy—vasectomy, tubal ligation, and hysterectomy—because producing pregnancy is a natural function of the bodies of men and women. The principle also forbids cosmetic surgery solely to change one's appearance, such as breast reduction, breast augmentation, rhinoplasty, and liposuction.

This principle is more deeply embedded in our thinking than we may at first think. When a news photograph in 1996 showed a mouse whose genetic system had been altered to grow a human ear on its back, many people felt disgust at seeing this mouse-with-human-ear. This disgust arose from a sense that the creation of this being had violated the bodily integrity of both humans and mice.

## SOCIAL CONTRACT THEORIES

Social contract theory, or contractarianism, is essentially secular, independent of belief in God. Contractarians assume that people are fundamentally self-interested and that moral rules have evolved for humans to get along with one another. It is rational for humans to agree to such rules because otherwise, everyone will pick up the sword and be worse off.

Social contract theory does not separate ethics from politics. Indeed, hypothetical political bargaining is viewed as the foundation of the kind of behavior that is allowed as ethical. (*Hypothetical* because contractarians do not believe people ever came together to make the basic social contract.) Plato described one early kind of hypothetical social contract in *The Republic,* but the philosopher who really gave this theory weight was the Englishman, Thomas Hobbes (1588–1679).

Hobbes believed that the most detestable condition for humans was the state of nature, a premoral agglomeration of self-interested individuals for whom life was (he said, famously) "solitary, poor, nasty, brutish, and short." By the use of their reason, people realize that each is better off in a society of moral and legal rules backed by the force of opinion and law. They therefore form a social contract to create "society" to better themselves.

Contractarianism can support both minimal and maximal government. To oversimplify, let us contrast two extreme champions of contractarianism: Libertarians and Rawlsians.

*Libertarians* favor government for defense and for very limited public works, perhaps not even including national parks or a public interstate road system (we could have private, toll roads). They disfavor government programs such as Medicare, Medicaid, disability insurance, food stamps, and welfare. Libertarians oppose forced taxation by the government, especially when it redistributes property and income from rich to poor. They champion the property rights of the status quo, but tend to be silent about how those enjoying the status quo acquired their property. Libertarian philosophers such as Harvard's Robert Nozick see forced taxation as equivalent to forced labor, that is, to slavery.

Accordingly, Libertarians oppose mandatory F.I.C.A. taxes on all workers' pay for Medicare and for the Hospital Insurance Trust Fund. Even though federal programs such as Medicare have made American physicians rich, libertarian physicians would rather have no government control over their business. Presumably, in a libertarian society, physicians would be reimbursed only in cash.

Critics say that in such a system, fewer hospitals would be built, elderly patients would frequently forgo procedures for lack of money (as never happens under Medicare), and physicians would earn far less money. It is also true that in such a system physicians would be controlled by no federal regulations.

*Rawlsians* are named for John Rawls, a Harvard colleague of Nozick. Rawls believes that the social contract should have moral restraints imposed on it. The most important restraint is what Rawls called "the veil of ignorance," meaning that in the hypothetical social contract, no one would know his or her age, gender, race, health, number of children, income, wealth, or other arbitrary personal information. Rawls' theory is contractarian in that it assumes that people are self-interested and are forced to form a social contract to choose the basic institutions of their society; on the other hand, it is Kantian (as we shall see in the next section) in that it imposes impartiality on the choosers.

Rawls argues, controversially, that the only rational way to choose under the veil of ignorance is as if one might be the least well-off person in society (because a person doesn't know anything personal under the veil, he doesn't know what place in society he occupies). This justifies the choice of his famous *difference principle:* choosers should opt for institutions creating equality unless a difference favors the least well-off group. Everyone should be trained in medicine unless training only a few is better for the least well-off. The choice of the difference principle, as the archprinciple of this theory of justice, can be seen as the imposition of the golden rule on the choice of the structure of society.

Rawlsian justice entails that every citizen should have equal access to medical care unless unequal access favored the poor (an unlikely prospect!). Rawlsian justice attempts to reduce the natural inequalities of fate; hence, it is especially important that children and those with genetic disease have good medical care. Let us consider these two classes combined: children with genetic disease. Their care takes up a large share of resources in children's hospitals, and costs for their care may be deliberately excluded in for-profit insurance plans. Nevertheless, for Rawls, such children deserve good medical care as a matter of justice.

Indeed, as genetics reveals new insights every year, we stand now under a real, not hypothetical, genetic veil of ignorance about our future illnesses and those of our children and grandchildren. The coming decade will identify much more precisely who is susceptible to genetic disease and who is not. In the future, it may be much more difficult for those with familial lines of genetic disease to purchase private medical insurance. Some of the people now attacking national medical plans may find themselves at risk.

Libertarians favor private medical insurance plans in which the healthy do not subsidize the unhealthy. Rawlsians see "healthy" and "unhealthy" as arbitrary distinctions, due more to genetics and fate than individual merit. Libertarians would allow for-profit companies to practice experience rating, whereby citizens with preexisting illness may be excluded (and genetic disease is increasingly being defined in this way). Rawlsians favor community rating, whereby risk and premium rates are spread over all members of a large community, such as a state or nation (for example, a federal, single-payer system).

# KANTIAN ETHICS

John Rawls is a modern Kantian using a social contract methodology. Immanuel Kant (1724–1804) published during the Enlightenment (that is, about the time of the American Revolution), and believed in the power of humans to use reason to solve their problems.

Kant was raised by conservative Protestant parents and was strongly oriented to conservative religious ethics until he studied science at his university, whereupon he became skeptical of his former beliefs. He continued to believe that many of the basic values and attitudes of Christian ethics were correct, but then he had a problem of how to justify those values. His solution was to base those values on abstract reason rather than on metaphysical beliefs about God or an afterlife.

The distinctive elements of Kantian ethics are these:

*a. Ethics is not a matter of consequences but of duty.*   Why an act is done is more important than its good or bad results. Specifically, an act must be done from the right motive, and the right motive is the desire to do one's moral duty. In its emphasis on motives and not consequences, Kant's ethics are Christian.

Kant's ethics are an ethics of duty (also called *deontological,* from *deontos,* duty) because they emphasize not having the right desires or feelings, but acting correctly according to obligation. Only acts done from duty, and not, say, from compassion, are praiseworthy. For Kant, the correct motive for treating a patient well is not because a physician feels like doing so, but because it is the right thing to do. When we act morally, Kant says, reason tells feelings what to do. Contrary to popular culture, we should not consult our feelings about what to do but reflect upon what is our duty.

Kant says the only thing valuable in the world is a good will, the trait of character indicating a willingness to choose the right act simply because it's right. But how do we know what is right? What is our duty? Kant gives two formulations.

*b. A right act has a maxim that is universalizable.*   An act is right if one can will its "maxim" or rule to be acted on by all others. "Lie to get out of keeping a promise" cannot be so willed because if everyone acted this way, promise-keeping would mean nothing.

*c. A right act always treats other humans as ends-in-themselves, never as a mere means.*   To treat another person as an "end in himself" is to treat him as having absolute, infinite moral worth, not relative worth. His welfare cannot be sacrificed to the good of others or to my own desires. So patients cannot unwittingly be used as guinea pigs in dangerous medical experiments to advance knowledge.

Consider the case of a pulmonary resident who discovers that he missed a small lesion three months previously on the X-ray of a 48-year-old patient. The patient now has level four untreatable cancer. The patient says, "I guess that cancer just grew out of nowhere because it wasn't there three months ago." Should the resident tell the patient the truth? A consequentialist might argue that he should not because it could do no good for the patient.

But for Kant, the answer is clear: the patient must be told the truth. Why? The only universalizable rule is "Always tell patients the truth." Such a rule is the basis of trust and of treating patients as "ends in themselves." If the physician was a patient, he would want to know the truth. The resident may *feel* that he shouldn't reveal the truth but his reason will tell him what his duty is.

**d. People are only free when they act rationally.** Kant would agree that much of how we act is governed by our emotions and other, nonrational parts of upbringing. But controversially, Kant denies that we are truly acting morally when we do the right thing because we are accustomed to it, because it feels right, or because our society favors the act. The only time a person can act morally is when she exercises her rational, free will to understand why certain rules are right and then chooses to bind her actions to those rules. Kant calls the capacity to act this way, *autonomy*. For him, it gives humans higher worth than animals.

It follows for Kant that very few people act morally. Kant accepts that fact. It was also true that in early Christianity, very few people were thought to be capable of salvation. The purity of Kant's view entails a moral elitism for the few who can successfully follow Kantian ethics.

Kantian ethics has several problems. First, Kant is regarded as the supreme rationalist in ethics because he claimed that anyone who disagreed with his view was guilty of a logical contradiction. But the utilitarian lifeboat commander, when he will not let everyone board to save those in the boat, does not contradict himself (he can will the maxim, *All those in control of lifeboats should maximize survivors, even if it means denying access to some in the water.*)

Kant is generally regarded as failing in his Enlightenment project. His critic and contemporary, the Scottish skeptic, David Hume, came close to arguing that ethics is nothing more than inculcated, socially valuable, feelings. This view in ethics is called *emotivism*. Charles Darwin and the father of psychiatry, Sigmund Freud, later agreed with Hume that reason is the tip of the moral iceberg because much of ethical life is emotional and not changeable by reason. Emotivism and Kant's rationalism are the two extreme views on the issue of the place of reason in ethics: the truth undoubtedly lies somewhere in between.

Other problems of Kantian ethics remain. For one thing, it fails to tell us how to resolve conflicts between competing, universalizable maxims. Its best answer is to try to universalize whatever ad-hoc solution to the conflict seems appropriate. But then our sense of what is appropriate, not our ability to universalize without contradiction, is the test of an act's morality. For another thing, it seems ridiculous to imply that consequences never count morally. Many critics believe that Kantians indirectly appeal to consequences in thinking about what to universalize. Finally, the ideal of treating each person as if he had infinite value is not always practical: it does not tell us how to deliberate about tradeoffs when, by definition, some humans will die in triage situations and cannot be treated as "ends in themselves."

Nevertheless, Kant provides useful insights to medical ethics. He would favor using a lottery to distribute a lifesaving but expensive new drug that most patients will be unable to obtain. His emphasis on people as "ends in themselves" explains the outrage that people have felt when learning of scandals involving medical experimentation, such as research done by Nazi physicians. Finally, perhaps Kant's most important legacy to modern medical ethics is his emphasis on the "autonomous will" of the free, rational individual as the seat of moral value. Autonomy explains why informed consent is necessary to legitimate participation in an experiment. When combined with the emphasis on personal liberty in our democracies, Kant's emphasis on autonomy sets the stage for modern medical ethics.

## UTILITARIANISM

Utilitarianism originated in late 18th and early 19th century England as a secular replacement for Christian ethics. Jeremy Bentham (1748–1832) and John Stuart Mill (1806–1873) were its two chief theorists. The essential idea of utilitarianism is that right acts should produce the greatest amount of good for the greatest number of people, which is called "utility."

The Puritans in England and America wanted to organize society so that everyone had to obey their rules, but utilitarians saw morality as a human construct that should minimize harms of humans to each other and maximize group welfare. For Christians, Jews, or Muslims, morality is inconceivable without God's existence, but not so for utilitarians.

Likened to the counterculture movement of students in the 1960s and 1970s, utilitarianism was a reform movement intended to humanize outmoded institutions. Developed by social reformers Jeremy Bentham and James Mill (the father of John Stuart Mill), it focused on large, practical changes that could benefit the vast majority of people who were not aristocrats.

Utilitarianism did not urge people to turn the other cheek and hope for justice in another life, nor did it exalt those virtues so cherished by England's aristocracy: stylish dress and manners, personal honor, literacy, scientific and artistic accomplishment, and patriotism. The foundation for reform came in 1832 in eliminating pocket boroughs under the control of one great landlord and in extending the vote to the 20 percent of the adult male population who had some property (propertyless males and women still had no vote). Utilitarian reformers also campaigned against slavery in the British empire and the intolerable factory conditions made famous by Charles Dickens in novels such as *Hard Times*. (Their Factory Act forbade employment of children under age nine in cotton mills and declared that thirteen-year-olds could work no more than twelve hours a day.) Similar bills were passed to make mining and industrial machinery less lethal to workers.

They also attacked the penal system, passed the Corn Laws, ended debtor's prison, opposed capital punishment for petty thefts, and advocated the vote for women. They urged public hospitals for the poor, proper sewage disposal, the penny post so that everyone could send and get mail, and created a central board of health, so that municipalities could create facilities for clean water, waste disposal, and sewers.

Utilitarianism's essence can be summed up in four basic tenets:

1. *Consequentialism:* Consequences count, not motives or intentions.
2. *The maximization principle:* The number of people affected by consequences matters; the more people, the more important the effect.
3. *A theory of value* (or of "good"): Good consequences are defined by pleasure (*hedonic utilitarianism*) or what people prefer (*preference utilitarianism*).
4. *A scope-of-morality premise:* Each being's happiness is to count as one and no more.

For utilitarians, right acts produce the (2) greatest amount of (3) good (1) consequences for the (2) greatest number of (4) beings.

Each of these tenets can be controversial. Bentham emphasized that the meaning of the fourth tenet was whether a being could suffer, not whether it was human or animal. As such, utilitarianism includes animals in its calculations of the *greatest number*.

To the modern utilitarian Peter Singer (and author of the famous *Animal Liberation*), utilitarianism was in advance of its time in not differentiating between the sufferings of humans and those of animals. Utilitarianism also seems to imply that every being's happiness on the planet matters, not just beings of my society. Singer also says that morality doesn't stop at the borders of his country.

Virtue ethicists and Kantians regard a person's motives as a sign of his character. John Stuart Mill says that the drowning man doesn't care why the lifeguard is swimming out to sea to rescue him, just that the lifeguard is coming. Utilitarians think motives only count insofar as they tend to produce the greatest good.

In medicine, it makes a difference whether a physician listens because she really cares about patients or because she's found that having satisfied patients is an effective way to maximize income. A utilitarian might argue that if the physician's techniques are good enough, whether she really cares about her patients matters very little; in either case, the behavior produces good consequences to real people.

Utilitarianism is also a theory of value (that is, a theory about what is a harmful consequence and about what is a good one). The simplest theory of value is *hedonic utilitarianism,* which equates a good consequence with pleasure, and harm with pain. *Negative utilitarianism* focuses on relieving the greatest misery for the greatest number, as in famine relief. *Positive utilitarianism* focuses on benefiting humanity. Utilitarian theorists debate whether some things are intrinsically valuable, such as pride and honor, or whether they are good only because they create good feelings in people over the longrun. A compromise view is called *preference utilitarianism,* and its adherents believe that utility is maximized by furthering the actual preferences that people have. Preference utilitarianism is compatible with a base of subjective feelings in ethics, whereas intrinsic value utilitarianism is not.

The maximization tenet can get utilitarians into trouble. Wouldn't utilitarianism be willing to violate the traditional sanctity-of-life principle to save many people? Here, utilitarians bite the bullet. They think that the Nazi generals who tried to kill Hitler in 1944 at Wolf's Lair were justified. They think that on the expedition to the South Pole, commander Robert Scott should have allowed his crew member with the gangrenous leg to die, rather than slowing down the whole party by carrying the injured man, which resulted in the death of all. They think that if an FBI sniper saw a terrorist about to detonate a bomb in a skyscraper full of innocent people, the sniper should shoot the terrorist.

These are the easy cases. The hard ones come in population policy. If more happiness is better than less, why shouldn't we create the maximal number of people on the planet? So long as each new life has more happiness than misery, and so long as everyone else's life has at least the same, shouldn't we produce more? This "total view" of utilitarianism is universally seen as what philosopher Derek Parfit calls "The Repugnant Conclusion," because we think the average happiness is more important. But it is difficult to see why utilitarianism entails maximizing average happiness and not the total good, so it may be stuck with this counterintuitive implication.

More specifically to medical ethics, wouldn't utilitarianism permit the sacrifice of an innocent, healthy person to transfer his organs to four patients who needed them to live? Aren't four people alive better than one? If consequences and number of lives define morality, what's morally wrong with doing so? Yet it certainly seems morally wrong to chop up an innocent patient this way.

One traditional reply among utilitarians is to distinguish between *act* and *rule* utilitarianism. Rule utilitarians believe that normal moral rules, such as "First, do no harm" in medicine, maximize utility over the decades. Act utilitarians advocate judging each act's utility. Some act utilitarians think rule utilitarianism has a dilemma: if there are exceptions, then you ultimately have act utilitarianism (since you never know in advance whether a particular situation needs to be judged as an exception); if there are no exceptions, then you are close to a Kantian and only a nominal utilitarian. If "First, do no harm" has no exceptions in medical ethics, it may explain why it is wrong to chop up an innocent person to transplant his organs to four others.

In medicine, the two areas where utilitarianism applies most powerfully are public health and triage situations. It is likely that improvements in public health have helped more people live longer (created more "utility") than all the drugs and surgeries ever invented. The English physician John Snow might have agreed: in 1849 he advocated clean water to prevent cholera epidemics, which were spread by contaminated water. (It took forty years and many more cholera epidemics for Snow's ideas to prevail.) It doesn't matter why Snow improved the water supply, only that he did and that many millions of people now live decades longer.

Triage involves the apportionment of scarce resources during emergencies when circumstances preordain that not all victims will live. Because consequences count, utilitarianism says a physician should not treat each patient equally, but should focus only on those whom he can actually benefit. Rigorous application of this principle gives utilitarianism its famous hard edge: a physician should abandon those who will *die* even if he helps and, just as ruthlessly, abandon those who will *live* without his help. He should help only those who waver between life and death and for whom he can make the difference. The goal is to save the maximal number of lives.

This point illustrates an ambiguity in sanctity-of-life ethics. Traditionally, sanctity-of-life ethics such as Kant's emphasize the absolute value of each individual, implying that the physician should at least comfort those who are beyond his help. But utilitarian-triage ethics maximizes the value of life in saving the maximal number of people who will eventually live.

## PRINCIPLES AND MEDICAL ETHICS

One modern method of analysis is to analyze a dilemma or case of medical ethics in terms of four powerful principles. According to advocates of this method, deciding what is the right thing to do in a particular case involves applying and balancing all four principles. These principles are clearly chosen as a distillation of the ethical theories described above.

What do each of the principles mean? *Autonomy* refers to the right to make decisions about one's own life and body without coercion by others. This principle celebrates the value that democracies place on allowing individuals to make their own decisions about whom to marry, whether to have children, how many children to have, what kind of career to pursue, and what kind of life they want to live. Insofar as is possible in a democracy, and to the extent that their decisions do not harm others, individuals should be left alone to make fundamental medical decisions that affect their own bodies and lives.

John Stuart Mill was a political theorist as well as an ethical theorist. In his most famous work of politics, *On Liberty* (1859), he defends "one very simple principle," his so-called *harm principle*: that "the only purpose for which power can rightfully be exercised over any member of a civilized community, against his will, is to prevent harm to others. His own good, either physical or moral, is not a sufficient warrant . . . Over himself, over his own body and mind, the individual is sovereign."

Such political individualism corresponds to personal autonomy in ethics. Since the beginnings of modern medical ethics in the early 1960s, autonomy has meant the patient's right to make her own decisions about her body, including dying and reproduction.

The ethics of autonomy evolved as a rejection of paternalistic ethics. During the patient rights movement in the early 1960s in America, paternalistic physicians were scorned as sexist octogenarians who would impose their rigid traditions on a more enlightened, freethinking, younger generation. Both secular and religious versions of virtue ethics tend to be paternalistic, especially when they emphasize the physician's greater wisdom and when they teach young physicians to follow the lead of older physicians in ignoring wishes of patients. These traditional, somewhat rigid, secular and religious roles of good physicians contrast starkly with the dominant value of more universal, modern theories of ethics, including the principle of individual autonomy.

In the first two decades of bioethics (1962–1982), autonomy was considered by many bioethicists to be the supreme value above all others, grounding the right of competent adults to end their lives when they choose and to decline to participate in dangerous experiments. Since then, bioethicists have realized that other values are also important, which must be weighed with autonomy in dictating answers in particular cases.

*Beneficence,* "doing good to others," is clearly tied to the Judaeo-Christian-Muslim virtue of compassion and helping others. The application of the principle of beneficence comes to the fore in efforts to distinguish therapeutic from nontherapeutic experiments on patients. If a physician means to help diabetic patients, an experiment on diabetic patients (with their consent) is justified by this principle. If the experiment is nontherapeutic, some other justification is required.

Beneficence can be seen both as a principle and as a virtue for physicians. Physicians receive special powers, income, and prestige from society. In return they are asked to dedicate their careers to helping others. Medical training requires this trait as demands on a student increase between premedical years and residency. Self-sacrifice is part of medicine. Ideally, physicians should want to help others, but if the internal desire is lacking, they should still help others from a sense of duty. The principle of beneficence spells out this duty.

Beneficence may sometimes come into conflict with autonomy (as, indeed, any of these principles may conflict with each of the others in a particular case). Consider the involuntary psychiatric commitment of schizophrenic, homeless people. Is it better to let such people wander the cold streets of a big city, or to incarcerate and medicate them against their will? Should we let them "die with their rights on" or inject them with sedatives and antipsychotic drugs "for their own good"? Maybe we should do nothing at all and not risk making them worseoff. After all, who are we to say that it is "beneficent" to do so? Maybe homeless schizophrenics want to stay as they are. How beneficence and autonomy are balanced in particular cases is not easy to understand. (Indeed, since John Stuart Mill advocated both utilitarianism and the value of autonomy, critics have wondered whether his views were actually consistent.)

*Nonmaleficence,* "not harming others," echoes an ancient maxim of professional medical ethics, "First, do not harm." Above all, this maxim implies that if a physician is not technically competent to do something, he shouldn't do it. So medical students should not harm a patient by practicing on them (unless the patient consents): patients are there to be helped, not to help students learn. At the very least, patients should not leave an encounter with a physician worse-off than they were before. This crucial principle of medical ethics prohibits corruption, incompetence, and dangerous, nontherapeutic experiments.

The principle of nonmaleficence also accords with Mill's harm principle and contractarianism: both of these are minimalist moralities implying that the state and society should not attempt to shape all citizens' lives for the goals of one worldview. In a fundamental sense, the first obligation we have is to leave one another alone, especially those who do not want our help, advice, or even concern. That means, above all else, not harming others by unsolicited intrusions.

The last principle, *justice,* has both a social and a political interpretation. Socially, it means treating similar kinds of people similarly (this is the so-called "formal element" of the larger principle). A just physician treats each patient the same, regardless of his insurance coverage.

Politically, the principle amounts to distributive justice, and thus in medicine, to the allocation of scarce medical resources. Because there are many theories of justice, this principle is not self-evident. For example, Rawls' theory of justice demands that medicine serve the worseoff people. But another view equates justice with simple egalitarianism: medicine is just if it treats each patient equally. Of course, that goal would not be easy to achieve either, and doing so would go a long way towards realizing Rawls's ideal. At the very least, it would mean a guarantee of equal access to medical care for every citizen, such that insurance coverage would not be a factor (as it is now) in selection of which patient receives an organ transplant. Finally, justice can be interpreted in a libertarian sense of treating anyone with the ability to pay the same. In this sense, it means not treating people who can not pay.

It is obvious that interpretation of the principle of justice is difficult, especially when an interpretation of this principle must be used with the three other principles in a particular case. However, in the most normal sense, justice requires physicians to treat patients impartially, without bias on account of gender, race, sexuality, or wealth. Even in such a minimal sense, justice requires a high standard of behavior among physicians.

## FEMINIST ETHICS: THE ETHICS OF CARE

In the early 1970s a modern version of feminism shook American medicine to its foundations and buttressed its sister movement, the patient's rights movement. Both movements attempted to take patients' decisions about their bodies and lives away from physicians—especially male physicians—and give women and patients control.

The landmark book was *Our Bodies, Ourselves,* by a group of dissatisfied women patients in Boston who had access to one of the grandest—some would say, most self-satisfied—medical centers in the world, Harvard. Because they couldn't get the information they wanted in down-to-earth, patient-friendly language, they published a "how-to" manual covering everything from breast cancer to abortions. Successive editions sold millions upon millions of copies and gave rise to the areas of publishing now called "alternative medicine" and "self-help."

During the 1980s feminist philosophers began to question whether many ways of knowing were *the* ways or merely *male* ways. Contractarianism, Kantianism, and utilitarianism all looked like male theories, too abstract, too intellectual, and largely false to the ordinary experience of many women. What was missing was emphasis on values such as cooperation, nurturing, and bonding.

Harvard education professor Carol Gilligan showed that many women analyzed ethical dilemmas differently from men. Subsequently, feminist theorists articulated theories of ethics whose central notions were not rights or universalization but caring, trust, and relationships. This so-called "ethics of care" may be considered a branch of virtue ethics that promotes the "female" virtues of caring, nurturing, trust, intimate friendship, and love. Even among feminist theorists, this statement is controversial because some theorists believe that such virtues are not inherent in women by nature but exist only because they are encouraged in most women by traditional, sexist, gender roles.

One might view the ethics of care as a corrective to the previous emphasis in ethical theory on abstract, semilegalistic concepts. Alternately, one might consider the ethics of care as reflecting a modern turning inward to the family and to those around one, fighting battles close at hand and letting far-off concerns such as world hunger take care of themselves. Finally, one might view this approach as taking a more modest, minimalist approach to morality—a kind of "within-my-circle-of-relationships" approach—in which moral concerns usually arise among those one knows.

Perhaps the ethics of care is best seen as an antidote to moral views that are cast only in terms of rights, utility, and duty. It is not yet a complete ethical theory, for it does not tell us how to treat people we do not know or care about. This is an important criticism in medical ethics because much of medicine is about treating strangers, at least when patients first meet a physician. It may be retorted that good physicians should care for all their patients, but the meaning of "care" gets too diluted when someone claims they care about everyone they meet. Nor does this theory yet tell us how to resolve conflicts among those we care about, such as when a female physician is torn between checking on a patient and being with her daughter at the birth of her first grandchild. This theory, however, is still very young and over coming decades, may have more to offer.

## CASE-BASED REASONING

Many physicians and medical ethicists do not find any of the theories described above very useful to their practice of medicine. To force the complexities of many medical cases into a preconceived, abstract frame-work is often to be guilty of oversimplification, and when that happens, the truth is rarely discovered.

In the past decade a new approach has been articulated that bases moral reasoning on paradigms or model cases. These paradigmatic cases serve as a basis from which a person can generalize to other, similar cases. For example, both Karen Quinlan and Nancy Cruzan were young women who went into lifelong comas called "persistent vegetative states" after, respectively, a drug overdose in 1975 and an automobile accident in 1983. In both cases, parents de-cided after many months that their daughter's biography was over and wanted to end the mere life of the remaining body. Karen Quinlan's case focused on re-moval of a respirator; Nancy Cruzan's on removal of a feeding tube. Both cases resulted in landmark legal decisions in, respectively, 1976 and 1990.

Advocates of case-based reasoning believe that study of these two famous cases can teach us a lot about how ethics in medicine has actually worked over the last two decades. Paradigms are bedrock cases from which we generalize in ever-expanding circles of similarity. By understanding and analyzing argu-ments on both sides—about killing and letting die, ordinary versus extraordi-nary treatment, forgoing versus withdrawing treatment, standards of brain death, and models of proxy consent for making decisions about incompetent patients—we can hope to increase our understanding of related issues in med-ical ethics.

Because thousands of patients may end up in comas like those of Karen Quinlan and Nancy Cruzan, studying how decisions were handled in their fa-mous cases can teach us how to handle future cases better. Case-based reason-ing is very similar to the method of case-analysis of some famous business schools and the traditional teaching on rounds in medical schools. It is much the same as an ancient method of theological reasoning called "casuistry," and some bioethicists with theological training today use this word to describe this orientation.

Case-based reasoning does not deny that ethical theories and moral rea-soning play roles in moral life. When these are relevant to a case, they must be discussed. It is just that when they are relevant, we need not study ethical the-ory to see their relevance. If a patient has been abused in a nontherapeutic, psychiatric experiment, we do not need to understand much about the princi-ple of justice to understand that the patient has been abused. In short, how all the different ingredients of the "ethical recipe" go together to bake a good re-sult can be judged only in terms of the complex details of each case, not in terms of preset formulas.

Case-based reasoning does deny that any overarching ethical principle of morality can guide us in making day-to-day ethical decisions in medicine. Each situation or case will present a unique array of people, interests, conflicting principles, incompatible role-duties, strong passions, and concerns about the larger good, about resources, about institutional policies, and about political consequences. Each set of circumstances will require what the Greeks called *phronesis*, or practical judgment, to find the optimal solution for all parties.

## CONCLUSION

The study of ethical theories enlightens the study of modern medical ethics, but the study of modern medical ethics is not the same as merely applying one ethical theory to a case. The study of these theories does not give us a definitive, absolute answer to each case in medical ethics. Our society has inherited many different ethical theories from the past, the most important of which have been sketched above. Although each theory has its champions who believe that it alone is completely correct, most sophisticated people today believe that the best part of each of these theories needs to guide us in a particular case, such that in analyzing some cases, we will use parts of many different theories together.

The study of how these theories originated and continue today gives us insights about how to solve some problems in medical ethics. Although this may seem a weak conclusion about the importance of ethical theories, it has the advantage of being true. Given our limited tools of reasoning in ethics, any valuable tool is welcome, and knowledge of such ethical theories is certainly one such tool.

## PART ONE

# Allowing Death to Occur in Incompetent Patients

# Active and Passive Euthanasia

## James Rachels

*One of the most controversial questions of the past few decades has been about how active physicians can be in bringing about the deaths of their terminal patients. Most physicians want to help the dying, but without transgressing ethical boundaries.*

*The following selection by James Rachels, first published a few months before the famous case of Karen Ann Quinlan in 1975, strongly influenced this debate. The piece, probably the first by a philosopher ever to appear in* The New England Journal of Medicine, *demonstrated how a non-physician could contribute to the debate. Since then, this essay has become one of the most widely reprinted in collections about general ethics or medical ethics.*

*Here, Rachels challenges the claim that "passive" euthanasia (or letting die) is always more humane than "active" euthanasia (or direct killing). In some situations, he argues, it may be more humane to kill.*

*He has written* The End of Life *and* Created from Animals *(Oxford University Press). His textbooks,* The Elements of Moral Philosophy *and* The Right Thing to Do *(McGraw-Hill), have undergone many editions and set standards for clear writing and thinking in the field. His most recent book,* Can Ethics Provide Answers? and Other Essays in Moral Philosophy *collects his best essays in one book.*

The distinction between active and passive euthanasia is thought to be crucial for medical ethics. The idea is that it is permissible, at least in some cases, to withhold treatment and allow a patient to die, but it is never permissible to take any direct action designed to kill the patient. This doctrine seems to be accepted by most doctors, and it is endorsed in a statement

*Source:* "Active and Passive Euthanasia" *New England Journal of Medicine* 292 no. 2 (January 9, 1975), pp. 79–80. Reprinted by permission of *The New England Journal of Medicine,* Copyright 1975, Massachusetts Medical Society and the author.

adopted by the House of Delegates of the American Medical Association on December 4, 1973:

> The intentional termination of the life of one human being by another—mercy killing—is contrary to that for which the medical profession stands and is contrary to the policy of the American Medical Association.
>
> The cessation of the employment of extraordinary means to prolong the life of the body when there is irrefutable evidence that biological death is imminent is the decision of the patient and/or his immediate family. The advice and judgment of the physician should be freely available to the patient and/or his immediate family.

However, a strong case can be made against this doctrine. In what follows I will set out some of the relevant arguments, and urge doctors to reconsider their views on this matter.

To begin with a familiar type of situation, a patient who is dying of incurable cancer of the throat is in terrible pain, which can no longer be satisfactorily alleviated. He is certain to die within a few days, even if present treatment is continued, but he does not want to go on living for those days since the pain is unbearable. So he asks the doctor for an end to it, and his family joins in the request.

Suppose the doctor agrees to withhold treatment, as the conventional doctrine says he may. The justification for his doing so is that the patient is in terrible agony, and since he is going to die anyway, it would be wrong to prolong his suffering needlessly. But now notice this. If one simply withholds treatment, it may take the patient longer to die, and so he may suffer more than he would if more direct action were taken and a lethal injection given. This fact provides strong reason for thinking that, once the initial decision not to prolong his agony has been made, active euthanasia is actually preferable to passive euthanasia, rather than the reverse. To say otherwise is to endorse the option that leads to more suffering rather than less, and is contrary to the humanitarian impulse that prompts the decision not to prolong his life in the first place.

Part of my point is that the process of being "allowed to die" can be relatively slow and painful, whereas being given a lethal injection is relatively quick and painless. Let me give a different sort of example. In the United States about one in 600 babies is born with Down's syndrome. Most of these babies are otherwise healthy—that is, with only the usual pediatric care, they will proceed to an otherwise normal infancy. Some, however, are born with congenital defects such as intestinal obstructions that require operations if they are to live. Sometimes, the parents and the doctor will decide not to operate, and let the infant die. Anthony Shaw describes what happens then:

> When surgery is denied [the doctor] must try to keep the infant from suffering while natural forces sap the baby's life away. As a surgeon whose natural inclination is to use the scalpel to fight off death, standing by and watching a salvageable baby die is the most emotionally exhausting experience I know. It is easy at a conference, in a theoretical discussion, to decide that such infants

should be allowed to die. It is altogether different to stand by in the nursery and watch as dehydration and infection wither a tiny being over hours and days. This is a terrible ordeal for me and the hospital staff—much more so than for the parents who never set foot in the nursery.[1]

I can understand why some people are opposed to all euthanasia, and insist that such infants must be allowed to live. I think I can also understand why other people favor destroying these babies quickly and painlessly. But why should anyone favor letting "dehydration and infection wither a tiny being over hours and days"? The doctrine that says that a baby may be allowed to dehydrate and wither, but may not be given an injection that would end its life without suffering, seems so patently cruel as to require no further refutation. The strong language is not intended to offend, but only to put the point in the clearest possible way.

My second argument is that the conventional doctrine leads to decisions concerning life and death made on irrelevant grounds.

Consider again the case of the infants with Down's syndrome who need operations for congenital defects unrelated to the syndrome to live. Sometimes, there is no operation, and the baby dies, but when there is no such defect, the baby lives on. Now, an operation such as that to remove an intestinal obstruction is not prohibitively difficult. The reason why such operations are not performed in these cases is, clearly, that the child has Down's syndrome and the parents and doctor judge that because of that fact it is better for the child to die.

But notice that this situation is absurd, no matter what view one takes of the lives and potentials of such babies. If the life of such an infant is worth preserving, what does it matter if it needs a simple operation? Or, if one thinks it better that such a baby should not live on, what difference does it make that it happens to have an unobstructed intestinal tract? In either case, the matter of life and death is being decided on irrelevant grounds. It is the Down's syndrome, and not the intestines, that is the issue. The matter should be decided, if at all, on that basis, and not be allowed to depend on the essentially irrelevant question of whether the intestinal tract is blocked.

What makes this situation possible, of course, is the idea that when there is an intestinal blockage, one can "let the baby die," but when there is no such defect there is nothing that can be done, for one must not "kill" it. The fact that this idea leads to such results as deciding life or death on irrelevant grounds is another good reason why the doctrine should be rejected.

One reason why so many people think that there is an important moral difference between active and passive euthanasia is that they think killing someone is morally worse than letting someone die. But is it? Is killing, in itself, worse than letting die? To investigate this issue, two cases may be considered that are exactly alike except that one involves killing whereas the other involves letting someone die. Then, it can be asked whether this difference makes any difference to the moral assessments. It is important that the cases be exactly alike, except for this one difference, since otherwise one cannot be confident that it is this difference and not some other that accounts for any variation in the assessments of the two cases. So, let us consider this pair of cases:

In the first, Smith stands to gain a large inheritance if anything should happen to his six-year-old cousin. One evening while the child is taking his bath, Smith sneaks into the bathroom and drowns the child, and then arranges things so that it will look like an accident.

In the second, Jones also stands to gain if anything should happen to his six-year-old cousin. Like Smith, Jones sneaks in planning to drown the child in his bath. However, just as he enters the bathroom Jones sees the child slip and hit his head, and fall face down in the water. Jones is delighted; he stands by, ready to push the child's head back under if it is necessary, but it is not necessary. With only a little thrashing about, the child drowns all by himself, "accidentally," as Jones watches and does nothing.

Now Smith killed the child, whereas Jones "merely" let the child die. That is the only difference between them. Did either man behave better, from a moral point of view? If the difference between killing and letting die were in itself a morally important matter, one should say that Jones's behavior was less reprehensible than Smith's. But does one really want to say that? I think not. In the first place, both men acted from the same motive, personal gain, and both had exactly the same end in view when they acted. It may be inferred from Smith's conduct that he is a bad man, although that judgment may be withdrawn or modified if certain further facts are learned about him—for example, that he is mentally deranged. But would not the very same thing be inferred about Jones from his conduct? And would not the same further considerations also be relevant to any modification on this judgment? Moreover, suppose Jones pleaded, in his own defense, "After all, I didn't do anything except just stand there and watch the child drown. I didn't kill him; I only let him die." Again, if letting die were in itself less bad than killing, this defense should have at least some weight. But it does not. Such a "defense" can only be regarded as a grotesque perversion of moral reasoning. Morally speaking, it is no defense at all.

Now, it may be pointed out, quite properly, that the cases of euthanasia with which doctors are concerned are not like this at all. They do not involve personal gain or the destruction of normal healthy children. Doctors are concerned only with cases in which the patient's life is of no further use to him, or in which the patient's life has become or will soon become a terrible burden. However, the point is the same in these cases: the bare difference between killing and letting die does not, in itself, make a moral difference. If a doctor lets a patient die, for humane reasons, he is in the same moral position as if he had given the patient a lethal injection for humane reasons. If his decision was wrong—if, for example, the patient's illness was in fact curable—the decision would be equally regrettable no matter which method was used to carry it out. And if the doctor's decision was the right one, the method used is not in itself important.

The AMA policy statement isolates the crucial issue very well: the crucial issue is "the intentional termination of the life of one human being by another." But after identifying this issue, and forbidding "mercy killing," the statement goes on to deny that the cessation of treatment is the intentional termination of a life. This is where the mistake comes in, for what is the cessation of treatment, in these circumstances, if it is not "the intentional termination of the life of one human being by another"? Of course it is exactly that, and if it were not, there would be no point to it.

Many people will find this judgment hard to accept. One reason, I think, is that it is very easy to conflate the question of whether killing is, in itself, worse than letting die, with the very different question of whether most actual cases of killing are more reprehensible than most actual cases of letting die. Most actual cases of killing are clearly terrible (think, for example, of all the murders reported in the newspapers), and one hears of such cases every day. On the other hand, one hardly ever hears of a case of letting die, except for the actions of doctors who are motivated by humanitarian reasons. So one learns to think of killing in a much worse light than of letting die. But this does not mean that there is something about killing that makes it in itself worse than letting die, for it is not the bare difference between killing and letting die that makes the difference in these cases. Rather, the other factors—the murderer's motive of personal gain, for example, contrasted with the doctor's humanitarian motivation—account for different reactions to the different cases.

I have argued that killing is not in itself any worse than letting die; if my contention is right, it follows that active euthanasia is not any worse than passive euthanasia. What arguments can be given on the other side? The most common, I believe, is the following:

"The important difference between active and passive euthanasia is that, in passive euthanasia, the doctor does not do anything to bring about the patient's death. The doctor does nothing, and the patient dies of whatever ills already afflict him. In active euthanasia, however, the doctor does something to bring about the patient's death: he kills him. The doctor who gives the patient with cancer a lethal injection has himself caused his patient's death; whereas if he merely ceases treatment, the cancer is the cause of the death."

A number of points need to be made here. The first is that it is not exactly correct to say that in passive euthanasia the doctor does nothing, for he does do one thing that is very important: he lets the patient die. "Letting someone die" is certainly different, in some respects, from other types of action—mainly in that it is a kind of action that one may perform by way of not performing certain other actions. For example, one may let a patient die by way of not giving medication, just as one may insult someone by way of not shaking his hand. But for any purpose of moral assessment, it is a type of action nonetheless. The decision to let a patient die is subject to moral appraisal in the same way that a decision to kill him would be subject to moral appraisal: it may be assessed as wise or unwise, compassionate or sadistic, right or wrong. If a doctor deliberately let a patient die who was suffering from a routinely curable illness, the doctor would certainly be to blame for what he had done, just as he would be to blame if he had needlessly killed the patient. Charges against him would then be appropriate. If so, it would be no defense at all for him to insist that he didn't "do anything." He would have done something very serious indeed, for he let his patient die.

Fixing the cause of death may be very important from a legal point of view, for it may determine whether criminal charges are brought against the doctor. But I do not think that this notion can be used to show a moral difference between active and passive euthanasia. The reason why it is considered bad to be the cause of someone's death is that death is regarded as a great evil—and so it is. However, if it has been decided that euthanasia—even passive euthanasia—is desirable in a given case, it has also been decided that in this instance death is no greater an evil than the patient's continued existence. And if this is true, the usual reason for not wanting to be the cause of someone's death simply does not apply.

Finally, doctors may think that all of this is only of academic interest—the sort of thing that philosophers may worry about but that has no practical bearing on their own work. After all, doctors must be concerned about the legal consequences of what they do, and active euthanasia is clearly forbidden by the law. But even so, doctors should also be concerned with the fact that the law is forcing upon them a moral doctrine that may well be indefensible, and has a considerable effect on their practices. Of course, most doctors are not now in the position of being coerced in this matter, for they do not regard themselves as merely going along with what the law requires. Rather, in statements such as the AMA policy statement that I have quoted, they are endorsing this doctrine as a central point of medical ethics. In that statement, active euthanasia is condemned not merely as illegal but as "contrary to that for which the medical profession stands," whereas passive euthanasia is approved. However, the preceding considerations suggest that there is really no moral difference between the two, considered in themselves (there may be important moral differences in some cases in their *consequences,* but, as I pointed out, these differences may make active euthanasia, and not passive euthanasia, the morally preferable option). So, whereas doctors may have to discriminate between active and passive euthanasia to satisfy the law, they should not do any more than that. In particular, they should not give the distinction any added authority and weight by writing it into official statements of medical ethics.

## NOTE

1. Shaw A: "Doctor, Do We Have a Choice?" The New York Times Magazine, January 30, 1972, p. 54[sic].

SELECTION 2

# On Killing Patients with Kindness: An Appeal for Caution

## Alan J. Weisbard and Mark Siegler

*Since the cases of Karen Quinlan in 1976 and Nancy Cruzan in 1990, there has been an increasing trend to let formerly competent but now incompetent patients die, especially if they are in long-term comas or have a chronic, debilitating condition.*

*In classic ethical theories, acts tend to be judged either by their motives or by their consequences. In this selection, Alan Weisbard and Mark Siegler ask us to be clear about the motives for "allowing" incompetent patients to die. Usually, justification for such a decision proceeds from the* substituted judgment *standard. This standard makes an assumption about what the patient would have decided, when competent, about what should be done to him if he later became incompetent. A different standard,* best interests, *stresses what is in the best interests now of the incompetent patient.*

*Do these standards reflect the reality of decision-making in such cases? Some legal commentators believe they do not, claiming they merely mask the family's desire for the financial and emotional ordeal to end. Some physicians agree, admitting that they feel relief when they no longer need to attend to such uncommunicative patients whose conditions can very rarely be improved.*

*Weisbard and Siegler warn that families and physicians may have mixed motives for wanting a quick death for such patients. They recommend that society and physicians give these patients the benefit of every doubt.*

*Alan Weisbard, JD, is associate professor of law and medical ethics at the University of Wisconsin Schools of Law and Medicine, Madison. Mark Siegler, MD, is professor of medicine and director of the Center for Clinical Medical Ethics at the University of Chicago, as well as coauthor of* Clinical Ethics.

Source: By No Extraordinary Means, ed. Joanne Lynne, Bloomington: Indiana University Press. Reprinted by permission of the publisher.

The powerful rhetoric of "death with dignity" has gained much intellectual currency and increasing practical import in recent years.[1] Beginning as a plea for more humane and individualized treatment in the face of the sometimes cold and impersonal technological imperatives of modern medicine, this rhetoric brought needed attention to the plight of dying patients not wishing to "endure the unendurable."[2] It has prompted legal and clinical changes empowering such patients (and sometimes their representatives) to assert some control over the manner, if not the fact, of their dying. The "death with dignity" movement has now advanced to a new frontier: the termination or withdrawal of fluids and nutritional support.

The increasing acceptability in respected forums of proposals to permit avoidable deaths by dehydration or malnutrition—proposals which, a few years ago, would almost certainly have been repudiated by the medical community as medically objectionable, legally untenable, and morally unthinkable—is evidenced by a slew of recent contributions to the medical and bioethics literature,[3] and by a sprinkling of court decisions.[4] This new stream of emerging opinion, supporting the explicit ethical and legal legitimation of this practice, is typically couched in comforting language of caution and compassion, by persons of undoubted sincerity and good faith. But the underlying analysis is, we fear, unlikely to long remain within these cautious bounds.

Careful scrutiny suggests what is ultimately at stake in this controversy: that for an increasing number of incompetent patients, the benefits of continued life are perceived as insufficient to justify the burden and cost of care; that death is seen as the desired outcome; and—critically—that the role of the health care professional is to participate in bringing this outcome about. Fearful that this development bodes ill for patients, health care professionals, the patient-physician relationship, and other vital societal values, we feel compelled to speak out against the all-too-rapid acceptance of withdrawal of fluids or nutritional support as accepted or standard medical practice. While recognizing that particular health care professionals, for reasons of compassion and conscience and with full knowledge of the personal legal risks involved, may on occasion elect to discontinue fluids and nutritional support, we nonetheless believe that such actions should generally be proscribed, pending much fuller debate and discussion than has yet taken place.

## QUALIFICATIONS

We do not intend to address here the deep philosophic issues posed by the moral status of the permanently unconscious. There is much philosophic dispute concerning whether the permanently unconscious are living persons who possess rights and interests, whether the obligation of care fully extends to such patients, and whether such patients should and eventually will be encompassed within a broadened understanding of brain death. The present authors take somewhat different views on these questions and present no joint

position here on the withdrawal of fluids and nutritional support from patients reliably diagnosed as permanently unconscious.

Nor is our principal concern with decisions by competent, adult, terminally ill patients who contemporaneously or through advance directives (living wills, durable powers of attorney, or carefully considered, reliably witnessed, oral statements) direct that their process of dying not be prolonged
through such techniques as those required to maintain life-sustaining nourishment and hydration. We encourage fuller discussion of these issues among patients, families, and medical professionals at a time the patient is able to participate in an informed and thoughtful fashion. We caution only that patients
should be made aware that some "artificial" techniques may be useful in making them more comfortable and in easing the dying process, and should not be
rejected unthinkingly by those seeking a more "natural" death. Further, as the
much publicized case of Elizabeth Bouvia[5] reminds us, neither physicians nor
health care institutions may be compelled to assist in, or to preside over, the
suicides of patients, especially those who are not terminally ill.

Nor, finally, do we mean to be understood as necessarily advocating the
use of that modality of providing hydration or nutritional support considered
most likely to extend survival time maximally without regard to other relevant factors, including the intrusiveness of the technology to the patient in
comparison with the plausible alternatives, or the nature and likelihood of serious side effects. Our position is intended as neither vitalist nor absolutist, except with regard to our insistence on providing sufficient assistance to preclude painful hunger or thirst and to avoid directly causing death (as
perceived by health care professionals and the wider society) by failing to provide food and water minimally necessary to preclude death by starvation or
dehydration.

## CRITIQUE

Our focus, then, is primarily on the withdrawal of fluids and nutrition from
patients possessing the capacity for consciousness who have not competently
rejected such support. While concerns may seem premature in light of the
qualifications and thoughtful discussions of both substantive and procedural
safeguards expressed in several recent contributions to the literature,[6] we remain troubled that the underlying analysis, once accepted by clinicians and
courts, will not long be confined within the limits initially set forth.

What, then, is the underlying analysis, and why do we find it so potentially troubling? The argument rests on the dual propositions that, first, the
provision of fluids and nutritional support by "artificial" means constitutes
"medical interventions guided by considerations similar to those governing
other treatment methods,"[7] and that, second, judgments regarding the withdrawal of such interventions should be based on calculations of the "burdens
and benefits" associated with the treatment (sometimes also referred to as

"proportionality"). These propositions are rooted in the work of the President's Commission for the Study of Ethical Problems in Medicine,[8] were adopted by the California appellate court in the *Barber* and *Nejdl*[9] case, and play a central role in the analyses set forth by several recent commentators.[10]

We do not dispute that the "benefits and burdens" formulation is useful in a number of contexts and marks a clear analytic improvement over unconsidered references to "extraordinary measures" or "artificial means," terms which have introduced much unnecessary confusion and provide little real assistance in decisionmaking. What we find troublesome is the assertion that physicians, families, courts, or other third parties can properly conclude that the "burdens" of [providing] fluids and nutrition—a generally unconvincing catalogue of potential "complications" or "side effects"—outweigh the benefit, sustaining life. (We recognize that, in rare cases, the provision of fluids and, particularly, nutritional support may be medically futile or counterproductive in sustaining life, and we do not here recommend that such futile or counterproductive steps be mandated.)

Advocates of withdrawing fluids and nutritional support that are effective in, and necessary for, sustaining life justify their position by arguing that a speedy and painless death is in the patient's "best interests" (a claim with little foundation in existing law, which has traditionally viewed the preservation of life, at least for noncomatose patients, as a core component of "best interests"). While the argument is compassionately made, and may be persuasive in certain cases, it fails to acknowledge explicitly that its objective may be attained more swiftly, more directly, more honestly, through the administration of lethal injections. Homicide is, in this setting, the ultimate analgesic. But to the extent active euthanasia is rejected—we think wisely—by existing law and medical ethics, we believe a similar conclusion is generally mandated for withdrawal of fluids and nutrition, and for much the same reasons.

If active euthanasia has found little support thus far in either medical or legal circles, the reasons are not confined to an exclusive concern with prolonging the life of the patient. The courts have made clear that respirators and dialysis machines are not legally mandated in all cases of respiratory or renal failure, even where their withdrawal is thought likely to result in death. In this sense, the withdrawal of fluids and nutrition is subject to a similar analysis. But in another and—we believe—more powerful sense, the result is quite different, at least in terms of our society's moral perceptions and self-image.

Withdrawal of respirators and dialysis machines can be seen, and *is* seen and emotionally understood, as the removal of artificial impediments to "letting nature take its course." Death can be understood in such cases as the natural result of the disease process. In cases where death may indeed be the desired (and ultimately unavoidable) outcome, it can be allowed to come without imposing a heavy burden of guilt and moral responsibility on physicians or family members for acting to bring it about, and without challenging important social barriers against killing.[11] And sometimes, as in the case of Karen Quinlan, nature can surprise us: the patient can survive despite some experts' predictions to the contrary.

The case of withdrawing fluids and nutritional supports is different in critical respects. Although the techniques for providing such supports may be medical, and thus logically associated with other medical interventions, the underlying obligations of providing food and drink to those who hunger or thirst transcend the medical context, summoning up deep human responses of caring, of nurturing, of human connectedness, and of human community. Social scientists and humanists have only begun to explore the deeper social meanings and ramifications of depriving patients of "food and water," of permitting deaths from starvation or dehydration. While sophisticated observers may argue that the image of "starvation" or "thirst" may be misleading in the cases of some patients, particularly the unconscious, or that limited nutritional intake may slow the progress of a cancer, it is far from clear that such explanations will be compelling to the public, or even, perhaps, to many members of the health professions, particularly if the practice of withholding fluids and nutritional supports takes root and is applied to an ever broader class of patients.

Further, unlike withdrawal of respirators or dialysis machines, withdrawal of fluids and nutrition cannot so readily be seen as "letting nature take its course." Dehydration or lack of nutrition become[s] the direct cause of death for which moral responsibility cannot be avoided. The psychological and social ramifications of bringing death about in this fashion will, in our view, be difficult or impossible to distinguish from those accompanying lethal injections or other modes of active euthanasia. There will be no surprises: withdrawal of all food and water from helpless patients must necessarily result in their deaths.

Given the demographic trends in our society—the dramatically increasing pool of those characterized as the "superannuated, chronically ill, physically marginal elderly," those Daniel Callahan has labeled "the biologically tenacious"—denial of fluids and nutrition may well become "the nontreatment of choice."[12] The process is tellingly illustrated by two recent court cases. Clarence Herbert, the patient whose death gave rise to the homicide prosecution in *Barber*, was initially understood, at least by his wife, to be brain dead. In fact, Herbert was comatose but not brain dead, although the quickness of diagnosis and the subsequent nontreatment decisions led to some troubling questions of the adequacy of both diagnosis and prognosis. The sequence of decisions is instructive. First the respirator was removed. When Herbert failed to succumb as predicted, intravenous feeding was discontinued. Only then—a week later—did Herbert "comply" with the course desired, and expire.[13]

Similarly, in the *Conroy* case, the patient's nephew had previously refused to authorize surgery for his aunt's gangrene.[14] When that condition proved not to be terminal, the nephew apparently expressed his disinclination to authorize other life-extending measures.[15] Only when this decision failed to bring about the desired result—death—did the nephew and physicians contemplate the next step: termination of fluids and nutrition supplied by nasogastric tube.

Both these cases illustrate a troubling dynamic, one much like a self-fulfilling prophecy. Once a determination has been reached—perhaps for understandable and humanitarian reasons—that death is the desired outcome, decisionmakers become increasingly less troubled by the choice of means to be employed to achieve that outcome. The line between "allowing to die" and "actively killing" can be elusive, and we are skeptical that any logical or psychological distinction between "allowing to die" by starvation and actively killing, as by lethal injection, will prove viable. If we as a society are to retain the prohibition against actively killing, the admittedly wavering line demarcating permissible "allowing to die" must exclude death by avoidable starvation. We frankly acknowledge that our concern here extends beyond a solicitude for the outcome for the patient to include our fears for the impact of decisions and actions on family members, health care professionals, and societal values, which will survive the death of the patient. If these separate and additional concerns are to be discounted, we are hard-pressed to understand the remaining justifications for prohibition of active euthanasia in the perceived "best interests" of the incompetent patient.

We have witnessed too much history to disregard how easily society disvalues the lives of the "unproductive"—the retarded, the disabled, the senile, the institutionalized, the elderly—of those who in another time and place were referred to as "useless eaters."[16] The confluence of the emerging stream of medical and ethical opinion favoring legitimation of withholding fluids and nutrition with the torrent of public and governmental concern over the costs of medical care (and the looming imposition of cost-containment strategies which may well impose significant financial penalties on the prolonged care of the impaired elderly) powerfully reinforces our discomfort. In the current environment, it may well prove convenient—and all too easy—to move from recognition of an individual's "right to die" (to us, an unfortunate rephrasing of the legally more limited right to refuse medical treatment) to a climate enforcing a socially obligatory "duty to die," preferably quickly and cheaply.[17] The recent suggestions that all new applicants for Medicare be provided copies of "living wills" or similar documents illustrate how this process may unfold.[18] Our concern here is not with the encouragement of patient self-determination regarding medical care, including decisions about dying, which we vigorously support, but rather with the incorporation of such strategies *as a method of cost control.*

Finally, we would urge that efforts in this field be rechanneled from demonstrating that some patients' quality of life is too poor, too "meaningless," to justify the burdens of continued life, toward the challenge of finding better ways to improve the comfort and quality of life of such patients. In particular, we hope the current debate will stimulate further discussion of the merits of different modalities of providing fluids and nutrition. For example, with the development of endoscopic placement techniques for gastronomy tubes, this superficially more invasive "surgical" procedure may prove safer and more comfortable for many patients than the nonsurgical insertion of nasogastric tubes, which are sometimes a source of continuing discomfort for patients and are more likely to elicit the use of restraints to prevent the deliberate or accidental removal of the tubes. More attention must be paid to the clinical, institutional, economic, and legal implications of these and other alternatives.

## CONCLUSION

When coupled with powerful economic forces and with the disturbing tendency, both among professionals and in the broader society, to disvalue the lives of the "unproductive," the compassionate call for withdrawing or withholding fluids and nutrition in a few, selected cases bears the seeds of great potential abuse. Little is to be lost, and much potentially gained, by slowing down the process of legitimation, taking stock of where we have come and where we are going, improving our methods of comforting and caring for the dying without necessarily hurrying to dispatch them on their way, and deferring any premature legal, ethical, or professional approval and legitimation of this new course. The movement for "death with dignity" arose in response to deficiencies on the caring side of medicine; it would be sadly ironic if this latest manifestation served to undercut the image of physician as caring and nurturing servant and to undermine deep human values of caring and nurturance throughout society.

## NOTES

1. Portions of this paper appeared, in a somewhat different form, in Mark Siegler and Alan J. Weisbard, "Against the Emerging Stream: Should Fluids and Nutritional Support Be Discontinued?" *Arch. Intern. Med.* 145:129–132 (January 1985).
2. *In re Quinlan,* 70 N.J. 10, 355 A.2d 647, *cert. denied,* 429 U.S. 922, 97 S. Ct. 319, 50 L. Ed. 2d 289 (1976).
3. See, e.g., David W. Meyers, "Legal Aspects of Withdrawing Nourishment from an Incurably Ill Patient," *Arch. Intern. Med.* 145:125–128 (January 1985); Rebecca S. Dresser and Eugene V. Boisaubin, Jr., "Ethics, Law and Nutritional Support," *Arch. Intern. Med.* 145:122–124 (January 1985); Joanne Lynn and James F. Childress, "Must Patients Always Be Given Food and Water?" *Hastings Cent. Rep.* 13:17–21 (October 1983); S. H. Wanzer et al., "The Physician's Responsibility Toward Hopelessly Ill Patients," *N. Engl. J. Med.* 310:955–959 (1984).
4. *Barber* v. *Superior Court of the State of California,* 195 Cal. Rptr. 484 (Cal. App. 2 Dist. 1983); *In re Conroy,* 98 N.J. 321, 486 A.2d 1209 (1985). *In the Matter of Mary Hier,* 18 Mass. App. 200, 464 N.E.2d 959, *app. den.,* 392 Mass. 1102 (1984).
5. *Bouvia* v. *County of Riverside,* Superior Ct. of St. of Calif., Riverside County, No. 159780 (1984).
6. See note 3.
7. Lynn and Childress, *supra* note 3, at 18.
8. President's Commission for the Study of Ethical Problems in Medicine and Biomedical and Behavioral Research, *Deciding to Forego Life-Sustaining Treatment.* Washington, D.C.: U.S. Government Printing Office (1983).

9. See note 4, *supra*.
10. See note 3, *supra*.
11. See generally, Alan J. Weisbard, "On the Bioethics of Jewish Law: The Case of Karen Quinlan," *Israel L. Rev.* 14:337–368 (1979); Robert A. Burt, "Authorizing Death for Anomalous Newborns," in Aubrey Milunsky and George J. Annas (eds.), *Genetics and the Law*, New York: Plenum Press (1975); Robert A. Burt, "The Ideal of Community in the Work of the President's Commission," *Cardozo L. Rev.* 6:267–286 (1985).
12. Daniel Callahan, "On Feeding the Dying," *Hastings Cent. Rep.* 13:22 (October 1983).
13. See *Barber, supra* note 4, and Bonnie Steinbock, "The Removal of Mr. Herbert's Feeding Tube," *Hastings Cent. Rep.* 13:13–16 (October 1983).
14. *Conroy, supra* note 4.
15. Personal communications to author.
16. The reference is to the Nazi euthanasia program. While the authors have been unable to locate an explicit reference to "useless eaters," Nazi usage of the phrase "useless mouths" is documented by Nora Levin, *The Holocaust: The Destruction of European Jewry: 1933–1945.* New York: Shocken (1968), 302.
17. Recent remarks on "the duty to die" attributed to Colorado Governor Richard Lamm are illustrative, *New York Times,* March 29, 1984 at A16, col. 5.
18. Proceedings of the House of Delegates, American Medical Association 133rd Annual Meeting, June 1984 at 177 (commenting on recommendations of Advisory Council on Social Security).

# The Cognitive Criterion of Personhood

## Joseph Fletcher

*The late Joseph Fletcher was a founder of the modern field of medical ethics. His 1954 book,* Morals and Medicine, *examined the ethics of truthtelling, contraception, euthanasia, and assisted reproduction two decades before they became subjects of academic and popular interest.*

*An Episcopal priest by training, he was a philosopher in his thinking and is said to have renounced belief in God in 1960 (although he remained a priest). His 1966 book,* Situation Ethics, *caused a sensation when he defended an ethic much like utilitarianism in judging acts right according to their consequences and not according to whether they agreed with the received interpretation of divine will.*

*Fletcher was both a deeply humanist scholar and a practical one, and his writings reflect these traits. He was married for sixty years to the former Forrest Hatfield, a friend of Margaret Sanger, the spiritual founder of Planned Parenthood. He belonged to the board of directors of the Euthanasia Educational Council and advocated reproductive freedom for couples.*

*In this selection, he lays out a pioneering argument, claiming that what makes life valuable is not people's biological form but their mental capacities. Although he uses the term "humanhood" in his article, this term later came to be called "personhood" such that "human" later denoted the mere biological form of humans and "person" denoted a human with mental capacities and a right to life. So what this early piece is advocating is what later came to be called the "cognitive criterion of personhood." (On this topic, see also selections by Michael Tooley, Don Marquis, and Mary Anne Warren.)*

*Fletcher died in 1991 at age 86. Before then, he was the Robert Treat Paine Professor at the Episcopal Theological School at Harvard University and visiting scholar in medical ethics at the University of Virginia.*

*Source: Hastings Center Report.* 4 (December, 1975), pp. 4–7. Reprinted by permission of the publisher and the estate of Joseph Fletcher.

Jean Rostand describes a meeting of French Catholic intellectuals: they spoke of a prosecution for infanticide following the thalidomide disaster of the Sixties.[1] Morvan Lebesque: "After centuries of morality, we still cannot answer questions like those raised by the trial in Liège. Should malformed babies be killed? Where does man begin?" Father Jolif: "No one knows what man is any longer."

That is the situation, exactly. Whether or not we ever knew in the past what man is, in the sense of having a consensus about it, we do not know now. To realize this, make only a quick scan of the wild confusion and variety on the subject gathered together by Erich Fromm and Ramon Xirau in their historical compendium.[2]

## FIRST THERE WAS ONE

Yet it is this question, how we are to define the *humanum,* which lies at the base of all serious talk about the quality of life. We cannot appraise quality or enumerate human values if we cannot first say what a human being is. The *Hastings Center Report* (November 1972) published a shortened version of an essay of mine in which I made a stab at this problem, under the title "Indicators of Humanhood: A Tentative Profile of Man."[3]

### The Original Indicators of Humanhood: A Tentative Profile of Man

#### Positive Human Criteria
1. Minimal intelligence
2. Self-awareness
3. Self-control
4. A sense of time
5. A sense of futurity
6. A sense of the past
7. The capability to relate to others
8. Concern for others
9. Communication
10. Control of existence
11. Curiosity
12. Change and changeability
13. Balance of rationality and feeling
14. Idiosyncrasy
15. Neo-cortical function

#### Negative Human Criteria
1. Man is not non- or anti-artificial
2. Man is not essentially parental
3. Man is not essentially sexual
4. Man is not a bundle of rights
5. Man is not a worshiper

In substance I contended that the acute question is what is a *person*: that rights (such as survival) attach only to persons; that out of some twenty criteria one (neocortical function) is the cardinal or hominizing trait upon which all the other human traits hinge; and then I invited those concerned to add or subtract, agree or disagree as they may. This was intended to keep the investigation going forward, and it worked; the issue has been vigorously discussed pro and con.

What crystals have precipitated? Without trying to explore them in any detail, as each of them deserves to be, four different traits have been nominated to date as the singular *esse* of humanness: neocortical function, self-consciousness, relational ability, and happiness—the last being included more in a light than a heavy vein. Various additional criteria of the optimal or *bene esse* kind are mentioned in a growing correspondence, but no argument *against* any one of them has been offered: e.g., one correspondent (Robert Morison) wants concern for the meek and dependent stipulated under my eighth trait, "concern for others."

But on the question which one of the optimal traits and capabilities is the *sine qua non*, the essential one without which no combination of the others can add up to humanhood, there are now four contenders in the running. It should be noted at the outset that of the four discrete cardinal criteria thus far entered, none of them is mutually exclusive of any of the others, any more than the optimal indicators are (sense of time, curiosity, ideomorphous identity, obligation, reason-feeling balance, self-control, changeability, etc.). The decisive question therefore appears to be about precondition. Which one of these traits, if any, is required for the presence of the others? To answer this is to find *the* criterion among the criteria.

## NOW THERE ARE FOUR

I. Michael Tooley of Stanford contends that the real precondition to "having a serious right to life" or to being the kind of moral entity we call a person, as in the Sixteenth Amendment sense, is subjectivity or self-awareness (no. 2 in my original list). He called it "the self-consciousness requirement."[4] As he points out, fetuses and infants lack that requirement. Machines have no consciousness at all, and therefore may be sacrificed in a competing values situation. Animals are probably not self-conscious, although a few pet lovers claim they are. Once a growing baby's neurological "switchboard" gets hooked up, allowing consciousness of self to emerge, he or she is a person. (Mind is, as Dubos points out, a verb—not a noun; it is not something given but acquired, a process rather than an event.[5] It is what the mind does, not what it is.) So runs Tooley's thesis.

II. Richard McCormick of the Kennedy Center for Bioethics at Georgetown University, on another tack, says "the meaning, substance, and consummation of life is found in human relationships," so that when we try to make quality of life judgments ("and we must"), as in cases of diseased or defective newborns, "life is a value to be preserved only insofar as it contains some potentiality for human relationships."[6] On this basis anencephalics certainly, and idiots probably, lack personal status, with a consequent lack of claim upon rights. If you lack what he calls "the relational potential" (what I call "the capability to relate to others," no. 7) you cannot be human. "If that potential is simply nonexistent or would be utterly submerged and undeveloped in the mere struggle to survive, that life has achieved its potential" and we need not save it from death's approach.

III. When a pediatrician at the Texas Medical Center (Houston), whose work takes her daily into a service for retarded children, heard me at a grand rounds expound my suggestion that minimal intelligence or cerebral function is the essential factor in being human, she rejected it: "I know a little four-year-old boy, certainly 20 minus or an idiot on any measurement scale and untrainable, but just the same he is a human being and nobody is going to tell me different. He is happy and that makes him human, as human as you or I." By "human" she meant morally, not only biologically. She described the child's affectionate responses to caresses and his constant euphoria. I thought of my neighbor's kitten and recalled the euphoria symptom as happiness without any reason for it, and I remembered Huxley's *Brave New World* where everybody was happy on drugs—except the rebellious intellectuals. I asked her if she really meant to say that euphoria qualifies us for humanhood. I took her silence to be an affirmative answer.

IV. As far as I can yet see, I will stand by my own thesis or hypothesis that neocortical function is the key to humanness, the essential trait, the human *sine qua non*. The point is that without the synthesizing function of the cerebral cortex (without thought or mind), whether before it is present or with its end, the person is nonexistent no matter how much the individual's brain stem and mid-brain may continue to provide feelings and regulate autonomic physical functions. To be truly Homo sapiens we must be sapient, however minimally. Only this trait or capability is necessary to *all* of the other traits which go into the fullness of humanness. Therefore this indicator, neocortical function, is the first-order requirement and the key to the definition of a human being. As Robert Williams of the University Medical Center (Seattle) puts it, "Without mentation the body is of no significant use."[7]

## DISCUSSION GOES ON

This search for a *shared* view of humanness, a consensus, may not find a happy ending. James Gustafson's (University of Chicago Divinity School) skepticism about reaching agreement has now been graduated into skepticism also about applying whatever criterion we might agree to.[8] He thinks now that "intuitive elements, grounded on beliefs and profound feelings," would color our judgments seriously. More sharply, Rostand warns us (p. 66) that looking for a single trait is "a temptation for the fanatics—and there are always fanatics everywhere—to think that his adversary is less human than himself because he lacks some mental or spiritual quality." In scientific and medical circles I find that a *biological* definition is thought to be feasible, but not a list of moral or psychological traits—to say nothing of picking out only one cardinal trait subsumed in all the rest.

One slant on the problem is to deny the problem itself, not as insoluble but as specious (no pun intended). For example, William May of Catholic University, trying to justify the prohibition of abortion, objects to "the thought of Fletcher, Tooley, and those who would agree with them" that membership in a *species* is of no moral significance.[9] He argues that we are human by virtue of what we are (our species), not by virtue of what we achieve or do. A member of the biological species is, as such, a human being. Thus, we would be human if we have opposable thumbs, are capable of face-to-face coitus and have a brain weighing 1,400 grams, whether a particular brain functions cerebrally or not. (I put in the thumbs and coitus to exclude elephants, whales and dolphins, the only other species having brains as big as or bigger than man's.) In this reasoning the term "human" slides back and forth between meaning sometimes the biological, sometimes the moral or personal, thus combining the fallacy of ambiguity with the fallacy of ostensive definition. ("He has opposable thumbs, therefore he is a person.")

Tristram Engelhardt of the Texas Medical Branch (Galveston) takes a different path: he renounces not the need to define humanhood but the attempt to single out any one crucial or essential indicator. Instead, he is synoptic in the same manner that René Dubos has so superbly shown us in *Man Adapting* and *So Human an Animal.* Engelhardt distinguishes the biological from personal life but follows a multifactorial, non-univocal line. Indeed, he points precisely to the traits elected in all three of the major univocal definitions discussed here; together they compose his own—cerebral function, self-consciousness, and relationship or the societal dimension. Yet it is difficult, studying his language, not to believe that he gives cerebral function the determinative place, as when he says that "for a person to be embodied and present in the world he must be conscious in it," but follows that up by adding, "The brain is the singular focus of the embodiment of the mind, and in its absence man as a person is absent."[10]

Being careful in all this is supremely important. Leonard Weber of Detroit urges "caution in adopting a neocortical definition of death" because this is tantamount to a definition of personhood, although he doesn't throw it out of court. He further asks us to make sure "the biological is not being undervalued as a component of human life."[11] On both scores I agree. I take "caution" to mean carefulness, which is always in order, and I certainly want to affirm our physical side, since why even talk of cerebral function apart from a cerebrum? "Mind is meat" may be too crass, but I agree that it contains a vital truth.

## RAPPROCHEMENT?

To Tooley and McCormick I would want to say, "You are on sound ground, so far." Of all the optimal traits of a full and authentic human life, I am inclined with you to give top importance to awareness of self (Tooley's cardinal and my optimal trait no. 2) and to the capacity for interpersonal and social relations (McCormick's cardinal and my optimal traits no. 7 and no. 8). But I still want to reason that *their* key indicators are only factors at all because of *my* key criterion—cerebral function. Is this not an issue to be carefully weighed?

Rizzo and Yonder of Canisius College, Buffalo, have argued the case for the neocortical definition.[12] Their conclusion is that "when there is incontrovertible evidence of neocortical death, the human life has ceased." To Professor Tooley and Father McCormick I would say, "Neocortical death means that both self-consciousness and other-orientedness are gone, whereas neither non-self-consciousness nor inability to relate to others means the end of neocortical activity." Just remember amnesia victims when self-consciousness is proposed as the key; just remember radically autistic and schizophrenic patients when the relational key is proposed. The amnesiac has lost his identity, his selfhood, and the psychotic is still *thinking,* no matter how falsely and in what disorder. On these grounds we cannot declare that such individuals are no longer persons, just as we cannot do so at some levels of mental retardation. Only irreversible coma or a decerebrate state is ground for such a serious determination. It seems that possibly the neocortical key is more conservative than some observers of the ethical debate suppose.

The importance of self-awareness is obvious. Abraham Maslow has taught this generation that much. Being able to recognize and respond to others is of the greatest importance to being truly human, as Gordon Allport's interpersonalism made plain. But as Julius Korein, the New York University neurologist, tells us, "Basic to the definition of the death of an individual is identification of the irreversible destruction of that critical component of the system which represents the essence of the person," and that essence, he says, is "cerebral death."[13] The "vegetable" patient, no matter how many spontaneous vital functions may be continuing, is dead, a nonperson, but not at the point he appears to be incapable of self-perception or of relational affect—only when neurologic diagnosis determines that cerebral function has ended permanently.

The non-neocortical theories (or paraneocortical) fail because they do not account for all cases. "Neocortical death," on the other hand, *necessarily* covers all other criteria, because they are by definition impossible criteria when neocortical function is gone. The key trait must be one that covers all cases, no matter how infrequently they are seen clinically. Incidentally but not unimportantly, the neocortical indicator is *medically* determinable, whereas Tooley's and McCormick's are not.

If it proves that very many ethicists feel these issues about a sound hypothesis for the *humanum* are crucial, those whose training has been in the humanities will need the help and advice of psychiatrists, psychologists, neurologists and brain specialists to teach us the limiting principles involved and expedite our discussion.

# NOTES

1. J. Rostand, *Humanly Possible: A Biologist's Notes on the Future of Mankind,* trans. L. Blair (New York: Saturday Review Press, 1973), p. 8.
2. E. Fromm and R. Xirau, *The Nature of Man* (New York: Macmillan, 1968).
3. The full text is "Medicine and the Nature of Man," in *The Teaching of Medical Ethics,* ed. R. M. Veatch, W. Gaylin, and C. Morgan (Hastings-on-Hudson, N.Y.: Institute of Society, Ethics and the Life Sciences, 1973), pp. 47–48. It appeared also in *Science, Medicine and Man* 1 (1973), pp. 93–102.
4. M. Tooley, "Abortion and Infanticide," *Philosophy and Public Affairs* 2 (Fall 1972), pp. 37–65.
5. R. Dubos, *Man Adapting* (New Haven: Yale University Press, 1965), p. 7n.
6. R. A. McCormick, "To Save or Let Die: The Dilemma of Modern Medicine," *Journal of the American Medical Association* 229 (July 8, 1974), pp. 172–76.
7. R. H. Williams, *To Live and to Die* (New York: Springer-Verlag, 1974), p. 18.
8. J. M. Gustafson, "Basic Ethical Issues in the Bio-Medical Fields," *Soundings* 53 (1970), 177; and "Mongolism, Parental Desires, and the Right to Live," *Perspectives in Biology and Medicine* 16 (Summer 1973), pp. 529–57.
9. W. May, "The Morality of Abortion," *Catholic Medical Quarterly* 26 (July 1974), pp. 116–28.
10. H. T. Engelhardt Jr., "The Beginnings of Personhood: Philosophical Considerations," *Perkins* (School of Theology) *Journal* 27 (1973), pp. 10, 20–27.
11. L. J. Weber, "Human Death or Neocortical Death: The Ethical Context," *Linacre Quarterly* 41 (May 1974), pp. 106–13.
12. R. F. Rizzo and J. M. Yonder, "Definition and Criteria of Clinical Death," *Linacre Quarterly* 40 (November 1973), pp. 223–33.
13. J. Korein, "On Cerebral, Brain, and Systemic Death," *Current Concepts of Cerebrovascular Disease* 8 (May–June 1973), p. 9.

## PART TWO

# Allowing Death to Occur in Competent Adults

# Voluntary Active Euthanasia

## Dan W. Brock

*In this selection, Dan Brock discusses first whether it is possible to support physician-assisted suicide but not "euthanasia," and second, whether there is a moral difference between a competent adult's giving herself a lethal overdose that has been prescribed to her by a physician and the physician's administering the overdose.*

*Brock discusses the argument that the latter course is wrong because it is the killing of an innocent person. He argues that many decisions about forgoing treatment at the end of life in medicine amount to the killing of innocent persons. (In this respect he agrees with James Rachels' main point in Selection 1.) The real issue, he claims, is whether euthanasia is unjustified killing and, if not, whether the psychological resistance of physicians to change is morally persuasive.*

*In a third section, Brock discusses the cost-benefit ratio of changing public policy to allow voluntary active euthanasia. He also discusses slippery-slope objections to the legalization of physician-assisted dying. (On this point, see also Selections 8 and 25.) He then discusses whether there would be a slide from legalization of voluntary active euthanasia to acceptance of involuntary active euthanasia, as well as the changing role of physicians in physician-assisted dying. He concludes by favoring a change to allow physicians to help competent dying adults end their lives.*

*Dan Brock, a philosopher, worked for one of the first congressional bioethics commissions, institutions that helped to legitimate and publicize the new field of medical ethics. Over two decades since, he has written many articles and books in this field in-*
*cluding* Life and Death: Philosophical Essays in Biomedical Ethics *(Cambridge,*

Source: Hastings Center Report, 22 (March–April 1992), 10–22. Reprinted by permission of the author and publisher. Earlier versions of this paper were presented at the American Philosophical Association Central Division meetings (at which David Velleman provided extremely helpful comments), Massachusetts General Hospital, Yale University School of Medicine, Princeton University, Brown University, and as the Brin Lecture at The Johns Hopkins School of Medicine. The author is grateful to the audiences on each of these occasions, to several anonymous reviewers, and to Norman Daniels for helpful comments. The paper was completed while the author was a Fellow in the Program in Ethics and the Professions at Harvard University.

*1993). Today he is director of the Center for Bioethics and university professor in the
philosophy department at Brown University.*

Since the case of Karen Quinlan first seized public attention fifteen years ago,
no issue in biomedical ethics has been more prominent than the debate about
forgoing life-sustaining treatment. Controversy continues regarding some aspects of that debate, such as forgoing life-sustaining nutrition and hydration,
and relevant law varies some from state to state. Nevertheless, I believe it is
possible to identify an emerging consensus that competent patients, or the surrogates of incompetent patients, should be permitted to weigh the benefits
and burdens of alternative treatments, including the alternative of no treatment, according to the patient's values, and either to refuse any treatment or
to select from among available alternative treatments. This consensus is re-
flected in bioethics scholarship, in reports of prestigious bodies such as the
President's Commission for the Study of Ethical Problems in Medicine, The
Hastings Center, and the American Medical Association, in a large body of judicial decisions in courts around the country, and finally in the beliefs and
practices of health care professionals who care for dying patients.[1]
     More recently, significant public and professional attention has shifted
from life-sustaining treatment to euthanasia—more specifically, voluntary active euthanasia—and to physician-assisted suicide. Several factors have contributed to the increased interest in euthanasia. In the Netherlands, it has been
openly practiced by physicians for several years with the acceptance of the
country's highest court.[2] In 1988 there was an unsuccessful attempt to get the
question of whether it should be made legally permissible on the ballot in California. In November 1991 voters in the state of Washington defeated a widely
publicized referendum proposal to legalize both voluntary active euthanasia
and physician-assisted suicide. Finally, some cases of this kind, such as "It's
Over, Debbie," described in the *Journal of the American Medical Association,* the
"suicide machine" of Dr. Jack Kevorkian, and the cancer patient "Diane" of
Dr. Timothy Quill, have captured wide public and professional attention.[3] Unfortunately, the first two of these cases were sufficiently problematic that even
most supporters of euthanasia or assisted suicide did not defend the physicians' actions in them. As a result, the subsequent debate they spawned has
often shed more heat than light. My aim is to increase the light, and perhaps
as well to reduce the heat, on this important subject by formulating and evaluating the central ethical arguments for and against voluntary active euthanasia
and physician-assisted suicide. My evaluation of the arguments leads me,
with reservations to be noted, to support permitting both practices. My primary aim, however, is not to argue for euthanasia, but to identify confusions
in some common arguments, and problematic assumptions and claims that
need more defense or data in others. The issues are considerably more complex than either supporters or opponents often make out; my hope is to advance the debate by focusing attention on what I believe the real issues under
discussion should be.

In the recent bioethics literature some have endorsed physician-assisted suicide but not euthanasia.[4] Are they sufficiently different that the moral arguments for one often do not apply to the other? A paradigm case of physician-assisted suicide is a patient's ending his or her life with a lethal dose of a medication requested of and provided by a physician for that purpose. A paradigm case of voluntary active euthanasia is a physician's administering the lethal dose, often because the patient is unable to do so. The only difference that need exist between the two is the person who actually administers the lethal dose—the physician or the patient. In each, the physician plays an active and necessary causal role.

In physician-assisted suicide the patient acts last (for example, Janet Adkins herself pushed the button after Dr. Kevorkian hooked her up to his suicide machine), whereas in euthanasia the physician acts last by performing the physical equivalent of pushing the button. In both cases, however, the choice rests fully with the patient. In both the patient acts last in the sense of retaining the right to change his or her mind until the point at which the lethal process becomes irreversible. How could there be a substantial moral difference between the two based only on this small difference in the part played by the physician in the causal process resulting in death? Of course, it might be held that the moral difference is clear and important—in euthanasia—the physician kills the patient whereas in physician-assisted suicide the patient kills him- or herself. But this is misleading at best. In assisted suicide the physician and patient together kill the patient. To see this, suppose a physician supplied a lethal dose to a patient with the knowledge and intent that the patient will wrongfully administer it to another. We would have no difficulty in morality or the law recognizing this as a case of joint action to kill for which both are responsible.

If there is no significant, intrinsic moral difference between the two, it is also difficult to see why public or legal policy should permit one but not the other; worries about abuse or about giving anyone dominion over the lives of others apply equally to either. As a result, I will take the arguments evaluated below to apply to both and will focus on euthanasia.

My concern here will be with *voluntary* euthanasia only—that is, with the case in which a clearly competent patient makes a fully voluntary and persistent request for aid in dying. Involuntary euthanasia, in which a competent patient explicitly refuses or opposes receiving euthanasia, and nonvoluntary euthanasia, in which a patient is incompetent and unable to express his or her wishes about euthanasia, will be considered here only as potential unwanted side-effects of permitting voluntary euthanasia. I emphasize as well that I am concerned with *active* euthanasia, not withholding or withdrawing life-sustaining treatment, which some commentators characterize as "passive euthanasia." Finally, I will be concerned with euthanasia where the motive of those who perform it is to respect the wishes of the patient and to provide the patient with a "good death," though one important issue is whether a change in legal policy could restrict the performance of euthanasia to only those cases.

A last introductory point is that I will be examining only secular arguments about euthanasia, though of course many people's attitudes to it are inextricable from their religious views. The policy issue is only whether euthanasia should be permissible, and no one who has religious objections to it should be required to take any part in it, though of course this would not fully satisfy some opponents.

## THE CENTRAL ETHICAL ARGUMENT FOR VOLUNTARY ACTIVE EUTHANASIA

The central ethical argument for euthanasia is familiar. It is that the very same two fundamental ethical values supporting the consensus on patient's rights to decide about life-sustaining treatment also support the ethical permissibility of euthanasia. These values are individual self-determination or autonomy and individual well-being. By self-determination as it bears on euthanasia, I mean people's interest in making important decisions about their lives for themselves according to their own values or conceptions of a good life, and in being left free to act on those decisions. Self-determination is valuable because it permits people to form and live in accordance with their own conception of a good life, at least within the bounds of justice and consistent with others doing so as well. In exercising self-determination people take responsibility for their lives and for the kinds of persons they become. A central aspect of human dignity lies in people's capacity to direct their lives in this way. The value of exercising self-determination presupposes some minimum of decisionmaking capacities or competence, which thus limits the scope of euthanasia supported by self-determination; it cannot justifiably be administered, for example, in cases of serious dementia or treatable clinical depression.

Does the value of individual self-determination extend to the time and manner of one's death? Most people are very concerned about the nature of the last stage of their lives. This reflects not just a fear of experiencing substantial suffering when dying, but also a desire to retain dignity and control during this last period of life. Death is today increasingly preceded by a long period of significant physical and mental decline, due in part to the technological interventions of modern medicine. Many people adjust to these disabilities and find meaning and value in new activities and ways. Others find the impairments and burdens in the last stage of their lives at some point sufficiently great to make life no longer worth living. For many patients near death, maintaining the quality of one's life, avoiding great suffering, maintaining one's dignity, and insuring that others remember us as we wish them to become of paramount importance and outweigh merely extending one's life. But there is no single, objectively correct answer for everyone as to when, if at all, one's life becomes all things considered a burden and unwanted. If self-determination is a fundamental value, then the great variability among people on this question makes it especially important that individuals control the manner, circumstances, and timing of their dying and death.

The other main value that supports euthanasia is individual well-being. It might seem that individual well-being conflicts with a person's self-determination when the person requests euthanasia. Life itself is commonly taken to be a central good for persons, often valued for its own sake, as well as necessary for pursuit of all other goods within a life. But when a competent patient decides to forgo all further life-sustaining treatment then the patient, either explicitly or implicitly, commonly decides that the best life possible for him or her with treatment is of sufficiently poor quality that it is worse than no further life at all. Life is no longer considered a benefit by the patient, but has now become a burden. The same judgment underlies a request for euthanasia: continued life is seen by the patient as no longer a benefit, but now a burden. Especially in the often severely compromised and debilitated states of many critically ill or dying patients, there is no objective standard, but only the competent patient's judgment of whether continued life is no longer a benefit.

Of course, sometimes there are conditions, such as clinical depression, that call into question whether the patient has made a competent choice, either to forgo life-sustaining treatment or to seek euthanasia, and then the patient's choice need not be evidence that continued life is no longer a benefit for him or her. Just as with decisions about treatment, a determination of incompetence can warrant not honoring the patient's choice; in the case of treatment, we then transfer decisional authority to a surrogate, though in the case of voluntary active euthanasia a determination that the patient is incompetent means that choice is not possible.

The value or right of self-determination does not entitle patients to compel physicians to act contrary to their own moral or professional values. Physicians are moral and professional agents whose own self-determination or integrity should be respected as well. If performing euthanasia became legally permissible, but conflicted with a particular physician's reasonable understanding of his or her moral or professional responsibilities, the care of a patient who requested euthanasia should be transferred to another.

Most opponents do not deny that there are some cases in which the values of patient self-determination and well-being support euthanasia. Instead, they commonly offer two kinds of arguments against it that on their view outweigh or override this support. The first kind of argument is that in any individual case where considerations of the patient's self-determination and well-being do support euthanasia, it is nevertheless always ethically wrong or impermissible. The second kind of argument grants that in some individual cases euthanasia may *not* be ethically wrong, but maintains nonetheless that public and legal policy should never permit it. The first kind of argument focuses on features of any individual case of euthanasia, while the second kind focuses on social or legal policy. In the next section I consider the first kind of argument.

# EUTHANASIA IS THE DELIBERATE KILLING
# OF AN INNOCENT PERSON

The claim that any individual instance of euthanasia is a case of deliberate killing of an innocent person is, with only minor qualifications, correct. Unlike forgoing life-sustaining treatment, commonly understood as allowing to die, euthanasia is clearly killing, defined as depriving of life or causing the death of a living being. While providing morphine for pain relief at doses where the risk of respiratory depression and an earlier death may be a foreseen but unintended side effect of treating the patient's pain, in a case of euthanasia the patient's death is deliberate or intended even if in both the physician's ultimate end may be respecting the patient's wishes. If the deliberate killing of an innocent person is wrong, euthanasia would be nearly always impermissible.

In the context of medicine, the ethical prohibition against deliberately killing the innocent derives some of its plausibility from the belief that nothing in the currently accepted practice of medicine is deliberate killing. Thus, in commenting on the "It's Over, Debbie" case, four prominent physicians and bioethicists could entitle their paper "Doctors Must Not Kill."[5] The belief that doctors do not in fact kill requires the corollary belief that forgoing life-sustaining treatment, whether by not starting or by stopping treatment, is allowing to die, not killing. Common though this view is, I shall argue that it is confused and mistaken.

Why is the common view mistaken? Consider the case of a patient terminally ill with ALS disease. She is completely respirator dependent with no hope of ever being weaned. She is unquestionably competent but finds her condition intolerable and persistently requests to be removed from the respirator and allowed to die. Most people and physicians would agree that the patient's physician should respect the patient's wishes and remove her from the respirator, though this will certainly cause the patient's death. The common understanding is that the physician thereby allows the patient to die. But is that correct?

Suppose the patient has a greedy and hostile son who mistakenly believes that his mother will never decide to stop her life-sustaining treatment and that even if she did her physician would not remove her from the respirator. Afraid that this inheritance will be dissipated by a long and expensive hospitalization, he enters his mother's room while she is sedated, extubates her, and she dies. Shortly thereafter the medical staff discovers what he has done and confronts the son. He replies, "I didn't kill her. I merely allowed her to die. It was her ALS disease that caused her death." I think this would rightly be dismissed as transparent sophistry—the son went into his mother's room and deliberately killed her. But, of course, the son performed just the same physical actions, did just the same thing, that the physician would have done. If that is so, then doesn't the physician also kill the patient when he extubates her?

I underline immediately that there are important ethical differences between what the physician and the greedy son do. First, the physician acts with the patient's consent whereas the son does not. Second, the physician acts with a good motive—to respect the patient's wishes and self-determination—whereas the son acts with a bad motive—to protect his own inheritance. Third, the physician acts in a social role through which he is legally authorized to carry out the patient's wishes regarding treatment whereas the son has no such authorization. These and perhaps other ethically important differences show that what the physician did was morally justified whereas what the son did was morally wrong. What they do *not* show, however, is that the son killed while the physician allowed to die. One can either kill or allow to die with or without consent, with a good or bad motive, within or outside of a social role that authorizes one to do so.

The difference between killing and allowing to die that I have been implicitly appealing to here is roughly that between acts and omissions resulting in death.[6] Both the physician and the greedy son act in a manner intended to cause death, do cause death, and so both kill. One reason this conclusion is resisted is that on a different understanding of the distinction between killing and allowing to die, what the physician does is allow to die. In this account, the mother's ALS is a lethal disease whose normal progression is being held back or blocked by the life-sustaining respiratory treatment. Removing this artificial intervention is then viewed as standing aside and allowing the patient to die of her underlying disease. I have argued elsewhere that this alternative account is deeply problematic, in part because it commits us to accepting that what the greedy son does is to allow to die, not kill.[7] Here, I want to note two other reasons why the conclusion that stopping life support is killing is resisted.

The first reason is that killing is often understood, especially within medicine, as unjustified causing of death; in medicine it is thought to be done only accidentally or negligently. It is also increasingly widely accepted that a physician is ethically justified in stopping life support in a case like that of the ALS patient. But if these two beliefs are correct, then what the physician does cannot be killing, and so must be allowing to die. Killing patients is not, to put it flippantly, understood to be part of physicians' job description. What is mistaken in this line of reasoning is the assumption that all killings are *unjustified* causings of death. Instead, some killings are ethically justified, including many instances of stopping life support.

Another reason for resisting the conclusion that stopping life support is often killing is that it is psychologically uncomfortable. Suppose the physician had stopped the ALS patient's respirator and had made the son's claim, "I didn't kill her, I merely allowed her to die. It was her ALS disease that caused her death." The clue to the psychological role here is how naturally the "merely" modifies "allowed her to die." The characterization as allowing to die is meant to shift felt responsibility away from the agent—the physician—and to the lethal disease process. Other language common in death and dying contexts plays a similar role; "letting nature take its course" or "stopping prolonging the dying process" both seem to shift responsibility from the physician who stops life support to the fatal disease process. However psychologically helpful these conceptualizations may be in making the difficult responsibility of a physician's role in the patient's death bearable, they nevertheless are confusions. Both physicians and family members can instead be helped to understand that it is the patient's decision and consent to stopping treatment that limits their responsibility for the patient's death and that shifts that responsibility to the patient.

Many who accept the difference between killing and allowing to die as the distinction between acts and omissions resulting in death have gone on to argue that killing is not in itself morally different from allowing to die.[8] In this account, very roughly, one kills when one performs an action that causes the death of a person (we are in a boat, you cannot swim, I push you overboard, and you drown), and one allows to die when one has the ability and opportunity to prevent the death of another, knows this, and omits doing so, with the result that the person dies (we are in a boat, you cannot swim, you fall overboard, I don't throw you an available life ring, and you drown). Those who see no moral difference between killing and allowing to die typically employ the strategy of comparing cases that differ in these and no other potentially morally important respects. This will allow people to consider whether the mere difference that one is a case of killing and the other of allowing to die matters morally, or whether instead it is other features that make most cases of killing worse than most instances of allowing to die. Here is such a pair of cases:

**Case 1**   A very gravely ill patient is brought to a hospital emergency room and sent up to the ICU. The patient begins to develop respiratory failure that is likely to require intubation very soon. At that point the patient's family members and long-standing physician arrive at the ICU and inform the ICU staff that there had been extensive discussion about future care with the patient when he was unquestionably competent. Given his grave and terminal illness, as well as his state of debilitation, the patient had firmly rejected being placed on a respirator under any circumstances, and the family and physician produce the patient's advance directive to that effect. The ICU staff do not intubate the patient, who dies of respiratory failure.

**Case 2**   The same as Case 1 except that the family and physician are slightly delayed in traffic and arrive shortly after the patient has been intubated and placed on the respirator. The ICU staff extubate the patient, who dies of respiratory failure.

In Case 1 the patient is allowed to die, in Case 2 he is killed, but it is hard to see why what is done in Case 2 is significantly different morally than what is done in Case 1. It must be other factors that make most killings worse than most allowings to die, and if so, euthanasia cannot be wrong simply because it is killing instead of allowing to die.

Suppose both my arguments are mistaken. Suppose that killing is worse than allowing to die and that withdrawing life support is not killing, although euthanasia is. Euthanasia still need not for that reason be morally wrong. To see this, we need to determine the basic principle for the moral evaluation of killing persons. What is it that makes paradigm cases of wrongful killing wrongful? One very plausible answer is that killing denies the victim something that he or she values greatly—continued life or a future. Moreover, since continued life is necessary for pursuing any of a person's plans and purposes, killing brings the frustration of all of these plans and desires as well. In a nutshell, wrongful killing deprives a person of a valued future, and of all the person wanted and planned to do in that future.

A natural expression of this account of the wrongness of killing is that people have a moral right not to be killed.[9] But in this account of the wrongness of killing, the right not to be killed, like other rights, should be waivable when the person makes a competent decision that continued life is no longer wanted or a good, but is instead worse than no further life at all. In this view, euthanasia is properly understood as a case of a person having waived his or her right not to be killed.

This rights view of the wrongness of killing is not, of course, universally shared. Many people's moral views about killing have their origins in religious views that human life comes from God and cannot be justifiably destroyed or taken away, either by the person whose life it is or by another. But in a pluralistic society like our own with a strong commitment to freedom of religion, public policy should not be grounded in religious beliefs which many in that society reject. I turn now to the general evaluation of public policy on euthanasia.

## WOULD THE BAD CONSEQUENCES OF EUTHANASIA OUTWEIGH THE GOOD?

The argument against euthanasia at the policy level is stronger than at the level of individual cases, though even here I believe the case is ultimately unpersuasive, or at best indecisive. The policy level is the place where the main issues lie, however, and where moral considerations that might override arguments in favor of euthanasia will be found, if they are found anywhere. It is important to note two kinds of disagreement about the consequences for public policy of permitting euthanasia. First, there is empirical or factual disagreement about what the consequences would be. This disagreement is greatly exacerbated by the lack of firm data on the issue. Second, since on any reasonable assessment there would be both good and bad consequences, there are moral disagreements about the relative importance of different effects. In addition to these two sources of disagreement, there is also no single, well-specified policy proposal for legalizing euthanasia on which policy assessments can focus. But without such specification, and especially without explicit procedures for protecting against well-intentioned misuse and ill-intentioned abuse, the consequences for policy are largely speculative. Despite these difficulties, a preliminary account of the main likely good and bad consequences is possible. This should help clarify where better data or more moral analysis and argument are needed, as well as where policy safeguards must be developed.

## Potential Good Consequences of Permitting Euthanasia

What are the likely good consequences? First, if euthanasia were permitted it would be possible to respect the self-determination of competent patients who want it, but now cannot get it because of its illegality. We simply do not know how many such patients and people there are. In the Netherlands, with a population of about 14.5 million (in 1987), estimates in a recent study were that about 1,900 cases of voluntary active euthanasia or physician-assisted suicide occur annually. No straightforward extrapolation to the United States is possible for many reasons, among them, that we do not know how many people here who want euthanasia now get it, despite its illegality. Even with better data on the number of persons who want euthanasia but cannot get it, significant moral disagreement would remain about how much weight should be given to any instance of failure to respect a person's self-determination in this way.

One important factor substantially affecting the number of persons who would seek euthanasia is the extent to which an alternative is available. The widespread acceptance in the law, social policy, and medical practice of the right of a competent patient to forgo life-sustaining treatment suggests that the number of competent persons in the United States who would want euthanasia if it were permitted is probably relatively small.

A second good consequence of making euthanasia legally permissible benefits a much larger group. Polls have shown that a majority of the American public believes that people should have a right to obtain euthanasia if they want it.[10] No doubt the vast majority of those who support this right to euthanasia will never in fact come to want euthanasia for themselves. Nevertheless, making it legally permissible would reassure many people that if they ever do want euthanasia they would be able to obtain it. This reassurance would supplement the broader control over the process of dying given by the right to decide about life-sustaining treatment. Having fire insurance on one's house benefits all who have it, not just those whose houses actually burn down, by reassuring them that in the unlikely event of their house burning down, they will receive the money needed to rebuild it. Likewise, the legalization of euthanasia can be thought of as a kind of insurance policy against being forced to endure a protracted dying process that one has come to find burdensome and unwanted, especially when there is no life-sustaining treatment to forgo. The strong concern about losing control of their care expressed by many people who face serious illness likely to end in death suggests that they give substantial importance to the legalization of euthanasia as a means of maintaining this control.

A third good consequence of the legalization of euthanasia concerns patients whose dying is filled with severe and unrelievable pain or suffering. When there is a life-sustaining treatment that, if forgone, will lead relatively quickly to death, then doing so can bring an end to these patients' suffering without recourse to euthanasia. For patients receiving no such treatment, however, euthanasia may be the only release from their otherwise prolonged suffering and agony. This argument from mercy has always been the strongest argument for euthanasia in those cases to which it applies.[11]

The importance of relieving pain and suffering is less controversial than is the frequency with which patients are forced to undergo untreatable agony that only euthanasia could relieve. If we focus first on suffering caused by physical pain, it is crucial to distinguish pain that *could* be adequately relieved with modern methods of pain control, though it in fact is not, from pain that is relievable only by death.[12] For a variety of reasons, including some physicians' fear of hastening the patient's death, as well as the lack of a publicly accessible means for assessing the amount of the patient's pain, many patients suffer pain that could be, but is not, relieved.

Specialists in pain control, as for example the pain of terminally ill cancer patients, argue that there are very few patients whose pain could not be adequately controlled, though sometimes at the cost of so sedating them that they are effectively unable to interact with other people or their environment. Thus, the argument from mercy in cases of physical pain can probably be met in a large majority of cases by providing adequate measures of pain relief. This should be a high priority, whatever our legal policy on euthanasia—the relief of pain and suffering has long been, quite properly, one of the central goals of medicine. Those cases in which pain could be effectively relieved, but in fact is not, should only count significantly in favor of legalizing euthanasia if all reasonable efforts to change pain management techniques have been tried and have failed.

Dying patients often undergo substantial psychological suffering that is not fully or even principally the result of physical pain.[13] The knowledge about how to relieve this suffering is much more limited than in the case of relieving pain, and efforts to do so are probably more often unsuccessful. If the argument from mercy is extended to patients experiencing great and unrelievable psychological suffering, the numbers of patients to which it applies are much greater.

One last good consequence of legalizing euthanasia is that once death has been accepted, it is often more humane to end life quickly and peacefully, when that is what the patient wants. Such a death will often be seen as better than a more prolonged one. People who suffer a sudden and unexpected death, for example by dying quickly or in their sleep from a heart attack or stroke, are often considered lucky to have died in this way. We care about how we die in part because we care about how others remember us, and we hope they will remember us as we were in "good times" with them and not as we might be when disease has robbed us of our dignity as human beings. As with much in the treatment and care of the dying, people's concerns differ in this respect, but for at least some people, euthanasia will be a more humane death than what they have often experienced with other loved ones and might otherwise expect for themselves.

Some opponents of euthanasia challenge how much importance should be given to any of these good consequences of permitting it, or even whether some would be good consequences at all. But more frequently, opponents cite a number of bad consequences that permitting euthanasia would or could produce, and it is to their assessment that I now turn.

## Potential Bad Consequences of Permitting Euthanasia

Some of the arguments against permitting euthanasia are aimed specifically against physicians, while others are aimed against anyone being permitted to perform it. I shall first consider one argument of the former sort. Permitting physicians to perform euthanasia, it is said, would be incompatible with their fundamental moral and professional commitment as healers to care for patients and to protect life. Moreover, if euthanasia by physicians became common, patients would come to fear that a medication was intended not to treat or care, but instead to kill, and would thus lose trust in their physicians. This position was forcefully stated in a paper by Willard Gaylin and his colleagues:

> The very soul of medicine is on trial . . . This issue touches medicine at its moral center; if this moral center collapses, if physicians become killers or are even licensed to kill, the profession—and, therewith, each physician—will never again be worthy of trust and respect as healer and comforter and protector of life in all its frailty.

These authors go on to make clear that, while they oppose permitting anyone to perform euthanasia, their special concern is with physicians doing so:

> We call on fellow physicians to say that they will not deliberately kill. We must also say to each of our fellow physicians that we will not tolerate killing of patients and that we shall take disciplinary action against doctors who kill. And we must say to the broader community that if it insists on tolerating or legalizing active euthanasia, it will have to find nonphysicians to do its killing.[14]

If permitting physicians to kill would undermine the very "moral center" of medicine, then almost certainly physicians should not be permitted to perform euthanasia. But how persuasive is this claim? Patients should not fear, as a consequence of permitting *voluntary* active euthanasia, that their physicians will substitute a lethal injection for what patients want and believe is part of their care. If active euthanasia is restricted to cases in which it is truly voluntary, then no patient should fear getting it unless she or he has voluntarily requested it. (The fear that we might in time also come to accept nonvoluntary, or even involuntary, active euthanasia is a slippery slope worry I address below.) Patients' trust of their physicians could be increased, not eroded, by knowledge that physicians will provide aid in dying when patients seek it.

Might Gaylin and his colleagues nevertheless be correct in their claim that the moral center of medicine would collapse if physicians were to become killers? This question raises what at the deepest level should be the guiding aims of medicine, a question that obviously cannot be fully explored here. But I do want to say enough to indicate the direction that I believe an appropriate response to this challenge should take. In spelling out above what I called the positive argument for voluntary active euthanasia, I suggested that two principal values—respecting patients' self-determination and promoting their well-being—underlie the consensus that competent patients, or the surrogates of incompetent patients, are entitled to refuse any life-sustaining treatment and to choose from among available alternative treatments. It is the commitment to these two values in guiding physicians' actions as healers, comforters, and protectors of their patients' lives that should be at the "moral center" of medicine, and these two values support physicians' administering euthanasia when their patients make competent requests for it.

What should not be at that moral center is a commitment to preserving patients' lives as such, without regard to whether those patients want their lives preserved or judge their preservation a benefit to them. Vitalism has been rejected by most physicians, and despite some statements that suggest it, is almost certainly not what Gaylin and colleagues intended. One of them, Leon Kass, has elaborated elsewhere the view that medicine is a moral profession whose proper aim is "the naturally given end of health," understood as the wholeness and well-working of the human being; "for the physician, at least, human life in living bodies commands respect and reverence—*by its very nature.*" Kass continues, "the deepest ethical principle restraining the physician's power is not the autonomy or freedom of the patient; neither is it his own compassion or good intention. Rather, it is the dignity and mysterious power of human life itself."[15] I believe Kass is in the end mistaken about the proper account of the aims of medicine and the limits on physicians' power, but this difficult issue will certainly be one of the central themes in the continuing debate about euthanasia.

A second bad consequence that some foresee is that permitting euthanasia would weaken society's commitment to provide optimal care for dying patients. We live at a time in which the control of health care costs has become, and is likely to continue to be, the dominant focus of health care policy. If euthanasia is seen as a cheaper alternative to adequate care and treatment, then we might become less scrupulous about providing sometimes costly support and other services to dying patients. Particularly if our society comes to embrace deeper and more explicit rationing of health care, frail, elderly, and dying patients will need to be strong and effective advocates for their own health care and other needs, although they are hardly in a position to do this. We should do nothing to weaken their ability to obtain adequate care and services.

This second worry is difficult to assess because there is little firm evidence about the likelihood of the feared erosion in the care of dying patients. There are at least two reasons, however, for skepticism about this argument. The first is that the same worry could have been directed at recognizing patients' or surrogates' rights to forgo life-sustaining treatment, yet there is no persuasive evidence that recognizing the right to refuse treatment has caused a serious erosion in the quality of care of dying patients. The second reason for skepticism about this worry is that only a very small proportion of deaths would occur from euthanasia if it were permitted. In the Netherlands, where euthanasia under specified circumstances is permitted by the courts, though not authorized by statute, the best estimate of the proportion of overall deaths that result from it is about 2 percent.[16] Thus, the vast majority of critically ill and dying patients will not request it, and so will still have to be cared for by physicians, families, and others. Permitting euthanasia should not diminish people's commitment and concern to maintain and improve the care of these patients.

A third possible bad consequence of permitting euthanasia (or even a public discourse in which strong support for euthanasia is evident) is to threaten the progress made in securing the rights of patients or their surrogates to decide about and to refuse life-sustaining treatment.[17] This progress has been made against the backdrop of a clear and firm legal prohibition of euthanasia, which has provided a relatively bright line limiting the dominion of others over patients' lives. It has therefore been an important reassurance to concerns about how the authority to take steps ending life might be misused, abused, or wrongly extended.

Many supporters of the right of patients or their surrogates to refuse treatment strongly oppose euthanasia, and if forced to choose might well withdraw their support of the right to refuse treatment rather than accept euthanasia. Public policy in the last fifteen years has generally let life-sustaining treatment decisions be made in health care settings between physicians and patients or their surrogates, and without the involvement of the courts. However, if euthanasia is made legally permissible greater involvement of the courts is likely, which could in turn extend to a greater court involvement in life-sustaining treatment decisions. Most agree, however, that increased involvement of the courts in these decisions would be undesirable, as it would make sound decisionmaking more cumbersome and difficult without sufficient compensating benefits.

As with the second potential bad consequence of permitting euthanasia, this third consideration too is speculative and difficult to assess. The feared erosion of patients' or surrogates' rights to decide about life-sustaining treatment, together with greater court involvement in those decisions, are both possible. However, I believe there is reason to discount this general worry. The legal rights of competent patients and, to a lesser degree, surrogates of incompetent patients to decide about treatment are very firmly embedded in a long line of informed consent and life-sustaining treatment cases, and are not likely to be eroded by a debate over, or even acceptance of, euthanasia. It will not be accepted without safeguards that reassure the public about abuse, and if that debate shows the need for similar safeguards for some life-sustaining treatment decisions they should be adopted there as well. In neither case are the only possible safeguards greater court involvement, as the recent growth of institutional ethics committees shows.

The fourth potential bad consequence of permitting euthanasia has been developed by David Velleman and turns on the subtle point that making a new option or choice available to people can sometimes make them worse off, even if once they have the choice they go on to choose what is best for them.[18]

Ordinarily, people's continued existence is viewed by them as given, a fixed condition with which they must cope. Making euthanasia available to people as an option denies them the alternative of staying alive by default. If people are offered the option of euthanasia, their continued existence is now a choice for which they can be held responsible and which they can be asked by others to justify. We care, and are right to care, about being able to justify ourselves to others. To the extent that our society is unsympathetic to justifying a severely dependent or impaired existence, a heavy psychological burden of proof may be placed on patients who think their terminal illness or chronic infirmity is not a sufficient reason for dying. Even if they otherwise view their life as worth living, the opinion of others around them that it is not can threaten their reason for living and make euthanasia a rational choice. Thus the existence of the option becomes a subtle pressure to request it.

This argument correctly identifies the reason why offering some patients the option of euthanasia would not benefit them. Velleman takes it not as a reason for opposing all euthanasia, but for restricting it to circumstances where there are "unmistakable and overpowering reasons for persons to want the option of euthanasia," and for denying the option in all other cases. But there are at least three reasons why such restriction may not be warranted. First, polls and other evidence support that most Americans believe euthanasia should be permitted (though the recent defeat of the referendum to permit it in the state of Washington raises some doubt about this support). Thus, many more people seem to want the choice than would be made worse off by getting it. Second, if giving people the option of ending their life really makes them worse off, then we should not only prohibit euthanasia, but also take back from people the right they now have to decide about life-sustaining treatment. The feared harmful effect should already have occurred from securing people's right to refuse life-sustaining treatment, yet there is no evidence of any such widespread harm or any broad public desire to rescind that right. Third, since there is a wide range of conditions in which reasonable people can and do disagree about whether they would want continued life, it is not possible to restrict the permissibility of euthanasia as narrowly as Velleman suggests without thereby denying it to most persons who would want it; to permit it only in cases in which virtually everyone would want it would be to deny it to most who would want it.

A fifth potential bad consequence of making euthanasia legally permissible is that it might weaken the general legal prohibition of homicide. This prohibition is so fundamental to civilized society, it is argued, that we should do nothing that erodes it. If most cases of stopping life support are killing, as I have already argued, then the court cases permitting such killing have already in effect weakened this prohibition. However, neither the courts nor most people have seen these cases as killing and so as challenging the prohibition of homicide. The courts have usually grounded patients' or their surrogates' rights to refuse life-sustaining treatment in rights to privacy, liberty, self-determination, or bodily integrity, not in exceptions to homicide laws.

Legal permission for physicians or others to perform euthanasia could not be grounded in patients' rights to decide about medical treatment. Permitting euthanasia would require qualifying, at least in effect, the legal prohibition against homicide, a prohibition that in general does not allow the consent of the victim to justify or excuse the act. Nevertheless, the very same fundamental basis of the right to decide about life-sustaining treatment—respecting a person's self-determination—does support euthanasia as well. Individual self-determination has long been a well-entrenched and fundamental value in the law, and so extending it to euthanasia would not require appeal to novel legal values or principles. That suicide or attempted suicide is no longer a criminal offense in virtually all states indicates an acceptance of individual self-determination in the taking of one's own life analogous to that required for voluntary active euthanasia. The legal prohibition (in most states) of assisting in suicide and the refusal in the law to accept the consent of the victim as a possible justification of homicide are both arguably a result of difficulties in the legal process of establishing the consent of the victim after the fact. If procedures can be designed that clearly establish the voluntariness of the person's request for euthanasia, it would under those procedures represent a carefully circumscribed qualification on the legal prohibition of homicide. Nevertheless, some remaining worries about this weakening can be captured in the final potential bad consequence, to which I will now turn.

This final potential bad consequence is the central concern of many opponents of euthanasia and, I believe, is the most serious objection to a legal policy permitting it. According to this "slippery slope" worry, although active euthanasia may be morally permissible in cases in which it is unequivocally voluntary and the patient finds his or her condition unbearable, a legal policy permitting euthanasia would inevitably lead to active euthanasia being performed in many other cases in which it would be morally wrong. To prevent those other wrongful cases of euthanasia we should not permit even morally justified performance of it.

Slippery slope arguments of this form are problematic and difficult to evaluate.[19] From one perspective, they are the last refuge of conservative defenders of the status quo. When all the opponent's objections to the wrongness of euthanasia itself have been met, the opponent then shifts ground and acknowledges both that it is not in itself wrong and that a legal policy which resulted only in its being performed would not be bad. Nevertheless, the opponent maintains, it should still not be permitted because doing so would result in its being performed in other cases in which it is not voluntary and would be wrong. In this argument's most extreme form, permitting euthanasia is the first and fateful step down the slippery slope to Nazism. Once on the slope we will be unable to get off.

Now it cannot be denied that it is *possible* that permitting euthanasia could have these fateful consequences, but that cannot be enough to warrant prohibiting it if it is otherwise justified. A similar *possible* slippery slope worry could have been raised to securing competent patients' rights to decide about life support, but recent history shows such a worry would have been

unfounded. It must be relevant how likely it is that we will end with horren-
dous consequences and an unjustified practice of euthanasia. How *likely* and
*widespread* would the abuses and unwarranted extensions of permitting it be?
By abuses, I mean the performance of euthanasia that fails to satisfy the conditions required for voluntary active euthanasia, for example, if the patient has
been subtly pressured to accept it. By unwarranted extensions of policy, I
mean later changes in legal policy to permit not just voluntary euthanasia, but
also euthanasia in cases in which, for example, it need not be fully voluntary.
Opponents of voluntary euthanasia on slippery slope grounds have not provided the data or evidence necessary to turn their speculative concerns into
well-grounded likelihoods.

It is at least clear, however, that both the character and likelihood of
abuses of a legal policy permitting euthanasia depend in significant part on
the procedures put in place to protect against them. I will not try to detail fully
what such procedures might be, but will just give some examples of what they
might include:

1. The patient should be provided with all relevant information about
   his or her medical condition, current prognosis, available alternative
   treatments, and the prognosis of each.
2. Procedures should ensure that the patient's request for euthanasia is
   stable or enduring (a brief waiting period could be required) and fully
   voluntary (an advocate for the patient might be appointed to ensure
   this).
3. All reasonable alternatives must have been explored for improving
   the patient's quality of life and relieving any pain or suffering.
4. A psychiatric evaluation should ensure that the patient's request is not
   the result of a treatable psychological impairment such as depression.[20]

These examples of procedural safeguards are all designed to ensure that
the patient's choice is fully informed, voluntary, and competent, and so a true
exercise of self-determination. Other proposals for euthanasia would restrict
its permissibility further—for example, to the terminally ill—a restriction that
cannot be supported by self-determination. Such additional restrictions might,
however, be justified by concern for limiting potential harms from abuse. At
the same time, it is important not to impose procedural or substantive safeguards so restrictive as to make euthanasia impermissible or practically infea-
sible in a wide range of justified cases.

These examples of procedural safeguards make clear that it is possible to
substantially reduce, though not to eliminate, the potential for abuse of a policy
permitting voluntary active euthanasia. Any legalization of the practice should
be accompanied by a well-considered set of procedural safeguards together
with an ongoing evaluation of its use. Introducing euthanasia into only a few
states could be a form of carefully limited and controlled social experiment that
would give us evidence about the benefits and harms of the practice. Even then
firm and uncontroversial data may remain elusive, as the continuing controversy over what has taken place in the Netherlands in recent years indicates.[21]

## The Slip into Nonvoluntary Active Euthanasia

While I believe slippery slope worries can largely be limited by making necessary distinctions both in principle and in practice, one slippery slope concern is legitimate. There is reason to expect that legalization of voluntary active euthanasia might soon be followed by strong pressure to legalize some nonvoluntary euthanasia of incompetent patients unable to express their own wishes. Respecting a person's self-determination and recognizing that continued life is not always of value to a person can support not only voluntary active euthanasia, but some nonvoluntary euthanasia as well. These are the same values that ground competent patients' right to refuse life-sustaining treatment. Recent history here is instructive. In the medical ethics literature, in the courts since Quinlan, and in norms of medical practice, that right has been extended to incompetent patients and exercised by a surrogate who is to decide as the patient would have decided in the circumstances if competent.[22] It has been held unreasonable to continue life-sustaining treatment that the patient would not have wanted just because the patient now lacks the capacity to tell us that. Life-sustaining treatment for incompetent patients is today frequently forgone on the basis of a surrogate's decision, or less frequently on the basis of an advance directive executed by the patient while still competent. The very same logic that has extended the right to refuse life-sustaining treatment from a competent patient to the surrogate of an incompetent patient (acting with or without a formal advance directive from the patient) may well extend the scope of active euthanasia. The argument will be, why continue to force unwanted life on patients just because they have now lost the capacity to request euthanasia from us?

A related phenomenon may reinforce this slippery slope concern. In the Netherlands, what the courts have sanctioned has been clearly restricted to voluntary euthanasia. In itself, this serves as some evidence that permitting it need *not* lead to permitting the nonvoluntary variety. There is some indication, however, that for many Dutch physicians euthanasia is no longer viewed as a special action, set apart from their usual practice and restricted only to competent persons.[23] Instead, it is seen as one end of a spectrum of caring for dying patients. When viewed in this way it will be difficult to deny euthanasia to a patient for whom it is seen as the best or most appropriate form of care simply because that patient is now incompetent and cannot request it.

Even if voluntary active euthanasia should slip into nonvoluntary active euthanasia, with surrogates acting for incompetent patients, the ethical evaluation is more complex than many opponents of euthanasia allow. Just as in the case of surrogates' decisions to forgo life-sustaining treatment for incompetent patients, so also surrogates' decisions to request euthanasia for incompetent persons would often accurately reflect what the incompetent person would have wanted and would deny the person nothing that he or she would have considered worth having. Making nonvoluntary active euthanasia legally permissible, however, would greatly enlarge the number of patients on whom it might be performed and substantially enlarge the potential for misuse and abuse. As noted above, frail and debilitated elderly people, often demented or otherwise incompetent and thereby unable to defend and assert their own interests, may be especially vulnerable to unwanted euthanasia.

For some people, this risk is more than sufficient reason to oppose the legalization of voluntary euthanasia. But while we should in general be cautious about inferring much from the experience in the Netherlands to what our own experience in the United States might be, there may be one important lesson that we can learn from them. One commentator has noted that in the Netherlands families of incompetent patients have less authority than do families in the United States to act as surrogates for incompetent patients in making decisions to forgo life-sustaining treatment.[24] From the Dutch perspective, it may be we in the United States who are *already* on the slippery slope in having given surrogates broad authority to forgo life-sustaining treatment for incompetent persons. In this view, the more important moral divide, and the more important with regard to potential for abuse, is not between forgoing life-sustaining treatment and euthanasia, but instead between voluntary and nonvoluntary performance of either. If this is correct, then the more important issue is ensuring the appropriate principles and procedural safeguards for the exercise of decisionmaking authority by surrogates for incompetent persons in *all* decisions at the end of life. This may be the correct response to slippery slope worries about euthanasia.

I have cited both good and bad consequences that have been thought likely from a policy change permitting voluntary active euthanasia, and have tried to evaluate their likelihood and relative importance. Nevertheless, as I noted earlier, reasonable disagreement remains both about the consequences of permitting euthanasia and about which of these consequences are more important. The depth and strength of public and professional debate about whether, all things considered, permitting euthanasia would be desirable or undesirable reflects these disagreements. While my own view is that the balance of considerations supports permitting the practice, my principal purpose here has been to clarify the main issues.

## THE ROLE OF PHYSICIANS

If euthanasia is made legally permissible, should physicians take part in it? Should only physicians be permitted to perform it, as in the case in the Netherlands? In discussing whether euthanasia is incompatible with medicine's commitment to curing, caring for, and comforting patients, I argued that it is not at odds with a proper understanding of the aims of medicine, and so need not undermine patients' trust in their physicians. If that argument is correct, then physicians probably should not be prohibited, either by law or by professional norms, from taking part in a legally permissible practice of euthanasia (nor, of course, should they be compelled to do so if their

personal or professional scruples forbid it). Most physicians in the Netherlands appear not to understand euthanasia to be incompatible with their professional commitments.

Sometimes patients who would be able to end their lives on their own
nevertheless seek the assistance of physicians. Physician involvement in such
cases may have important benefits to patients and others beyond simply assuring the use of effective means. Historically, in the United States suicide has
carried a strong negative stigma that many today believe unwarranted. Seeking a physician's assistance, or what can almost seem a physician's blessing,
may be a way of trying to remove that stigma and show others that the decision for suicide was made with due seriousness and was justified under the
circumstances. The physician's involvement provides a kind of social approval, or more accurately helps counter what would otherwise be unwarranted social disapproval.

There are also at least two reasons for restricting the practice of euthanasia
to physicians only. First, physicians would inevitably be involved in some of
the important procedural safeguards necessary to a defensible practice, such
as seeing to it that the patient is well-informed about his or her condition,
prognosis, and possible treatments, and ensuring that all reasonable means
have been taken to improve the quality of the patient's life. Second, and probably more important, one necessary protection against abuse of the practice is
to limit the persons given authority to perform it, so that they can be held accountable for their exercise of that authority. Physicians, whose training and
professional norms give some assurance that they would perform euthanasia
responsibly, are an appropriate group of persons to whom the practice may be
restricted.

## NOTES

1. President's Commission for the Study of Ethical Problems in Medicine
   and Biomedical and Behavioral Research, *Deciding to Forego Life-Sustaining
   Treatment [sic]* (Washington, DC: US Government Printing Office, 1983);
   The Hastings Center, *Guidelines on the Termination of Life-Sustaining Treat-
   ment and Care of the Dying* (Bloomington: Indiana University Press, 1987);
   *Current Opinions of the Council on Ethical and Judicial Affairs of the American
   Medical Association—1989: Withholding or Withdrawing Life-Prolonging Treat-
   ment* (Chicago: American Medical Association, 1989); George Annas and
   Leonard Glantz, "The Right of Elderly Patients to Refuse Life-Sustaining
   Treatment," *Millbank Memorial Quarterly* 64, suppl. 2 (1986), pp. 95–162;
   Robert F. Weir, *Abating Treatment with Critically Ill Patients* (New York: Ox-
   ford University Press, 1989); Sidney J. Wanzer et al., "The Physician's Responsibility toward Hopelessly Ill Patients." *New England Journal of Medicine* 310 (1984), pp. 955–59.

2. M. A. M. de Wachter, "Active Euthanasia in the Netherlands," *JAMA* 262 (1989), pp. 3315–19.
3. Anonymous, "It's Over, Debbie," *JAMA* 259 (1988), p. 272; Timothy E. Quill, "Death and Dignity," *New England Journal of Medicine* 322 (1990), pp. 1881–83.
4. Wanzer et al., "The Physician's Responsibility toward Hopelessly Ill Patients: A Second Look," *New England Journal of Medicine* 320 (1989), pp. 844–49.
5. Willard Gaylin, Leon R. Kass, Edmund D. Pellegrino, and Mark Siegler, "Doctors Must Not Kill," *JAMA* 259 (1988), pp. 2139–40.
6. Bonnie Steinbock, ed., *Killing and Allowing to Die* (Englewood Cliffs, NJ: Prentice Hall, 1980).
7. Dan W. Brock, "Forgoing Food and Water: Is It Killing?" in *By No Extraordinary Means: The Choice to Forgo Life-Sustaining Food and Water,* ed. Joanne Lynn (Bloomington: Indiana University Press, 1986), pp. 117–31.
8. James Rachels, "Active and Passive Euthanasia," *New England Journal of Medicine* 292 (1975), pp. 78–80; Michael Tooley, *Abortion and Infanticide* (Oxford: Oxford University Press, 1983). In my paper, "Taking Human Life," *Ethics* 95 (1985), pp. 851–65, I argue in more detail that killing in itself is not morally different from allowing to die and defend the strategy of argument employed in this and the succeeding two paragraphs in the text.
9. Dan W. Brock, "Moral Rights and Permissible Killing," in *Ethical Issues Relating to Life and Death,* ed. John Ladd (New York: Oxford University Press, 1979), pp. 94–117.
10. P. Painton and E. Taylor, "Love or Let Die," *Time,* March 19, 1990, pp. 62–71; *Boston Globe*/Harvard University Poll, *Boston Globe,* November 3, 1991.
11. James Rachels, *The End of Life* (Oxford: Oxford University Press, 1986).
12. Marcia Angell, "The Quality of Mercy," *New England Journal of Medicine* 306 (1982), pp. 98–99; M. Donovan, P. Dillon, and L. Mcguire, "Incidence and Characteristics of Pain in a Sample of Medical-Surgical Inpatients," *Pain* 30 (1987), pp. 69–78.
13. Eric Cassell, *The Nature of Suffering and the Goals of Medicine* (New York: Oxford University Press, 1991).
14. Gaylin et al., "Doctors Must Not Kill."
15. Leon R. Kass, "Neither for Love nor Money: Why Doctors Must Not Kill," *Public Interest* 94 (1989), pp. 25–46; cf. also his *Toward a More Natural Science: Biology and Human Affairs* (New York: Free Press, 1985), chaps. 6–9.
16. Paul J. Van der Maas et al., "Euthanasia and Other Medical Decisions Concerning the End of Life," *Lancet* 338 (1991), pp. 669–74.
17. Susan M. Wolf, "Holding the Line on Euthanasia," Special Supplement, *Hastings Center Report* 19, no. 1 (1989), pp. 13–15.
18. My formulation of this argument derives from David Velleman's statement of it in his commentary on an earlier version of this paper delivered

at the American Philosophical Association Central Division meetings; a similar point was made to me by Elisha Milgram in discussion on another occasion. For more general development of the point see Thomas Schelling, *The Strategy of Conflict* (Cambridge, Mass.: Harvard University Press, 1960); and Gerald Dworkin, "Is More Choice Better than Less?" in *The Theory and Practice of Autonomy* (Cambridge: Cambridge University Press, 1988).

19. Frederick Schauer, "Slippery Slopes," *Harvard Law Review* 99 (1985), pp. 361–83; Wibren van der Burg, "The Slippery Slope Argument," *Ethics* 102 (October 1991), pp. 42–65.

20. There is evidence that physicians commonly fail to diagnose depression. See Robert I. Misbin, "Physicians Aid in Dying," *New England Journal of Medicine* 325 (1991), pp. 1304–7.

21. Richard Fenigsen, "A Case against Dutch Euthanasia," Special Supplement, *Hastings Center Report* 19, no. 1 (1989), pp. 22–30.

22. Allen E. Buchanan and Dan W. Brock, *Deciding for Others: The Ethics of Surrogate Decisionmaking* (Cambridge: Cambridge University Press, 1989).

23. Van der Maas et al., "Euthanasia and Other Medical Decisions."

24. Margaret P. Battin, "Seven Caveats Concerning the Discussion of Euthanasia in Holland," *American Philosophical Association Newsletter on Philosophy and Medicine* 89, no. 2 (1990).

# The Right to Suicide: A Psychiatrist's View

## Jerome A. Motto

*John Stuart Mill argued famously in* On Liberty *that competent adults should be free to lead their lives as they see fit, unfettered by paternalistic physicians or government interference.*

*But what are "competent adults"? In the famous cases of Elizabeth Bouvia, Larry McAfee, and Donald Cowart in the 1980s, young patients, who did not have terminal diseases but who had suffered from congenital, vehicular or industrial accidents, struggled for a right to die but changed their minds when that right was finally granted. When they were empowered by having this right, they chose to live. Obviously, psychiatric issues figure prominently in the debate over the right to die, such as whether people wishing to die are irrationally depressed.*

*In the following pages, Jerome Motto, MD, argues that people wishing to commit suicide should have a realistic assessment of their situation and not be ambivalent about their decisions to die. Psychiatrists are trained to distinguish "rational suicides" from their irrational counterparts.*

*Jerome Motto is professor emeritus of psychiatry and attending psychiatry at the Psychiatric Consultation Service of the University of California at San Francisco. He is a past president of the American Association of Suicidology, past secretary general of the International Society for Suicide Prevention, and a member of the Ethics Committee of the American Association of Suicidology.*

To speak as a psychiatrist may suggest to some that psychiatrists have a certain way of looking at things. This would be a misconception, though a common one. I know of no professional group with more diverse approaches to those matters concerning it than the American psychiatric community. All physicians, however, including psychiatrists, share a tradition of commitment

*Source: Suicide and Life-Threatening Behavior* 2, no. 3 (Fall 1972), pp. 183–88. Reprinted by permission of the publisher.

**67**

to both the preservation and the quality of human life. With this one reservation, I speak as a psychiatrist strictly in the singular sense.

The emergence of thoughts or impulses to bring an end to life is a phenomenon observed in persons experiencing severe pain, whether that pain stems from physical or emotional sources. Thus physicians, to whom persons are inclined to turn for relief from suffering, frequently encounter suicidal ideas and impulses in their patients. Those who look and listen do, at least.

From a psychiatric point of view, the question as to whether a person has the right to cope with the pain in his world by killing himself can be answered without hesitation. He does have that right. With a few geographical exceptions the same can be said from the legal and social point of view as well. It is only when philosophical or theological questions are raised that one can find room for argument about the right to suicide, as only in these areas can restrictions on behavior be institutionalized without requiring social or legal support.

The problem we struggle with is not whether the individual *has* the right to suicide; rather, we face a twofold dilemma stemming from the fact that he does have it. Firstly, what is the extent to which the exercise of that right should be subject to limitations? Secondly, when the right is exercised, how can we eliminate the social stigma now attached to it?

Putting limitations on rights is certainly not a new idea, since essentially every right we exercise has its specified restrictions. It is generally taken for granted that certain limitations must be observed. In spite of this, it is inevitable that some will take the position that unless the right is unconditional it is not "really" granted.

I use two psychological criteria as grounds for limiting a person's exercise of his right to suicide: (*a*) the act must be based on a realistic assessment of his life situation, and (*b*) the degree of ambivalence regarding the act must be minimal. Both of these criteria clearly raise a host of new questions.


## REALISTIC ASSESSMENT OF LIFE SITUATION

What is reality? Who determines whether a realistic assessment has been made? Every person's perception is reality to *him,* and the degree of pain experienced by one can never be fully appreciated by another, no matter how empathic he is. Differences in capacity to *tolerate* pain add still another crucial yet unmeasurable element.

As formidable as this sounds, the psychiatrist is obliged to accept this task as his primary day-to-day professional responsibility, whether or not the issue of suicide is involved. With an acute awareness of how emotions can—like lenses—distort perceptions which in turn shape one's thoughts and actions, and with experience in understanding and dealing with this underlying substrate of emotion, he is constantly working with his patients on the process of differentiating between what is realistic and what is distorted. The former must be dealt with on a rational level; the latter must be explored and modified till the distortion is reduced at least to the point where it is not of handicapping severity. He is aware of the nature and extent of his own tendency to distort ("Physician, heal thyself"), and realizes that the entire issue is one of degree. Yet he must use his own perception of reality as a standard, shortcomings notwithstanding, realizing full well how much information must be carefully considered in view of the frailty of the human perceptual and reality-testing apparatus.

Some persons have a view of reality so different from mine that I do not hesitate to interfere with their right to suicide. Others' perceptions are so like mine that I cannot intercede. The big problem is that large group in between.

In the final analysis, then, when a decision has to be made, what a psychiatrist calls "realistic" is whatever looks realistic to *him*. At the moment of truth, that is all any person can offer. This inherent human limitation in itself is a reality that accounts for a great deal of inevitable chaos in the world; it is an article of faith that not to make such an effort would create even greater chaos. On a day-to-day operational level, one contemporary behavioral scientist expressed it this way: "No doubt the daily business of helping troubled individuals, including suicides, gives little time for the massive contemplative and investigative efforts which alone can lead to surer knowledge. And the helpers are not thereby to be disparaged. They cannot wait for the best answers conceivable. They must do only the best they can *now*."[1]

Thus if I am working with a person in psychotherapy, one limitation I would put on his right to suicide would be that his assessment of his life situation be realistic as *I* see it.

A related concept is that of "rational suicide," which has enjoyed a certain vogue since at least the seventeenth century, when the "Rationalist Era" saw sharp inroads being made into the domination of the church in determining ethical and social values.[2] According to one contemporary philosopher, "the degree of rationality of the [suicidal] act would depend on the degree of rationality of the philosophy which was guiding the person's deliberations." Rationality is defined as a means of problem solving, using "methods such as logical, mathematical, or experimental procedures which have gained men's confidence as reliable tools for guiding instrumental actions." The rationality of one's philosophy is determined by the degree to which it is free of mysticism. Further, "A person who is considering how to act in an intensely conflicting situation cannot be regarded as making the most rational decision, unless he has been as critical as possible of the philosophy that is guiding his decision. If the philosophy is institutionalized as a political ideology or a religious creed, he must think critically about the institution in order to acquire maximum rationality of judgment. This principle is clear enough, even if in practice it is enormously difficult to fulfill."[3]

The idea of "rational suicide" is a related yet distinctly different issue from the "realistic assessment of one's life situation" referred to above. Making this assessment involves assembling and understanding all the facts clearly, while the idea of a "rational suicide" can only be entertained after this assessment is done and the question is "what to do" in the light of those facts.

The role of the psychiatrist and the thinking of the rationalist tend to merge, at one point, however. In the process of marshaling all the facts and exploring their meaning to the person, the psychiatrist must ensure that the patient does indeed critically examine not only his perception of reality but his own philosophy. This often entails making that philosophy explicit for the first time (without ever using the term "philosophy"), and clarifying how it has influenced his living experience. The implication is clear that modification of the person's view of his world, with corresponding changes in behavior, may lead to a more satisfying life.

The rationalist concedes that where one's philosophy is simply an "intellectual channeling of emotional forces," rational guidelines have severe limitations, since intense emotional conflicts cut off rational guidance. These circumstances would characterize "irrational" grounds for suicide and would identify those persons whose suicide should be prevented.

The argument for "rational suicide" tends to apply principally to two sets of circumstances: altruistic self-sacrifice for what is perceived as a noble cause; and the severe, advanced physical illness with no new therapeutic agents anticipated in the foreseeable future. This does not help us very much because these circumstances generate relatively little real controversy among behavioral scientists. The former situations are not usually recognized till after the act, and the latter at present are receiving a great deal of well-deserved attention from the point of view of anticipating (and sometimes hastening) the foreseeable demise in comfort and dignity.

Our most difficult problem is more with the person whose pain is emotional in origin and whose physical health is good, or at most constitutes a minor impairment. For these persons, the discussion above regarding "rational" and "irrational" distinctions seems rather alien to the clinical situation. This is primarily due to the rationalist's emphasis on intellectual processes, when it is so clear (at least to the psychiatrist) that it is feelings of worthiness of love, of relatedness, of belonging, that have the strongest, stabilizing influence on the suicidal person.

I rarely hear a patient say, "I've never looked at it that way," yet no response is more frequently encountered than "Yes, I understand, but I don't feel any differently." It is after a continuing therapeutic effort during which feelings of acceptance and worthiness are generated that emotional pain is reduced and suicidal manifestations become less intense. Either exploring the philosophy by which one lives or carefully assessing the realities of one's life can provide an excellent means of accomplishing this, but it is rarely the influence of the philosophy or the perception of the realities per se that brings it about. Rather, it is through the influence of the therapeutic relationship that the modified philosophy or perception develops, and can then be applied to the person's life situation.

## MANIFESTATIONS OF AMBIVALENCE

The second criterion to be used as the basis for limiting a person's exercise of his right to suicide is minimal ambivalence about ending his life. I make the assumption that if a person has no ambivalence about suicide he will not be in my office, nor write to me about it, nor call me on the telephone. I interpret, rightly or wrongly, a person's calling my attention to his suicidal impulses as a request to intercede that I cannot ignore.

At times this call will inevitably be misread, and my assumption will lead me astray. However, such an error on my part can be corrected at a later time; meanwhile, I must be prepared to take responsibility for having prolonged what may be a truly unendurable existence. If the error is made in the other direction, no opportunity for correction may be possible.

This same principle regarding ambivalence applies to a suicide prevention center, minister, social agency, or a hospital emergency room. The response of the helping agency may be far from fulfilling the needs of the person involved, but in my view, the ambivalence expressed is a clear indication for it to limit the exercise of his right to suicide.

## REDUCING THE STIGMA OF SUICIDE

The second horn of our dilemma about the right to suicide is the fact that the suicidal act is not considered respectable in our society. It can be maintained that granting a right but stigmatizing the exercise of that right is tantamount to not having granted it in the first place. In order to develop a realistic approach to this problem it is necessary to reduce the negative social implications attached to it.

The first step is to talk about it freely—with each other, with doctors, ministers, patients, and families. Just as with past taboos—TB, cancer, sex (especially homosexuality), drug addiction, abortion—it will gradually lose the emotional charge of the forbidden. The second step is the continued institutionalization of supportive and treatment services for suicidal persons, through local, state, and federal support.

News media should be responsible for reporting suicidal deaths with dignity and simplicity, without attempting either to cover up or to sensationalize pertinent information. In an economically competitive field this would not be a reasonable expectation unless it were made part of an accepted ethical code.

Instruction regarding this problem should be provided as a matter of course in the education and training for all health care personnel, emergency services (police, firemen), behavioral sciences (psychology, sociology, anthropology), and those to whom troubled people most often turn, such as ministers, teachers, and counselors. In short, every person who completes the equivalent of a high school education would be provided with an orientation toward the problem of suicide, and those responsible for responding to others in stressful circumstances should be prepared to assist in providing—or at least locating—help when needed.

A question has been raised whether incorporating concern for suicide into our social institutions might depersonalize man to some extent. I would anticipate the contrary. The more our social institutions reflect awareness of and concern for man's inner life and provide means for improving it, the greater is the implied respect for that life—even if this takes the form of providing a dignified means of relinquishing it.

It seems inevitable to me that we must eventually establish procedures for the voluntary cessation of life, with the time, place, and manner largely controlled by the person concerned. It will necessarily involve a series of deliberate steps providing assurance that appropriate criteria are met, such as those proposed above, as we now observe specific criteria when a life is terminated by abortion or by capital punishment.

The critical word is "control." I would anticipate a decrease in the actual number of suicides when this procedure is established, due to the psychological power of this issue. If I know something is available to me and will remain available till I am moved to seize it, the chances of my seizing it now are thereby much reduced. It is only by holding off that I maintain the option of changing my mind. During this period of delay the opportunity for therapeutic effort—and the therapy of time itself—may be used to advantage.

Finally, we have to make sure we are not speaking only to the strong. It is too easy to formulate a way of dealing with a troublesome problem in such a manner, that if the person in question could approach it as we suggest, he would not be a person who would have the problem in the first place.

When we discuss—in the abstract—the right to suicide, we tend to gloss over the intricacies of words like "freedom," "quality of life," "choice," or even "help," to say nothing of "rational" and "realistic." Each of these concepts deserves a full inquiry in itself, though in practice we use them on the tacit assumption that general agreement exists as to their meaning.

Therefore it is we who, in trying to be of service to someone else, have the task of determining what is rational for us, and what our perception of reality is. And we must recognize that in the final analysis it will be not only the suicidal person but we who have exercised a choice, by doing what we do to resolve our feelings about this difficult human problem.

## NOTES

1. J. Diggory, "Suicide and Value," in *Suicidal Behaviors*, ed. H. Resnik (Boston: Little, Brown, 1968), p. 18.
2. S. C. Sprott, *The English Debate on Suicide—From Donne to Hume* (LaSalle, IL: Open Court, 1961).
3. S. Pepper, "Can a Philosophy Make One Philosophical?" in *Essays in Self-Destruction*, ed. E. S. Shneidman (New York: Science House, 1967), pp. 121, 123.

# Physician-Assisted Dying: Self-Determination Run Amok

## Daniel Callahan

*In this selection the philosopher Daniel Callahan tackles the issue of whether an ethical physician should take an active part in hastening the end of a patient's life. Callahan argues against a right to physician-assisted dying because it would put undue power into the hands of physicians. He supports a distinction that bans killing while allowing terminally ill patients to die. (See Selections 1 and 4 for a contrary view.)*

*Daniel Callahan is the cofounder and president from 1969 to 1996 of The Hastings Center, in Briarcliff Manor, New York, the first institute for medical ethics in the world. Along with Joseph Fletcher, he is one of the pioneering giants of the modern, interdisciplinary field of medical ethics. His many writings include* Abortion, Law, Choice, and Morality; Abortion: Understanding Differences; *and* Setting Limits: Medical Goals in an Aging Society.

The euthanasia debate is not just another moral debate, one in a long list of arguments in our pluralistic society. It is profoundly emblematic of three important turning points in Western thought. The first is that of the legitimate conditions under which one person can kill another. The acceptance of voluntary active euthanasia would morally sanction what can only be called "consenting adult killing." By that term I mean the killing of one person by another in the name of their mutual right to be killer and killed if they freely agree to play those roles. This [in] turn flies in the face of a long-standing effort to limit the circumstances under which one person can take the life of another, from efforts to control the free flow of guns and arms, to abolish capital punishment, and to more tightly control warfare. Euthanasia would add a whole new category of killing to a society that already has too many excuses to indulge itself in that way.

*Source: Hastings Center Report* 22 (March–April 1992), pp. 52–55. Reprinted by permission of the author and publisher.

The second turning point lies in the meaning and limits of self-determination. The acceptance of euthanasia would sanction a view of autonomy holding that individuals may, in the name of their own private, idiosyncratic view of the good life, call upon others, including such institutions as medicine, to help them pursue that life, even at the risk of harm to the common good. This works against the idea that the meaning and scope of our own right to lead our own lives must be conditioned by, and be compatible with, the good of the community, which is more than an aggregate of self-directing individuals.

The third turning point is to be found in the claim being made upon medicine: it should be prepared to make its skills available to individuals to help them achieve their private vision of the good life. This puts medicine in the business of promoting the individualistic pursuit of general human happiness and well-being. It would overturn the traditional belief that medicine should limit its domain to promoting and preserving human health, redirecting it instead to the relief of that suffering which stems from life itself, not merely from a sick body.

I believe that, at each of these three turning points, proponents of euthanasia push us in the wrong direction. Arguments in favor of euthanasia fall into four general categories, which I will take up in turn: (1) the moral claim of individual self-determination and well-being; (2) the moral irrelevance of the difference between killing and allowing to die; (3) the supposed paucity of evidence to show likely harmful consequences of legalized euthanasia; and (4) the compatibility of euthanasia and medical practice.

## SELF-DETERMINATION

Central to most arguments for euthanasia is the principle of self-determination. People are presumed to have an interest in deciding for themselves, according to their own beliefs about what makes life good, how they will conduct their lives. That is an important value, but the question in the euthanasia context is, What does it mean and how far should it extend? If it were a question of suicide, where a person takes her own life without assistance from another, that principle might be pertinent, at least for debate. But euthanasia is not that limited a matter. The self-determination in that case can only be effected by the moral and physical assistance of another. Euthanasia is thus no longer a matter only of self-determination, but of a mutual, social decision between two people, the one to be killed and the other to do the killing.

How are we to make the moral move from my right of self-determination to some doctor's right to kill me—from *my* right to *his* right? Where does the doctor's moral warrant to kill come from? Ought doctors to be able to kill anyone they want as long as permission is given by competent persons? Is our right to life just like a piece of property, to be given away or alienated if the price (happiness, relief of suffering) is right? And then to be destroyed with our permission once alienated?

In answer to all those questions, I will say this: I have yet to hear a plausible argument why it should be permissible for us to put this kind of power in the hands of another, whether a doctor or anyone else. The idea that we can waive our right to life, and then give to another the power to take that life, requires a justification yet to be provided by anyone.

Slavery was long ago outlawed on the ground that one person should not have the right to own another, even with the other's permission. Why? Because it is a fundamental moral wrong for one person to give over his life and fate to another, whatever the good consequences, and no less a wrong for another person to have that kind of total, final power. Like slavery, dueling was long ago banned on similar grounds: even free, competent individuals should not have the power to kill each other, whatever their motives, whatever the circumstances. Consenting adult killing, like consenting adult slavery or degradation, is a strange route to human dignity.

There is another problem as well. If doctors, once sanctioned to carry out euthanasia, are to be themselves responsible moral agents—not simply hired hands with lethal injections at the ready—then they must have their own *independent* moral grounds to kill those who request such services. What do I mean? As those who favor euthanasia are quick to point out, some people want it because their life has become so burdensome it no longer seems worth living.

The doctor will have a difficulty at this point. The degree and intensity to which people suffer from their diseases and their dying, and whether they find life more of a burden than a benefit, has very little directly to do with the nature or extent of their actual physical condition. Three people can have the same condition, but only one will find the suffering unbearable. People suffer, but suffering is as much a function of the values of individuals as it is of the physical causes of that suffering. Inevitably in that circumstance, the doctor will in effect be treating the patient's values. To be responsible, the doctor would have to share those values. The doctor would have to decide, on her own, whether the patient's life was "no longer worth living."

But how could a doctor possibly know that or make such a judgment? Just because the patient said so? I raise this question because [at a recent euthanasia conference in Holland] the doctors present agreed that there is no objective way of measuring or judging the claims of patients that their suffering is unbearable. And if it is difficult to measure suffering, how much more difficult to determine the value of a patient's statement that her life is not worth living?

However one might want to answer such questions, the very need to ask them, to inquire into the physician's responsibility and grounds for medical and moral judgment, points out the social nature of the decision. Euthanasia is not a private matter of self-determination. It is an act that requires two people to make it possible, and a complicit society to make it acceptable.

# KILLING AND ALLOWING TO DIE

Against common opinion, the argument is sometimes made that there is no moral difference between stopping life-sustaining treatment and more active forms of killing, such as lethal injection. Instead I would contend that the notion that there is no morally significant difference between omission and commission is just wrong. Consider in its broad implications what the eradication of the distinction implies: that death from disease has been banished, leaving only the actions of physicians in terminating treatment as the cause of death. Biology, which used to bring about death, has apparently been displaced by human agency. Doctors have finally, I suppose, thus genuinely become gods, now doing what nature and the deities once did.

What is the mistake here? It lies in confusing causality and culpability, and in failing to note the way in which human societies have overlaid natural causes with moral rules and interpretations. Causality (by which I mean the direct physical causes of death) and culpability (by which I mean our attribution of moral responsibility to human actions) are confused under three circumstances.

They are confused, first, when the action of a physician in stopping treatment of a patient with an underlying lethal disease is construed as *causing* death. On the contrary, the physician's omission can only bring about death on the condition that the patient's disease will kill him in the absence of treatment. We may hold the physician morally responsible for the death, if we have morally judged such actions wrongful omissions. But it confuses reality and moral judgment to see an omitted action as having the same causal status as one that directly kills. A lethal injection will kill both a healthy person and a sick person. A physician's omitted treatment will have no effect on a healthy person. Turn off the machine on me, a healthy person, and nothing will happen. It will only, in contrast, bring the life of a sick person to an end because of an underlying fatal disease.

Causality and culpability are confused, second, when we fail to note that judgments of moral responsibility and culpability are human constructs. By that I mean that we human beings, after moral reflection, have decided to call some actions right or wrong, and to devise moral rules to deal with them. When physicians could do nothing to stop death, they were not held responsible for it. When, with medical progress, they began to have some power over death—but only its timing and circumstances, not its ultimate inevitability—moral rules were devised to set forth their obligations. Natural causes of death were not thereby banished. They were, instead, overlaid with a medical ethics designed to determine moral culpability in deploying medical power.

To confuse the judgments of this ethics with the physical causes of death—which is the connotation of the word *kill*—is to confuse nature and human action. People will, one way or another, die of some disease; death will have dominion over all of us. To say that a doctor "kills" a patient by allowing this to happen should only be understood as a moral judgment about the licitness of his omission, nothing more. We can, as a fashion of speech only, talk about a doctor *killing* a patient by omitting treatment he should have provided. It is a fashion of speech precisely because it is the underlying disease that brings death when treatment is omitted; that is its cause, not the physician's omission. It is a misuse of the word *killing* to use it when a doctor stops a treatment he believes will no longer benefit the patient—when, that is, he steps aside to allow an eventually inevitable death to occur now rather than later. The only deaths that human beings invented are those that come from direct killing—when, with a lethal injection, we both cause death and are morally responsible for it. In the case of omissions, we do not cause death even if we may be judged morally responsible for it.

This difference between causality and culpability also helps us see why a doctor who has omitted a treatment he should have provided has "killed" that patient while another doctor—performing precisely the same act of omission on another patient in different circumstance—does not kill her, but only allows her to die. The difference is that we have come, by moral convention and conviction, to classify unauthorized or illegitimate omissions as acts of "killing." We call them "killing" in the expanded sense of the term: a culpable action that permits the real cause of death, the underlying disease, to proceed to its lethal conclusion. By contrast, the doctor who, at the patient's request, omits or terminates unwanted treatment does not kill at all. Her underlying disease, not his action, is the physical cause of death; and we have agreed to consider actions of that kind to be morally licit. He thus can truly be said to have "allowed" her to die.

If we fail to maintain the distinction between killing and allowing to die, moreover, there are some disturbing possibilities. The first would be to confirm many physicians in their already too-powerful belief that, when patients die or when physicians stop treatment because of the futility of continuing it, they are somehow both morally and physically responsible for the deaths that follow. The notion needs to be abolished, not strengthened. It needlessly and wrongly burdens the physician, to whom should not be attributed the powers of the gods. The second possibility would be that, in every case where a doctor judges medical treatment no longer effective in prolonging life, a quick and direct killing of the patient would be seen as the next, most reasonable step, on grounds of both humaneness and economics. I do not see how that logic could easily be rejected.

## CALCULATING THE CONSEQUENCES

When concerns about the adverse social consequences of permitting euthanasia are raised, its advocates tend to dismiss them as unfounded and overly speculative. On the contrary, recent data about the Dutch experience suggests [sic] that such concerns are right on target. From my own discussions in Holland, and from several recent articles on the subject . . . I believe we can now fully see most of the *likely* consequences of legal euthanasia.

Three consequences seem almost certain, in this or any other country: the inevitability of some abuse of the law; the difficulty of precisely writing, and then enforcing, the law; and the inherent slipperiness of the moral reasons for legalizing euthanasia in the first place.

Why is abuse inevitable? One reason is that almost all laws on delicate, controversial matters are to some extent abused. This happens because not everyone will agree with the law as written and will bend it, or ignore it, if they can get away with it. From explicit admissions to me by Dutch proponents of euthanasia, and from the corroborating information provided by the Remmelink Report and the outside studies of Carlos Gomez and John Keown, I am convinced that in the Netherlands there are a substantial number of cases of nonvoluntary euthanasia, that is, euthanasia undertaken without the explicit permission of the person being killed. The other reason abuse is inevitable is that the law is likely to have a low enforcement priority in the criminal justice system. Like other laws of similar status, unless there is an unrelenting and harsh willingness to pursue abuse, violations will ordinarily be tolerated. The worst thing to me about my experience in Holland was the casual, seemingly indifferent attitude toward abuse. I think that would happen everywhere.

Why would it be hard to precisely write, and then enforce, the law? The Dutch speak about the requirement of "unbearable" suffering, but admit that such a term is just about indefinable, a highly subjective matter admitting of no objective standards. A requirement for outside opinion is nice, but it is easy to find complaisant colleagues. A requirement that a medical condition be "terminal" will run aground on the notorious difficulties of knowing when an illness is actually terminal.

Apart from those technical problems there is a more profound worry. I see no way, even in principle, to write or enforce a meaningful law that can guarantee effective procedural safeguards. The reason is obvious yet almost always overlooked. The euthanasia transaction will ordinarily take place within the boundaries of the private and confidential doctor-patient relationship. No one can possibly know what takes place in that context unless the doctor chooses to reveal it. In Holland, less than 10 percent of the physicians report their acts of euthanasia and do so with almost complete legal impunity. There is no reason why the situation should be any better elsewhere. Doctors will have their own reasons for keeping euthanasia secret, and some patients will have no less a motive for wanting it concealed.

I would mention, finally, that the moral logic of the motives for euthanasia contain[s] within them the ingredients of abuse. The two standard motives for euthanasia and assisted suicide are said to be our right of self-determination, and our claim upon the mercy of others, especially doctors, to relieve our suffering. These two motives are typically spliced together and presented as a single justification. Yet if they are considered independently—and there is no inherent reason why they must be linked—they reveal serious problems. It is said that a competent, adult person should have a right to euthanasia for the relief of suffering. But why must the person be suffering? Does not that stipulation already compromise the principle of self-determination? How can self-determination have any limits? Whatever the person's motives may be, why are they not sufficient?

Consider next the person who is suffering but not competent, who is perhaps demented or mentally retarded. The standard argument would deny euthanasia to that person. But why? If a person is suffering but not competent, then it would seem grossly unfair to deny relief solely on the grounds of incompetence. Are the incompetent less entitled to relief from suffering than the competent? Will it only be affluent, middle-class people, mentally fit and savvy about working the medical system, who can qualify? Do the incompetent suffer less because of their incompetence?

Considered from these angles, there are no good moral reasons to limit euthanasia once the principle of taking life for that purpose has been legitimated. If we really believe in self-determination, then any competent person should have a right to be killed by a doctor for any reason that suits him. If we believe in the relief of suffering, then it seems cruel and capricious to deny it to the incompetent. There is, in short, no reasonable or logical stopping point once the turn has been made down the road to euthanasia, which could soon turn into a convenient and commodious expressway.

## EUTHANASIA AND MEDICAL PRACTICE

A fourth kind of argument one often hears both in the Netherlands and in this country is that euthanasia and assisted suicide are perfectly compatible with the aims of medicine. I would note at the very outset that a physician who participates in another person's suicide already abuses medicine. Apart from depression (the main statistical cause of suicide), people commit suicide because they find life empty, oppressive, or meaningless. Their judgment is a judgment about the value of continued life, not only about health (even if they are sick). Are doctors now to be given the right to make judgments about the kinds of life worth living and to give their blessing to suicide for those they judge wanting? What conceivable competence, technical or moral, could doctors claim to play such a role? Are we to medicalize suicide, turning judgments about its worth and value into one more clinical issue? Yes, those are rhetorical questions.

Yet they bring us to the core of the problem of euthanasia and medicine. The great temptation of modern medicine, not always resisted, is to move beyond the promotion and preservation of health into the boundless realm of general human happiness and well-being. The root problem of illness and mortality is both medical and philosophical or religious. "Why must I die?" can be asked as a technical, biological question or as a question about the meaning of life. When medicine tries to respond to the latter, which it is always under pressure to do, it moves beyond its proper role.

It is not medicine's place to lift from us the burden of that suffering which turns on the meaning we assign to the decay of the body and its eventual death. It is not medicine's place to determine when lives are not worth living or when the burden of life is too great to be borne. Doctors have no conceivable way of evaluating such claims on the part of patients, and they should have no right to act in response to them. Medicine should try to relieve human suffering, but only that suffering which is brought on by illness and dying as biological phenomena, not that suffering which comes from anguish or despair at the human condition.

Doctors ought to relieve those forms of suffering that medically accompany serious illness and the threat of death. They should relieve pain, do what they can to allay anxiety and uncertainty, and be a comforting presence. As sensitive human beings, doctors should be prepared to respond to patients who ask why they must die, or die in pain. But here the doctor and the patient are at the same level. The doctor may have no better an answer to those old questions than anyone else, and certainly no special insight from his training as a physician. It would be terrible for physicians to forget this, and to think that in a swift, lethal injection, medicine has found its own answer to the riddle of life. It would be a false answer, given by the wrong people. It would be no less a false answer for patients. They should neither ask medicine to put its own vocation at risk to serve their private interests, nor think that the answer to suffering is to be killed by another. The problem is precisely that, too often in human history, killing has seemed the quick, efficient way to put aside that which burdens us. It rarely helps, and too often simply adds to one evil still another. That is what I believe euthanasia would accomplish. It is self-determination run amok.

## PART THREE

# Assisted Reproduction: Embryos

# The Moral Status of the Embryo

## Peter Singer

*In the following selection philosopher Peter Singer argues that the moral status of the embryo is not the same as that of an adult person. His reasoning warrants comparison with Judith Thomson's in Selection 12. Both maintain that there are different senses of the term "right to life," and that some of these do not generate any duties on the part of other persons to fulfill such rights. For another use of this "argument from potential," but one leading to a different conclusion, see Selection 14.*

*Peter Singer is a clear, thought-provoking, and prolific writer of books and articles in many areas of bioethics. His books include* Practical Ethics *and, most recently,* The Sanctity of Life. *He has edited* A Companion to Ethics *and several anthologies on animal rights, and coedits the journal* Bioethics. *Peter Singer is professor of philosophy and director of the Centre for Human Bioethics, Monash University, Australia.*

### THE STANDARD ARGUMENT

The standard argument in favor of attributing a right to life to the embryo goes like this:

Every human being has a right to life.

A human embryo is a human being.

Therefore the embryo has a right to life.

To avoid questions about capital punishment, or killing in self-defense, it can be stipulated that the term "innocent" is assumed whenever we are talking of human beings and their rights.

*Source:* Peter Singer and Deane Wells, *Making Babies* (New York: Scribner's, 1985). Copyright 1984, 1985, Peter Singer and Deane Wells. Reprinted by permission.

The standard argument has a standard response. The standard response is to accept the first premise, that all human beings have a right to life, but to deny the second premise, that the human embryo is a human being. This standard response, however, runs into difficulties, because the embryo is clearly a being of some sort, and it can't possibly be of any other species than *Homo sapiens*. So it seems to follow that it must be a human being. Attempts to say that it only becomes a human being at viability, or at birth, are not entirely convincing. Viability is so closely tied to the state of development of neonatal intensive care that it is hardly the kind of thing that can determine when a being gets a right to live. As for birth, those who draw the line there must explain why an infant born premature at 26 weeks should have a right to life, whereas a fetus of 32 weeks, more developed in every respect, should not. Can location relative to the cervix really make so much difference to one's right to life?

## QUESTIONING THE FIRST PREMISE

So the standard argument for attributing a right to life to the embryo can withstand the standard response. It is not easy to mount a direct challenge to the claim that the embryo is a human being. What the standard argument cannot withstand, however, is a more critical examination of its first premise: the premise that every human being has a right to life. At first glance, this seems the stronger premise. Do we really want to deny that every (innocent) human being has a right to life? Are we about to condone murder? No wonder it is at the second premise that most of the fire has been directed. But the first premise is surprisingly vulnerable. Its vulnerability becomes apparent as soon as we cease to take "Every human being has a right to life" as some kind of unquestionable moral axiom, and instead inquire into the moral basis for our particular objection to killing human beings.

By "our particular objection to killing human beings" I mean the objection we have to killing human beings, over and above any objections we may have to killing other living beings, such as pigs and cows and dogs and cats, and even trees and lettuces. Why is it that we think killing human beings is so much more serious than killing these other beings?

The obvious answer is that human beings are different from other animals, and the greater seriousness of killing them is a result of these differences. But which of the many differences between humans and other animals justify such a distinction? Again, the obvious response is that the morally relevant differences are those based on our superior mental powers—our self-awareness, our rationality, our moral sense, our autonomy, or some combination of these. They are the kinds of thing, we are inclined to say, which make us "truly human." To be more precise, they are the kinds of thing which make us *persons*.

That the particular objection to killing human beings rests on such qualities is very plausible. To take the most extreme of the differences between living things, consider a person who is enjoying life, is part of a network of relationships with other people, is looking forward to what tomorrow may bring, and freely choosing the course her or his life will take for the years to come. Now think about a lettuce, which, we can safely assume, knows and feels nothing at all. One would have to be quite mad, or morally blind, or warped, not to see that killing the person is far more serious than killing the lettuce.

We shall postpone, for the present, asking just which of the mental qualities make the difference in the moral seriousness between the killing of a person and the killing of a lettuce. For our immediate purposes, all we need to note is that the plausibility of the assertion that human beings have a right to life depends on the fact that human beings generally possess mental qualities which other living beings do not possess. So should we accept the premise that every human being has a right to life? We may do so, but *only* if we bear in mind that by "human being" here we refer to those beings who have the mental qualities that generally distinguish members of our species from members of other species.

## TWO SENSES OF "HUMAN"

If this is the sense in which we can accept the first premise, however, what of the second premise? It is immediately clear that in the sense of the term "human being" which is required to make the first premise acceptable, the second premise is false. The embryo, especially the early embryo, is obviously not a being with the mental qualities which generally distinguish members of our species from members of other species. The early embryo has no brain, no nervous system. It is reasonable to assume that, so far as its mental life goes, it has no more awareness than a lettuce.

It is still true that the human embryo is a member of the species *Homo sapiens*. That is, as we saw, why it is difficult to deny that the human embryo is a human being. But we can now see that this is not the sense of "human being" we need to make the standard argument work. A valid argument cannot equivocate on the meanings of the central terms it uses. If the first premise is true when "human" means "a being with certain mental qualities" and the second premise is true when "human" means "member of the species *Homo sapiens*," the argument is based on a slide between the two meanings and is invalid.

## SPECIESISM

Can the argument be rescued? It obviously cannot be rescued by claiming that the embryo is a being with the requisite mental qualities. That *might* be arguable for some later stage of the development of the embryo or fetus, but it is impossible to make out the claim for the early embryo. If the second premise cannot be reconciled with the first in this way, can the first perhaps be defended in a form which makes it compatible with the second? Can it be argued that human beings have a right to life, not because of any moral qualities they may possess, but because they—and not pigs, cows, dogs, or lettuces—are members of the species *Homo sapiens?*

This is a desperate move. Those who make it find themselves having to defend the claim that species membership is *in itself* morally relevant to the wrongness of killing a being. But why should species membership in itself be morally crucial? If we are considering whether it is wrong to destroy something, surely we must look at its actual characteristics, not just the species to which it belongs. If ET and similar visitors from other planets turn out to be sensitive, thinking, planning beings, who get homesick just like we do, would it be acceptable to kill them simply because they are not members of our species? Should you be in any doubt, ask yourself the same kind of question, but with "race" substituted for "species." If we reject the claim that membership of a particular race is *in itself* morally relevant to the wrongness of killing a being, it is not easy to see how we could accept the same claim when based on species membership. Remember that the fact that other races, like our own, can feel, think, and plan for the future is not relevant to this question, for we are considering the simple fact of membership of the particular group— whether race or species—as the *sole* basis for distinguishing between the wrongness of killing those who belong to *our* group, and those who are of some *other* group. As long as we keep this in mind, I am sure that we will conclude that neither race nor species can, *in itself,* provide any justifiable basis for such a distinction.

So the standard argument fails. It fails not because of the standard response that the embryo is not a human being, but because the sense in which the embryo is a human being is not the sense in which we should accept that every human being has a right to life.

## THE ARGUMENT FROM POTENTIAL

At this point in the discussion, those who wish to defend the embryo's right to life often switch ground. We should not, they say, base our views of the status of the embryo on the mental qualities it *actually has while an embryo;* we must, rather, consider what it has the potential to *become.*

Indeed, we do need to consider the moral relevance of the embryo's potential. But this argument is not as easy to grasp as it may appear. If we attempt to set it out in an argument of standard form, as we did with the previous argument, we get

Every potential human being has a right to life.

The embryo is a potential human being.

Therefore the embryo has a right to life.

There is no equivocation in this argument, and its second premise is undoubtedly true. The problem is with the first premise. The claim that every potential human being has a right to life is by no means self-evidently true. We would need to be given good grounds for accepting it. What grounds could there be?

One might try to argue that since full-fledged human beings (those with at least some of the mental qualities I have been discussing) have a right to life, anything with the potential to become a full-fledged human being must also have a right to life. But there is no general rule that a potential X has the rights of an X. If there were, Prince Charles, who is a potential King of England, would now have the rights of a King of England. But he does not.

Another possible argument might go like this: there is nothing of greater moral significance than a thinking, choosing rational being. We value such beings above almost everything else. Therefore anything which can give rise to such a being has value because of what it can become.

What is this argument asserting? It suggests that the destruction of an embryo is wrong because it means that a person who might have existed will now not exist; and since we value people, the destruction of the embryo has caused us to lose something of value. But this proves too much. For destroying an embryo is not the only way of ensuring that a person who might have existed will not exist. If a couple decide, after their second, or third, or fourth child, that their family is complete, it is also the case that a person who might have existed—in fact, several people who might have existed—will not exist. Since some people who oppose abortion also oppose the use of contraceptives, it is worth pointing out that this is true whether the couple use contraceptives, or simply abstain from sexual intercourse during the woman's fertile periods (though admittedly the latter method gives the possible people a greater chance of existence). Yet those who condemn the destruction of embryos do not condemn with equal weight the use of contraceptives, and they generally do not condemn at all the use of sexual abstinence to limit the size of one's family. So it seems that the basis for their objection to the destruction of the embryo cannot be that a person who might have existed will now not exist.

Another example, more relevant to the question of embryo research, suggests the same conclusion. Suppose that a scientist has obtained two ripe eggs from two women, let us call them Jan and Maria. They are hoping to have their eggs fertilized with their husbands' sperm and transferred to their wombs. Jan had her laparoscopy first, her egg was put into a petri dish, and her husband's sperm added to it some hours ago. On checking it, the scientist finds that fertilization has taken place. In the case of Maria's egg the sperm has only just been added to the dish, so fertilization cannot yet have taken place, but the laboratory has a 90 percent success rate for achieving fertilization in these circumstances, and the scientist is reasonably confident that fertilization will take place within the next few hours. Some would say that to destroy Jan's embryo would be gravely wrong, but to destroy the egg and sperm from Maria and her husband would not be wrong at all, or would be much less seriously wrong. In terms of preventing a possible person from existing, however, the difference is only that there is a slightly higher probability of a person's resulting from what is in Jan's petri dish than there is of a person's resulting from what is in Maria's petri dish. If the difference in the wrongness of disposing of the contents of the two dishes is greater than this slightly higher probability would justify, it cannot be preventing the existence of a possible future person that makes such disposal wrong. To borrow a phrase from the Oxford philosopher Jonathan Glover, if it is cake we are after, it doesn't make much difference whether we throw away the ingredients separately or after they are mixed together.[1]

## UNIQUENESS

At this point some will say that it is wrong to destroy an embryo because the embryo already contains the unique genetic basis for a particular person. When a couple abstain from intercourse, or the scientist washes out the petri dish before fertilization has taken place, the genetic constitution of the person who might have existed has yet to be determined. This is true, of course, but does it matter? All human beings are genetically determinate, and all, except identical siblings, are genetically unique. Imagine that instead of just dropping lots of sperm into a petri dish containing a ripe egg, we carried out a program of artificial reproduction by singling out just *one* sperm and placing it with the egg. Then, once the sperm had been singled out and placed with the egg, the genetic constitution of the person who could develop from the egg-and-sperm would also have been uniquely determined. Suppose now that after the egg and sperm have been placed together, but before fertilization has taken place, the woman is found to have a medical condition which makes pregnancy inadvisable. Freezing is not available, and there are no patients interested in a donated embryo. Would it be wrong to throw out the egg and sperm at this stage? If you do not think that it would be wrong to dispose of the egg and the sperm in *this* situation (and worse than it would be if the usual procedure, involving millions of sperm, had been used) then you cannot be attributing much moral significance to the existence of a genetically unique entity.

I have pursued the will-o'-the-wisp of potential for a long time—not just today, but over the past five years in which I have been working on this topic. I can understand the view that fertilization is one step in the development of a person and that if potentiality is a matter of degree, the embryo is a degree closer to being a person than a collection of egg and sperm in a petri dish before fertilization has taken place. What I still cannot find is any basis for the view that this difference of degree makes an enormous difference in the moral status of what we have before us.

## A POSITIVE APPROACH

We have now seen the inadequacy of attempts to argue that the early embryo has a right to life. It remains only to say something positive about when in its development the embryo may acquire rights.

The answer must depend on the actual characteristics of the embryo. The minimal characteristic which is needed to give the embryo a claim to consideration is sentience, or the capacity to feel pain or pleasure. Until the embryo reaches that point, there is nothing we can do to the embryo which causes harm to *it*. We can, of course, damage it in such a way as to cause harm to the person it will become, if it lives, but if it never becomes a person, the embryo has not been harmed, because its total lack of awareness means that it can have no interest in becoming a person.

Once an embryo may be capable of feeling pain, there is a clear case for very strict controls over the experimentation which can be done with it. At this point the embryo ranks, morally, with other creatures who are conscious but not self-conscious. Many nonhuman animals come into this category, and in my view they have often been unjustifiably made to suffer in scientific research. We should have stringent controls over research to ensure that this cannot happen to embryos, just as we should have stringent controls to ensure that it cannot happen to animals.

## PRACTICAL IMPLICATIONS OF THE MORAL STATUS OF EMBRYOS

The conclusion to draw from this is that as long as the parents give their consent, there is no ethical objection to discarding a very early embryo. If the early embryo can be used for significant research, so much the better. What is crucial is that the embryo not be kept beyond the point at which it has formed a brain and a nervous system, and might be capable of suffering. Two government committees—the Warnock Committee in Britain and the Waller Committee in Victoria, Australia—have recently recommended that research on embryos should be allowed, but only up to 14 days after fertilization.[2] This is the period at which the so-called "primitive streak," the first indication of the development of a nervous system, begins to form, and up to this stage there is certainly no possibility of the embryo feeling anything at all. In fact, the 14-day limit is unnecessarily conservative. A limit of, say, 28 days would still be very much on the safe side of the best estimates of when the embryo may be able to feel pain; but such a limit would, in contrast to the 14-day limit, allow research on embryos at the stage at which some of the more specialized cells have begun to form. . . . [T]his research would, according to Robert Edwards, have the potential to cure such terrible diseases as sickle-cell anemia and leukemia.[3]

As for freezing the embryo with a view to later implantation, the question here is essentially one of risk. If freezing carries no special risk of abnormality, there seems to be nothing objectionable about it. With embryo freezing, this appears to be the case. The ethical objections some people have to freezing embryos has led to the suggestions that it would be better to freeze eggs;[4] for this and other reasons there has been a considerable research effort directed at freezing eggs. Human eggs are more difficult to freeze than human embryos, and until recently it had not proved possible to freeze them in a manner which allowed fertilization after thawing. In December 1985, however, an IVF [*in vitro* fertilization] team at Flinders University, in Adelaide, South Australia, announced that it had succeeded in obtaining a pregnancy from an egg which had been frozen and thawed before being fertilized.[5] The technique used involved stripping away a protective outer layer from the egg, so that it would take up a chemical which would protect it during the freezing process. This technique does overcome the ethical problems some find in freezing embryos, but it does so at the cost of introducing a new potential cause of risk to the offspring, the risk that the chemicals absorbed by the egg may have some harmful effect.[6] Whether or not this risk proves to be a real one, from the point of view of ethics, one may doubt whether the risk is worth running, if the primary reason for running it is to avoid objections, which we have now seen to be ill-founded, to the freezing of embryos. . . .

Going beyond the simple case does bring us into a more ethically controversial area, but there is no overall case against applying IVF outside the restricted ambit of the simple case. The essential point is to consider each additional step carefully before it is taken. Some steps will prove unwise, but others will be beneficial and not open to any well-grounded objections.

## THE FUTURE OF THE REPRODUCTION REVOLUTION

What lies ahead? IVF has opened the door to a wide range of further possibilities. In the near future we shall have to consider which of these possibilities to pursue, and which to reject. Here are some of the possibilities:

1. A surrogate could bear a child for another couple; the child would be the genetic child of the other couple, and would be returned to the genetic parents after birth. The genetic parents might be unable to conceive in the normal way, or they might simply find the surrogate arrangement more convenient. The surrogate might be paid for her services, or—in the case of otherwise infertile couples—she may have more altruistic motives.
2. Embryos may be used in order to provide "spare parts" for people who through accident or illness need some kind of transplant. It has been suggested that embryonic tissue could restore nerve function to paraplegics. Embryos might be grown to the point at which the organs begin to form, and then the organs could be separated and grown in culture until they were large enough to be used.
3. Several embryos could be produced, and some of their genetic characteristics identified; the one considered most desirable could then be implanted, and the remainder discarded; alternatively it will eventually be possible to modify the genetic properties of an embryo so as to eliminate defects and to build in desirable genetic qualities. . . .

The proposal that embryos be used for "spare parts" has already caused howls of protest from those who regard embryos as having the same rights as normal human beings. [This view, however,] cannot be defended by rational argument. As long as there are adequate safeguards to ensure that the embryo is at all times incapable of suffering in any way, it is difficult to find sound ethical reason against this proposal—and it is obvious that the possible benefits are considerable.

Of all the possible applications of IVF, however, it is genetic selection and genetic engineering which raise the most far-reaching questions. Should we tinker with the human genetic pool? If so, in what way? Here I will limit myself to pointing out that we already tinker with the genetic pool when we offer genetic counseling, amniocentesis, and abortion to those who are at special risk of producing genetically defective offspring. And this is nothing new, at least insofar as its impact on the genetic pool is concerned: other societies have practiced infanticide to the same end, and of course in the past, even if one tried to rear the defective child, in most cases nature used its own brutal methods to ensure that the genes were eliminated from the gene pool.

So genetic engineering differs only in its techniques from what is now going on, and has gone on for a long time. But this difference is a significant one, because the new techniques are so much more powerful, and because they would, in principle, allow us to select for desirable traits as well as to select against undesirable ones. Many fear that these techniques will place too much power in the hands of governments, who will not be able to resist the temptation of designing future generations to be docile and to vote for the governing party at every election.

The fear that genetic engineering will produce the ultimate in entrenched dictatorship is exaggerated. Most political leaders want quick results, and it would take at least 18 years for genetic engineering to have any effect at the polls. If we have succeeded in keeping our freedom in the age of television and state education, we should be able to cling to it in the age of genetic engineering as well.

But should we allow positive modifications, as distinct from the elimination of defects, at all? In time we might come to accept the desirability of positive modifications. One reason for accepting this is that, looking around us, there is reason to think that natural selection has left ample room for improvement. Another reason is that the distinction between eliminating a defect and making a positive modification is a difficult one to draw. If we learn how to eliminate a wide range of defects which predispose us to common diseases, we will have created an abnormally healthy person. If we learn how to affect intelligence, should we stop short at eliminating mental ability below the above-average range? If we eliminate abnormally depressive personalities, would it be wrong to try to produce people who tend to be a little more cheerful than most of us are now? If we eliminate tendencies toward criminal violence, might we not build just a little more kindness into the human constitution? If the risks of such an enterprise are great, so too are the potential rewards for us all.

## NOTES

1. Glover quoted in M. Warnock (chairperson), *Report of the Committee of Inquiry into Human Fertilisation and Embryology* (London: Her Majesty's Stationery Office, 1984), p. 66.
2. Ibid.; L. Waller (chairman), Victorian Government Committee to Consider the Social, Ethical, and Legal Issues Arising from In Vitro Fertilization, *Report on the Disposition of Embryos Produced by In Vitro Fertilization* (Melbourne: Victorian Government Printer, 1984), p. 47.
3. R. G. Edwards, paper presented at the Fourth World Congress on IVF, Melbourne, Australia, November 22, 1985.
4. Waller Committee, *Report on the Disposition of Embryos.*
5. *The Australian,* December 19, 1985.
6. A. Trounson, paper presented at the Fourth World Congress on IVF, Melbourne, Australia, November 22, 1985.

SELECTION 8

# "Making Babies" Revisited

## Leon R. Kass

*In this selection and the next, the cloning of the lamb Dolly gives new urgency to the question of whether physicians may create human beings through methods other than intercourse. Most physicians want to help infertile couples, but controversy persists about how far they should go with "assisted" reproduction.*

*In the following selection Leon Kass predicts practices of embryonic experimentation and genetic therapy on embryos. Of special interest is his emphasis on the "wedge" or "slippery slope" argument that what justifies one practice will also justify a very similar practice.*

*Leon Kass, PhD, MD, is the Addie Clark Harding Professor in the College and Committee on Social Thought at the University of Chicago. Trained both as a biologist and as a physician, Kass has written many important articles in bioethics, including "Is There a Right to Die?" and "Regarding the End of Medicine and the Pursuit of Health." He is also the author of* Toward a More Natural Science: Biology and Human Affairs.

*And the man knew not Eve his wife; but she conceived without him and bore Cain, and said: I have gotten a man with the help of Dr. Steptoe.*

Ectogenesis IV, 1

*And Isaac entreated the NIH for his wife, because she was barren; and the NIH let Itself be entreated of him, and Rebekah his wife conceived.*

Ectogenesis XXV, 21

Source: *Public Interest* 54 (Winter 1979), pp. 32–60. Reprinted by permission of the author and publisher.

I

Seven years ago [1972], in the pages of this journal, in an article entitled "Making Babies—the New Biology and the 'Old' Morality," I explored some of the moral and political questions raised by projected new powers to intervene in the processes of human reproduction. I concluded that it would be foolish to acquire and use these powers. The questions have since been debated in "bioethical" circles and in college classrooms, and they have received intermittent attention in the popular press and in sensational novels and movies. This past year they have gained the media limelight with the Del Zio suit against Columbia University, and more especially with the birth last summer in Britain of Louise Brown, the first identified human baby born following conception in the laboratory.

Back in 1975, after prolonged deliberations, the National Commission for the Protection of Human Subjects of Biomedical and Behavioral Research issued its report and recommendations for research on the human fetus. And in the *Federal Register* of August 8, 1975, the Secretary of Health, Education, and Welfare published regulations regarding research, development, and related activities involving fetuses, pregnant women, and *in vitro* fertilization. These provided that no federal monies should be used for *in vitro* fertilization of human eggs until a special Ethics Advisory Board reviews the special ethical issues and offers advice about whether government should support any such proposed research. There has been an effective moratorium on federal support for human *in vitro* fertilization research since that time. But now the whole matter has once again become the subject of an intensive policy debate, for such a board has been established by HEW to consider whether the United States government should finance research on human *in vitro* fertilization and embryo transfer.

The question has been placed on the policy table by a research proposal submitted to the National Institute of Child Health and Human Development by Dr. Pierre Soupart of Vanderbilt University. Dr. Soupart requested $465,000, over three years, for a study to define in part the genetic risk involved in obtaining early human embryos by tissue-culture methods. He proposes to fertilize about 450 human ova, obtained from donors undergoing gynecological surgery (i.e., not from women whom the research could be expected to help), with donor sperm, to observe their development for five to six days, and to examine them microscopically for chromosomal and other abnormalities before discarding them. In addition, Dr. Soupart proposes to study whether such laboratory-grown embryos can be frozen and stored without producing abnormalities; it is thought that temporary cold storage of human embryos might improve the success rate in the embryo-transfer procedure used to produce a child. Though Dr. Soupart does not now propose to do embryo transfers to women seeking to become pregnant, his research is intended to serve that goal: He seeks to reassure us that baby-making with the help of *in vitro* fertilization is safe; and he seeks to perfect the techniques introduced by Drs. Edwards and Steptoe in England.

Dr. Soupart's application was approved for funding by the National Institutes of Health review process in October 1977, but because of the administrative regulations it could not be funded without review by an Ethics Advisory Board. The Secretary of HEW, Joseph Califano, has constituted the 13-member Board, and charged it, not only with a decision on the Soupart proposal, but with an inquiry into all the scientific, ethical, and legal issues involved, urging it "to provide recommendations on broad principles to guide the Department in future decision making." The Board, comprising a distinguished group of physicians, academics, and laymen, has invited expert and public testimony on the widest range of questions. By the end of the first phase of its work, it will have held at least 11 meetings and public hearings all over the United States, offering all interested citizens or groups the chance to express their opinions.

I was asked by the Board to discuss the ethical issues raised by the proposed research on human *in vitro* fertilization, laboratory cultures of—and experimentation with—human embryos, and the intra-uterine transfer of such embryos for the purpose of assisting human generation. In addition, I was asked to comment on the appropriateness of federal funding of such research and on the implications of this work for the provision of health care. The present article is based largely on testimony given before the Ethics Advisory Board, at its Boston meeting, October 13–14, 1978.

## II

How should one think about the ethical issues, here and in general? There are many possible ways, and it is not altogether clear which way is best. For some people ethical issues are immediately matters of right and wrong, of purity and sin, of good and evil. For others, the critical terms are benefits and harms, risks and promises, gains and costs. Some will focus on so-called rights of individuals or groups, e.g., a right to life or childbirth; still others will emphasize so-called goods for society and its members, such as the advancement of knowledge and the prevention and cure of disease.

My own orientation here is somewhat different. I wish to suggest that before deciding what to do, one should try to understand the implications of doing or not doing. The first task, it seems to me, is not to ask "moral or immoral?" "right or wrong?" but to try to understand fully the meaning and significance of the proposed actions.

This concern with significance leads me to take a broad view of the matter. For we are concerned here not only with the proposed research of Dr. Soupart, and the narrow issues of safety and informed consent it immediately raises, but also with a whole range of implications including many that are tied to definitely foreseeable consequences of this research and its predictable extensions—and touching even our common conception of our own humanity. The very establishment of a special Ethics Advisory Board testifies that we are at least tacitly aware that more is at stake than in ordinary biomedical research, or in experimenting with human subjects at risk of bodily harm. At stake is the *idea* of the *humanness* of our human life and the meaning of our embodiment, our sexual being, and our relation to ancestors and descendants. In reaching the necessarily particular and immediate decision in the case at hand, we must be mindful of the larger picture and must avoid the great danger of trivializing this matter for the sake of rendering it manageable.

## III

What is the status of a fertilized human egg (i.e., a human zygote) and the embryo that develops from it? How are we to regard its being? How are we to regard it morally, i.e., how are we to behave toward it? These are, alas, all-too-familiar questions. At least analogous, if not identical, questions are central to the abortion controversy and are also crucial in considering whether and what sort of experimentation is properly conducted on living but aborted fetuses. Would that it were possible to say that the matter is simple and obvious, and that it has been resolved to everyone's satisfaction!

But the controversy about the morality of abortion continues to rage and to divide our nation. Moreover, many who favor or do not oppose abortion do so despite the fact that they regard the pre-viable fetus as a living human organism, even if less worthy of protection than a woman's desire not to give it birth. Almost everyone senses the importance of this matter of the decision about laboratory culture of, and experimentation with, human embryos. Thus, we are obliged to take up the question of the status of the embryos, in a search for the outlines of some common ground on which many of us can stand. To the best of my knowledge, the discussion which follows is not informed by any particular sectarian or religious teaching, though it may perhaps reveal that I am a person not devoid of reverence and the capacity for awe and wonder, said by some to be the core of the "religious" sentiment.

I begin by noting that the circumstances of laboratory-grown blastocysts (i.e., 3-to-6-day-old embryos) and embryos are not identical with those of the analogous cases of (1) living fetuses facing abortion and (2) living aborted fetuses used in research. First, the fetuses whose fates are at issue in abortion are unwanted, usually the result of "accidental" conception. Here, the embryos are wanted, and deliberately created, despite certain knowledge that many of them will be destroyed or discarded.[1] Moreover, the fate of these embryos is not in conflict with the wishes, interests, or alleged rights of the pregnant women. Second, though the HEW guidelines governing fetal research permit studies conducted on the not-at-all-viable aborted fetus, such research merely takes advantage of available "products" of abortions not themselves undertaken for the sake of the research. No one has proposed and no one would sanction the deliberate production of live fetuses to be aborted for the sake of research, even very beneficial research.[2] In contrast, we are here considering the deliberate production of embryos for the express purpose of experimentation.

The cases may also differ in other ways. Given the present state of the art, the largest embryo under discussion is the blastocyst, a spherical, relatively undifferentiated mass of cells, barely visible to the naked eye. In appearance it does not look human; indeed, only the most careful scrutiny by the most experienced scientist might distinguish it from similar blastocysts of other mammals. If the human zygote and blastocyst are more like the animal zygote and blastocyst than they are like the 12-week-old human fetus (which already has a humanoid appearance, differentiated organs, and electrical activity of the brain), then there would be a much-diminished ethical dilemma regarding their deliberate creation and experimental use. Needless to say, there are articulate and passionate defenders of all points of view. Let us try, however, to consider the matter afresh.

First of all, the zygote and early embryonic stages are clearly alive. They metabolize, respire, and respond to changes in the environment; they grow and divide. Second, though not yet organized into distinctive parts or organs, the blastocyst is an organic whole, self-developing, genetically unique and distinct from the egg and sperm whose union marked the beginning of its career as a discrete, unfolding being. While the egg and sperm are alive as cells, something new and alive *in a different sense* comes into being with fertilization. The truth of this is unaffected by the fact that fertilization takes time and is not an instantaneous event. For after fertilization is *complete,* there exists a new individual, with its unique genetic identity, fully potent for the self-initiated development into a mature human being, if circumstances are cooperative. Though there is some sense in which the lives of egg and sperm are continuous with the life of the new organism-to-be (or, in human terms, that the parents live on in the child or child-to-be), in the decisive sense there is a discontinuity, a new beginning, with fertilization. *After* fertilization, there is continuity of subsequent development, even if the locus of the embryo alters with implantation (or birth). Any honest biologist must be impressed by these facts, and must be inclined, at least on first glance, to the view that a human life begins at fertilization. Even Dr. Robert Edwards has apparently stumbled over this truth, perhaps inadvertently, in the remark about Louise Brown attributed to him in an article by Peter Gwynne in *Science Digest:* "The last time I saw *her, she* was just eight cells in a test-tube. *She* was beautiful *then,* and she's still beautiful *now!*"[3]

But granting that a human life begins at fertilization, and comes-to-be via a continuous process thereafter, surely—one might say—the blastocyst itself is hardly a human being. I myself would agree that a blastocyst is not, in a *full* sense, a human being—or what the current fashion calls, rather arbitrarily and without clear definition, a person. It does not look like a human being nor can it do very much of what human beings do. Yet, at the same time, I must acknowledge that the human blastocyst is (1) human in origin and (2) *potentially* a mature human being, if all goes well. This too is beyond dispute; indeed it is precisely because of its peculiarly human potentialities that people propose to study *it* rather than the embryos of other mammals. The human blastocyst, even the human blastocyst *in vitro,* is not humanly nothing; it possesses a power to become what everyone will agree is a human being.

Here it may be objected that the blastocyst *in vitro* has today no such power, because there is now no way *in vitro* to bring the blastocyst to that much later fetal stage at which it might survive on its own. There are no published reports of culture of human embryos past the blastocyst stage (though this has been reported for mice). The *in vitro* blastocyst, like the 12-week-old aborted fetus, is *in this sense* not viable (i.e., it is at a stage of maturation before the stage of possible independent existence). But if we distinguish, among the *not*-viable embryos, between the *pre*-viable and the *not-at-all* viable—on the basis that the former, though not yet viable is capable of *becoming* or *being made* viable[4]—we note a crucial difference between the blastocyst and the 12-week abortus. Unlike an aborted fetus, the blastocyst is possibly salvageable, and hence *potentially* viable *if it is transferred to a woman for implantation.* It is not strictly true that the *in vitro* blastocyst is *necessarily* not-viable. Until proven otherwise, by embryo transfer and attempted implantation, we are right to consider the human blastocyst *in vitro* as potentially a human being and, in this respect, not fundamentally different from a blastocyst *in utero.* To put the matter more forcefully, the blastocyst *in vitro* is *more* "viable," in the sense of more salvageable, than aborted fetuses at most later stages, up to say 20 weeks.

This is not to say that such a blastocyst is therefore endowed with a so-called right to life, that failure to implant it is negligent homicide, or that experimental touchings of such blastocysts constitute assault and battery. (I myself tend to reject such claims, and indeed think that the ethical questions are not best posed in terms of "rights.") But the blastocyst is not nothing; it is *at least* potential humanity, and as such it elicits, or ought to elicit, our feelings of awe and respect. In the blastocyst, even in the zygote, we face a mysterious and awesome power, a power governed by an immanent plan that may produce an indisputably and fully human being. It deserves our respect not because it has rights or claims or sentience (which it does not have at this stage), but because of what it is, now *and* prospectively.

Let us test this provisional conclusion by considering intuitively our response to two possible fates of such zygotes, blastocysts, and early embryos. First, should such an embryo die, will we be inclined to mourn its passing? When a woman we know miscarries, we are sad—largely for *her* loss and disappointment, but perhaps also at the premature death of a life that might have been. But we do not mourn the departed fetus, nor do we seek ritually to dispose of the remains. In this respect, we do not treat even the fetus as fully one of us.

On the other hand, we would I suppose recoil even from the thought, let alone the practice—I apologize for forcing it upon the reader—of eating such embryos, should someone discover that they would provide a great delicacy, a "human caviar." The human blastocyst would be protected by our taboo against cannibalism, which insists on the humanness of human flesh and which does not permit us to treat even the flesh of the dead as if it were mere meat. *The human embryo is not mere meat; it is not just stuff; it is not a thing.*[5] Because of its origin and because of its capacity, it commands a higher respect.

How much more respect? As much as for a fully developed human being? My own inclination is to say "probably not," but who can be certain? Indeed, there might be prudential and reasonable grounds for an affirmative answer, partly because the presumption of ignorance ought to err in the direction of never underestimating the basis for respect of human life, partly because so many people feel very strongly that even the blastocyst is protectably human. As a first approximation, I would analogize the early embryo *in vitro* to the early embryo *in utero* (because both are potentially viable and human). On this ground alone, *the most sensible policy is to treat the early embryo as a pre-viable fetus, with constraints imposed on early embryo research at least as great as those on fetal research.*

To some this may seem excessively scrupulous. They will argue for the importance of the absence of distinctive humanoid appearance or the absence of sentience. To be sure, we would feel more restraint in invasive procedures conducted on a five-month-old or even 12-week-old living fetus than on a blastocyst. But this added restraint on inflicting suffering on a "look-alike," feeling creature in no way denies the propriety of a prior restraint, grounded in respect for individuated, living, potential humanity. Before I would be persuaded to treat early embryos differently from later ones, I would insist on the establishment of a reasonably clear, naturally grounded boundary that separates "early" and "late," and which provides the basis for respecting "the early" less than "the late." This burden *must* be accepted by proponents of experimentation with human embryos *in vitro* if a decision to permit creating embryos for such experimentation is to be treated as ethically responsible.

## IV

Where does the above analysis lead in thinking about treatment of *in vitro* human embryos? I shall indicate, very briefly, the lines toward a possible policy, though that is not my major intent.

The *in vitro* fertilized embryo has four possible fates: (1) *implantation,* in the hope of producing from it a child; (2) *death,* by active "killing" or disaggregation, or by a "natural" demise; (3) use in *manipulative experimentation*— embryological, genetic, etc.; (4) use in attempts at *perpetuation in vitro* beyond the blastocyst stage, ultimately, perhaps, to viability. I will not now consider this fourth and future possibility, though I would suggest that full laboratory growth of an embryo into a viable human being (i.e., ectogenesis), while perfectly compatible with respect owed to its potential humanity as an individual, may be incompatible with the kind of respect owed to its humanity that is grounded in the bonds of lineage and the nature of parenthood.

On the strength of my analysis of the status of the embryo, and the respect due it, no objection would be raised to implantation. *In vitro* fertilization and embryo transfer to treat infertility, as in the case of Mr. and Mrs. Brown, is perfectly compatible with a respect and reverence for human life, including potential human life. Moreover, no disrespect is intended or practiced by the mere fact that several eggs are removed for fertilization, to increase the chance of success. Were it possible to guarantee successful fertilization and normal growth with a single egg, no more would need to be obtained. Assuming nothing further is done with the unimplanted embryos, there is nothing disrespectful going on. The demise of the unimplanted embryos would be analogous to the loss of numerous embryos wasted in the normal *in vivo* attempts to generate a child. It is estimated that over 50 percent of eggs successfully fertilized during unprotected sexual intercourse fail to implant, or do not remain implanted, in the uterine wall, and are shed soon thereafter, before a diagnosis of pregnancy could be made. Any couple attempting to conceive a child tacitly accepts such embryonic wastage as the perfectly acceptable price to be paid for the birth of a (usually) healthy child. Current procedures to initiate pregnancy with laboratory fertilization thus differ from the natural "procedure" in that what would normally be spread over four or five months *in vivo* is compressed into a single effort, using all at once a four or five months' supply of eggs.[6]

Parenthetically, we should note that the natural occurrence of embryo and fetal loss and wastage does not necessarily or automatically justify all deliberate, humanly caused destruction of fetal life. For example, the natural loss of embryos in early pregnancy cannot in itself be a warrant for deliberately aborting them or for invasively experimenting on them *in vitro,* any more than stillbirths could be a justification for newborn infanticide. There are many things that happen naturally that we ought not to do deliberately. It is curious how the same people who deny the relevance of nature as a guide for evaluating human interventions into human generation, and who deny that the term "unnatural" carries any ethical weight, will themselves appeal to "nature's way" when it suits their purposes.[7] Still, in this present matter, the closeness to natural procreation—the goal is the same, the embryonic loss is unavoidable and not desired, and the amount of loss is similar—leads me to believe that we do no more intentional or unjustified harm in the one case than in the other, and practice no disrespect.

But must we allow *in vitro* unimplanted embryos to die? Why should they not be either transferred for "adoption" into another infertile woman, or else used for investigative purposes, to seek new knowledge, say about gene action? The first option raises questions about the nature of parenthood and lineage to which I will return. But even on first glance, it would seem likely to raise a large objection from the original couple, who were seeking a child of their own and not the dissemination of their "own" biological children for prenatal adoption.

But what about experimentation on such blastocysts and early embryos? Is that compatible with the respect they deserve? This is the hard question. On balance, I would think not. Invasive and manipulative experiments involving such embryos very likely presume that they are things or mere stuff, and deny the fact of their possible viability. Certain observational and noninvasive experiments might be different. But on the whole, I would think that the respect for human embryos for which I have argued—I repeat, not their so-called right to life—would lead one to oppose most potentially interesting and useful experimentation. This is a dilemma, but one which cannot be ducked or defined away. Either we accept certain great restrictions on the permissible uses of human embryos or we deliberately decide to override—though I hope not deny—the respect due to the embryos.

I am aware that I have pointed toward a seemingly paradoxical conclusion about the treatment of the unimplanted embryos: Leave them alone, and do not create embryos for experimentation only. To let them die "naturally" would be the most respectful course, grounded on a reverence, generically, for their potential humanity, and a respect, individually, for their being the seed and offspring of a particular couple who were themselves seeking only to have a child of their own. An analysis which stressed a "right to life," rather than respect, would of course lead to different conclusions. Only an analysis of the status of the embryo which denied both its so-called rights *or* its worthiness of all respect would have no trouble sanctioning its use in investigative research, donation to other couples, commercial transactions, and other activities of these sorts.

V

The attempt to generate a child with the aid of *in vitro* fertilization constitutes an experiment upon the prospective child. As yet, we have no knowledge of the range of such risks. It thus raises a most peculiar question for the ethics of human experimentation: Can one ethically choose for a yet hypothetical, unconceived child-to-be the unknown hazards he must face, obviously without his consent, and simultaneously choose to give him life in which to face them? This question has been much debated, as it points to a serious and immediate ethical concern: the hazards of manipulating the embryo as it bears on the health of the child-to-be.

Everyone agrees that human-embryo transfer for the sake of generation should not be performed until prior laboratory research in animals has provided a sound basis for estimating the likely risks to any human beings who will be born as a result of this transfer and gestation. Argument centers on whether a sufficiently sound basis for estimating the likely risks to humans *can be* provided by animal experiments, and, if so, whether adequate experimentation has been done, and what level of risk is acceptable.

There is, it seems to me, good reason for insisting that risk of incidence and likely extent of possible harm be very, very low—lower, say, than in therapeutic experimentation in children or adults. But I do not think that the risk of harm must be positively excluded (and it certainly cannot be). It would suffice if those risks were equivalent to, or less than, the risks to the child from normal procreation. To insist on more rigorous standards, especially when we permit known carriers of genetic disease to reproduce, would seem a denial of equal treatment to infertile couples contemplating *in vitro* assistance. Moreover, it is to give undue weight to the importance of bodily harm over against risks of poor nurture and rearing after birth. Wouldn't the couple's great eagerness for the child count, in the promise of increased parental affection, toward offsetting even a slightly higher but unknown risk of mental retardation?

Finally, to insist on extrascrupulosity regarding risks in laboratory-assisted reproduction is to attach too much of one's concern to the wrong issue. True, everyone understands about harming children, while very few worry about dehumanization of procreation or problems of lineage. But those are the things that are distinctive about laboratory-assisted reproduction, not the risk of bodily harm to offspring. It should suffice that the risks be comparable to those for ordinary procreation, not greater but no less.

It remains a question whether we now know enough about these risks to go ahead with human-embryo transfer. Here I would defer to the opinions of the cautious experts—for caution is the posture of responsibility toward such prospective children. I would agree with Doctors Luigi Mastroianni, Benjamin Brackett, and Robert Short—all researchers in the field—that the risks for humans have not yet been sufficiently assessed, in large part because the risks in animals have been so poorly assessed (due to the small numbers of such births and to the absence of any *prospective* study to identify and evaluate deviations from the norm).

## VI

Many people rejoiced at the birth of Louise Brown. Some were pleased by the technical accomplishment, many were pleased that she was born apparently in good health. But most of us shared the joy of her parents, who, after a long, frustrating, and fruitless period, at last had the pleasure and blessing of a child of their own. The desire to have a child of one's own is acknowledged to be a powerful and deep-seated human desire—some have called it "instinctive"—and the satisfaction of this desire, by the relief of infertility, is said to be one major goal of continuing the work with *in vitro* fertilization and embryo transfer. That this is a worthy goal few, if any, would deny.

Yet let us explore what is meant by *"to have a child of one's own."* First, what is meant by "to *have*"? Is the crucial meaning that of gestating and bearing? Or is it "to have" as a possession? Or is it to nourish and to rear, the child being the embodiment of one's activity as teacher and guide? Or is it rather to provide someone who descends and comes after, someone who will replace oneself in the family line or preserve the family tree by new sproutings and branchings?

More significantly, what is meant by *"one's own"*? What sense of one's own is important? A scientist might define "one's own" in terms of carrying one's own genes. Though in some sense correct, this cannot be humanly decisive. For Mr. Brown or for most of us, it would not be a matter of indifference if the sperm used to fertilize the egg were provided by an identical twin brother—whose genes would be, of course, the same as his. Rather, the humanly crucial sense of "one's own," the sense that leads most people to choose their own, rather than to adopt, is captured in such phrases as "my seed," "flesh of my flesh," "sprung from my loins." More accurately, since "one's own" is not the own of one but of *two,* the desire to have a child of "one's own" is *a couple's desire* to embody, out of the conjugal union of their separate bodies, a child who is flesh of their separate flesh made one. This archaic language may sound quaint, but I would argue that this is precisely what is being celebrated by most people who rejoice at the birth of Louise Brown, whether they would articulate it this way or not. Mr. and Mrs. Brown, by the birth of their daughter, fulfill this aspect of their separate sexual natures and of their married life together, they acquire descendants and a new branch of their joined family tree, and the child Louise is given solid and unambiguous roots from which she has sprung and by which she will be nourished.

If this were to be the *only* use made of embryo transfer, and if providing *in this sense* "a child of one's own" were indeed the sole reason for the clinical use of the techniques, there could be no objection. Yet there will almost certainly be other uses, involving third parties, to satisfy the desire "to have" a child of "one's own" in different senses of "to have" and "one's own." I am not merely speculating about future possibilities. With the technology to effect human *in vitro* fertilization and embryo transfer comes the *immediate* possibility of egg donation (egg from donor, sperm from husband), embryo donation (egg and sperm from outside of the marriage), and foster pregnancy (host surrogate for gestation).

Nearly everyone agrees that these circumstances are morally and perhaps psychologically more complicated than the intramarital case. Here the meaning of "one's own" is no longer so unambiguous; neither is the meaning of motherhood and the status of pregnancy. On the one hand, it is argued that embryo donation, or "prenatal adoption," would be superior to present adoption, because the woman would have the experience of pregnancy and the child would be born of the "adopting" mother, rendering the maternal tie even more close. On the other hand, the mother-child bond rooted in pregnancy and delivery is held to be of little consequence by those who would endorse the use of surrogate gestational "mothers," say for a woman whose infertility is due to uterine disease rather than ovarian disease or oviduct obstruction. Clearly, the "need" and demand for extramarital embryo transfer are real and probably large, probably even greater than the intramarital ones. Already, the Chairman of the Ethics Advisory Board has testified in Congress about the need to define the responsibilities of *the donor* and the recipient "parents." Thus the new techniques will not only serve to ensure and preserve lineage, but will also serve to confound and complicate it. The principle truly at work here is not to provide married couples with a child of *their own,* but to provide anyone who wants one with a child, by whatever possible or convenient means.

"So what?" it will be said. First of all, we already practice and encourage adoption. Second, we have permitted artificial insemination—though we have, after some 40 years of this practice, yet to resolve questions of legitimacy. Third, what with the high rate of divorce and remarriage, identification of "mother," "father," and "child" is already complicated. Fourth, there is a growing rate of illegitimacy and husbandless parentages. Fifth, the use of surrogate mothers for foster pregnancy has already occurred, with the aid of artificial insemination.[8] Finally, our age in its enlightenment is no longer so certain about the virtues of family, lineage, and heterosexuality, or even about the taboos against adultery and incest. Against this background, it will be asked, why all the fuss about some little embryos that stray from the nest?

It is not an easy question to answer. Yet, consider. We practice adoption because there are abandoned children who need a good home. We do not, and would not, encourage people deliberately to generate children for others to adopt; partly we wish to avoid baby markets, partly we think it unfair to the child deliberately to deprive him of his natural ties. Recent years have seen a rise in our concern with roots, against the rootless and increasingly homogeneous background of contemporary American life. Adopted children, in particular, are pressing for information regarding their "real parents," and some states now require that such information be made available (on that typically modern ground of "freedom of information," rather than because of the profound importance of lineage for self-identity). The practice of artificial insemination has yet to be evaluated, the secrecy in which it is practiced being an apparent concession to the dangers of publicity.[9] Indeed, most physicians who practice artificial insemination routinely mix in some semen from the husband, to preserve some doubt about paternity—again, a concession to the importance of lineage and legitimacy. Finally, what about the changing mores of marriage, divorce, single-parent families, and sexual behavior? Do we applaud these changes? Do we want to contribute further to the confusion of thought, identity, and practice?[10]

Properly understood, the largely universal taboos against incest, and also the prohibition against adultery, suggest that clarity about who your parents are, clarity in the lines of generation, clarity about who is whose, are the indispensable foundations of a sound family life, itself the sound foundation of civilized community. Clarity about your origins is crucial for self-identity, itself important for self-respect. It would be, in my view, deplorable public policy further to erode such fundamental beliefs, values, institutions, and practices. This means, concretely, no encouragement of embryo adoption or especially of surrogate pregnancy. While it would be perhaps foolish to try to proscribe or outlaw such practices, it would not be wise for the federal government to foster them. The Ethics Advisory Board should carefully consider whether it should and can attempt to restrict the use of embryo transfer to the married couple from whom the embryo derives.

The case of surrogate wombs bears a further comment. While expressing no objection to the practice of foster pregnancy itself, some people object that it will be done for pay, largely because of their fear that poor women will be exploited by such a practice. But if there were nothing wrong with foster pregnancy, what would be wrong with making a living at it? Clearly, this objection harbors a *tacit* understanding that to bear another's child for pay is in some sense a degradation of oneself—in the same sense that prostitution is a degradation *primarily* because it entails the loveless surrender of one's body to serve another's lust, and *only derivatively* because the woman is paid. It is to deny the meaning and worth of one's body, to treat it as a mere incubator, divested of its human meaning. It is also to deny the meaning of the bond among sexuality, love, and procreation. The buying and selling of human flesh and the dehumanized uses of the human body ought not to be encouraged. To be sure, the practice of womb donation could be engaged in for love not money, as it apparently has been in the case in Michigan [in the original version of this selection]. A woman could bear her sister's child out of sisterly love. But to the degree that one escapes in this way from the degradation and difficulties of the *sale* of human flesh and bodily services, and the treating of the body as stuff (the problem of cannibalism), one approaches instead the difficulties of potential incest and near-incest.

## VII

Objections have been raised about the deliberate technological intervention into the so-called natural processes of human reproduction. Some would simply oppose such interventions as "unnatural," and therefore wrong. Others are concerned about the consequences of these interventions, and about their ends and limits. Again, I think it important to explore the meaning and possible significance of such interventions, present and projected, especially as they bear on fundamental beliefs, institutions, and practices. To do so requires that we consider likely future developments in the laboratory study of human reproduction. Indeed, I shall argue that we *must* consider such future developments in reaching a decision in the present case.

What can we expect in the way of new modes of reproduction, as an outgrowth of present studies? To be sure, prediction is difficult. One can never know with certainty what will happen, much less how soon. Yet uncertainty is not the same as simple ignorance. Some things, indeed, seem likely. They seem likely because (1) they are thought necessary or desirable, at least by some researchers and their sponsors, (2) they are probably biologically possible and technically feasible, and (3) they will be difficult to prevent or control (especially if no one anticipates their development or sees a need to worry about them). One of the things the citizenry, myself included, would expect from an Ethics Advisory Board and our policy makers generally is that they face up to reasonable projections of future accomplishments, consider whether they are cause for social concern, and see whether or not the principles *now* enunciated and the practices *now* established are adequate to deal with any such concerns.

I project at least the following:

1. The growth of human embryos in the laboratory will be extended beyond the blastocyst stage. Such growth must be deemed desirable under all the arguments advanced for developmental research *up to* the blastocyst

stage; research on gene action, chromosome segregation, cellular and organic differentiation, fetus-environment interaction, implantation, etc., cannot answer all its questions with the blastocyst. Such *in vitro* post-blastocyst differentiation has apparently been achieved in the mouse, in culture; the use of other mammals as temporary hosts for human embryos is also a possibility. How far such embryos will eventually be perpetuated is anybody's guess, but full-term ectogenesis cannot be excluded. Neither can the existence of laboratories filled with many living human embryos, growing at various stages of development.

2. Experiments will be undertaken to alter the cellular and genetic composition of these embryos, at first without subsequent transfer to a woman for gestation, perhaps later as a prelude to reproductive efforts. Again, scientific reasons now justifying Dr. Soupart's research already justify further embryonic manipulations, including formation of hybrids or chimeras (within species and between species); gene, chromosome, and plasmid insertion, excision, or alteration; nuclear transplantation or cloning, etc. The techniques of DNA recombination, coupled with the new skills of handling embryos, make prospects for some precise genetic manipulation much nearer than anyone would have guessed 10 years ago. And embryological and cellular research in mammals is making astounding progress. On the cover of a recent issue of *Science* is a picture of a hexaparental mouse, born after reaggregation of an early embryo with cells disaggregated from three separate embryos. (Note: That sober journal calls this a "handmade mouse"—i.e., literally a *manu-factured* mouse—and goes on to say that it was "manufactured by genetic engineering techniques.")[11]

3. Storage and banking of living human embryos (and ova) will be undertaken, perhaps commercially. After all, commercial sperm banks are already well-established and prospering.

Space does not permit me to do more than identify a few kinds of questions that must be considered in relation to such possible coming control over human heredity and reproduction: questions about the wisdom required to engage in such practices; questions about the goals and standards that will guide our interventions; questions about changes in the concepts of being human, including embodiment, gender, love, lineage, identity, parenthood, and sexuality; questions about the responsibility of power over future generations; questions about awe, respect, humility; questions about the kind of society we will have if we follow along our present course.[12]

Though I cannot discuss these questions now, I can and must face a serious objection to considering them at all. Most people would agree that the projected possibilities raise far more serious questions than do simple fertilization of a few embryos, their growth *in vitro* to the blastocyst stage, and their possible transfer to women for gestation. Why burden the present decision with these possibilities? Future "abuses," it is often said, do not disqualify present uses (though these same people also often say that "future benefits justify present questionable uses"). Moreover, there can be no certainty that "A" will lead to "B." This thin-edge-of-the-wedge argument has been open to criticism.

But such criticism misses the point, for two reasons. *First,* critics often misunderstand the wedge argument. The wedge argument is not primarily an argument of prediction, that A *will* lead to B, say on the strength of the empirical analysis of precedent and an appraisal of the likely direction of present research. It is primarily an argument about the *logic* of justification. Do the principles of justification *now* used to justify the current research proposal already justify *in advance* the further developments? Consider some of these principles:

1. It is desirable to learn as much as possible about the processes of fertilization, growth, implantation, and differentiation of human embryos and about human gene expression and its control.
2. It would be desirable to acquire improved techniques for *enhancing* conception and implantation, for *preventing* conception and implantation, for the treatment of genetic and chromosomal abnormalities, etc.
3. In the end, only research using *human* embryos can answer these questions and provide these techniques.
4. There should be no censorship or limitation of scientific inquiry or research.

This logic knows no boundary at the blastocyst stage or, for that matter, at any later stage. For these principles *not* to justify future extensions of current work, some independent additional principles, limiting such justification to particular stages of development, would have to be found. Here, the task is to find such a biologically defensible distinction that could be respected as reasonable and not arbitrary, a difficult—perhaps impossible—task, given the continuity of development after fertilization. The citizenry, myself included, will want to know *precisely* what grounds our policy makers will give for endorsing Soupart's research, and whether their principles have not already sanctioned future developments. If they do give such wedge-opening justifications, let them do so deliberately, candidly, and intentionally.

A better case to illustrate the wedge logic is the principle offered for the embryo-transfer procedures as treatment for infertility. Will we support the use of *in vitro* fertilization and embryo transfer because it provides a "child of *one's own*," in a strict sense of *one's own*, to a married couple? Or will we support the transfer because it is treatment of involuntary infertility, which deserves treatment in or out of marriage, hence endorsing the use of any available technical means (which would produce a healthy and normal child), including surrogate wombs or even ectogenesis?

*Second,* logic aside, the opponents of the wedge argument do not counsel well. It would be simply foolish to ignore what might come next, and to fail to make the *best possible* assessment of the implications of present action (or inaction). Let me put the matter very bluntly: the Ethics Advisory Board, in the decision it must now make, may very well be helping to decide whether human beings will eventually be produced in laboratories. I say this not to shock—and I do not mean to beg the question of whether that would be desirable or not. I say this to make sure that they and we face squarely the full import and magnitude of this decision. Once the genies let the babies into the bottle, it may be impossible to get them out again.

## VIII

So much, then, for the meaning of initiating and manipulating human embryos in the laboratory. These considerations still make me doubt the wisdom of proceeding with these practices, both in research and in their clinical application, notwithstanding that valuable knowledge might be had by continuing the research and identifiable suffering might be alleviated by using it to circumvent infertility. To doubt the wisdom of going ahead makes one at least a fellow traveller of the opponents of such research, but it does not, either logically or practically, require that one join them in trying to prevent it, say by legal prohibition. Not every folly can or should be legislated against. Attempts at prohibition here would seem to be both ineffective and dangerous—ineffective because impossible to enforce, dangerous because the costs of such precedent-setting interference with scientific research might be greater than the harm it prevents. To be sure, we already have legal restrictions on experimentation with human subjects, which restrictions are manifestly not incompatible with the progress of medical science. Neither is it true that science cannot survive if it must take some direction from the law. Nor is it the case that all research, because it is research, is or should be absolutely protected. But it does not seem to me that *in vitro* fertilization and embryo transfer deserve, *at least at present,* to be treated as sufficiently dangerous for legislative interference.

But if to doubt the wisdom does not oblige one to seek to outlaw the folly, neither does a decision *to permit* require a decision *to encourage or support.* A researcher's freedom to do *in vitro* fertilization, or a woman's right to have a child with laboratory assistance, in no way implies a public (or even a private) obligation to pay for such research or treatment. A right *against* interference is not an entitlement *for assistance.* The question before the Ethics Advisory Board and the Department of Health, Education, and Welfare is *not* whether to permit such research but whether the federal government should fund it. This is the policy question that needs to be discussed.

The arguments in favor of federal support are well known. *First,* the research is seen as continuous with, if not quite an ordinary instance of, the biomedical research which the federal government supports handsomely; roughly two-thirds of the money spent on biomedical research in the United States comes from Uncle Sam. Why is this research different from all other research? Its scientific merit has been attested to by the normal peer-review process at NIH. For some, that is a sufficient reason to support it.

*Second,* there are specific practical fruits expected from the anticipated successes of this new line of research. Besides relief for many cases of infertility, the research promises new birth-control measures based upon improved understanding of the mechanisms of fertilization and implantation, which in turn could lead to techniques unblocking these processes. Also, studies on early embryonic development hold forth the promise of learning how to prevent some congenital malformations and certain highly malignant tumors (e.g., hydatiform mole) that derive from aberrant fetal tissue.

*Third,* as he who pays the piper calls the tune, federal support would make easy the federal regulation and supervision of this research. For the government to abstain, so the argument runs, is to leave the control of research and clinical application in the hands of profit-hungry, adventurous, insensitive, reckless, or power-hungry private physicians, scientists, or drug companies; or, on the other hand, at the mercy of the vindictive, mindless, and superstitious civic groups that will interfere with this research through state and local legislation. Only through federal regulation—which, it is said, can only follow with federal funding—can we have reasonable, enforceable, and uniform guidelines.

*Fourth* is the chauvinistic argument that the United States should lead the way in this brave new research, especially as it will apparently be going forward in other nations. Indeed, one witness testifying before the Ethics Advisory Board deplored the fact that the first Louise Brown was British and not American, and complained, in effect, that the existing moratorium on federal support has already created what one might call an *"in vitro* fertilization gap." The preeminence of American science and technology, so the argument implies, is the center of our preeminence among the nations, a position which will be jeopardized if we hang back out of fear.

Let me respond to these arguments, in reverse order. Conceding the premise of the importance of American science for American prestige and strength, it is far from clear that failure to support *this* research would jeopardize American science. Certainly the use of embryo transfer to overcome infertility, though a vital matter for the couples involved, is hardly a matter of vital national interest—at least not unless and until the majority of American women are similarly infertile. The demands of international competition, admittedly often a necessary evil, should be invoked only for things that really matter; a missile gap and an embryo-transfer gap are chasms apart. In areas not crucial to our own survival, there will be many things we should allow other nations to develop, if that is their wish, without feeling obliged to join them. Moreover, one should not rush into potential folly to avoid being the last to commit it.

The argument about governmental regulation has much to recommend it. But it fails to consider that there are other safeguards against recklessness, at least in the clinical applications, known to the high-minded as the canons of medical ethics and to the cynical as liability for malpractice. Also, federal regulations attached to federal funding will not in any case regulate research done with private monies, say by the drug companies. Moreover, there are enough concerned practitioners of these new arts who would have a compelling interest in regulating their own practice, if only to escape the wrath and interference of hostile citizen groups in response to unsavory goings-on. The available evidence does not convince me that a sensible practice of *in vitro* experimentation requires regulation by the federal government.

In turning to the argument about anticipated technological powers, we face difficult calculations of unpredictable and more-or-less-likely costs and benefits, and the all-important questions of priorities in the allocation of scarce

resources. Here it seems useful to consider separately the techniques for generating children and the anticipated techniques for birth control or for preventing developmental anomalies and malignancies.

First, accepting that providing a child of their own to infertile couples is a
worthy goal—and it is both insensitive and illogical to cite the population
problem as an argument for ignoring the problem of infertility—one can nevertheless question its rank relative to other goals of medical research. One can
even wonder—and I have done so in print—whether it is indeed a *medical* goal
or a worthy goal for *medicine,* that is, whether alleviating infertility, especially
in this way, is part of the art of *healing*.[13] Just as abortion for genetic defect is a
peculiar innovation in medicine (or in preventive medicine) in which a disease
is treated by eliminating the patient (or, if you prefer, a disease is prevented
by "preventing" the patient), so laboratory fertilization is a peculiar treatment
for oviduct obstruction, in that it requires the creation of a new life to "heal"
an existing one. All this simply emphasizes the uniqueness of the reproductive
organs, in that their proper function involves other people, and calls attention
to the fact that infertility is not a "disease," like heart disease or stroke, even
though obstruction of a normally patent tube or vessel is the proximate cause
of each.

However this may be, there is a more important objection to this approach
to the problem. It represents yet another instance of our thoughtless preference for expensive, high-technology, therapy-oriented approaches to disease
and dysfunctions. What about spending this money on discovering the causes
of infertility? What about the prevention of tubal obstruction? We complain
about rising medical costs, but we insist on the most spectacular and the most
technological—and thereby the most costly—remedies.

The truth is that we do know a little about the causes of tubal obstruction—though much less than we should or could. For instance, it is estimated
that at least one-third of such cases are the aftermath of pelvic-inflammatory
disease, caused by that uninvited venereal guest, gonococcus. Leaving aside
any question about whether it makes sense for a federally funded baby to be
the wage of aphrodisiac indiscretion,[14] one can only look with wonder at a society that will have "petri-dish babies"[15] before it has found a vaccine against
gonorrhea.

True, there are other causes of blocked oviducts, and blocked oviducts are
not the only cause of female infertility. True, it is not logically necessary to
choose between prevention and cure. But *practically* speaking, with money
for research as limited as it is, research funds targeted for the relief of infertility should certainly go first to epidemiological and preventive measures—
especially where the costs in the high-technology cure are likely to be great.

What about these costs? I have already explored some of the nonfinancial
costs, in discussing the meaning of this research for our images of humanness.
Let us, for now, consider only the financial costs. How expensive was Louise
Brown? We do not know, partly because Drs. Edwards and Steptoe have yet to
publish their results, indicating how many failures preceded their success, how
many procedures for egg removal and for fetal monitoring were performed on

Mrs. Brown, and so on. One must add in the costs of monitoring the baby's development to check on her "normality" and, should it come, the costs of governmental regulation. A conservative estimate might place the costs of a successful pregnancy of this kind at between five and ten thousand dollars. If we use the conservative figure of 500,000 for estimating the number of infertile women *with* blocked oviducts in the United States whose *only* hope of having children lies in *in vitro* fertilization,[16] we reach a conservative estimated cost of $2.5 to $5 billion. Is it really even fiscally wise for the federal government to start down this road?

Clearly not, if it is also understood that the costs of providing the service, rendered possible by a successful technology, will also be borne by the taxpayers. Nearly everyone now agrees that the kidney-machine legislation, obliging the federal government to pay about $25,000–30,000 per patient per year for kidney dialysis for anyone in need (cost to the taxpayers in 1978 was nearly $1 billion), is an impossible precedent—notwithstanding that individual lives have been prolonged as a result. But once the technique of *in vitro* fertilization and embryo transfer is developed and available, how should the babymaking be paid for? Should it be covered under medical insurance? If a national health insurance program is enacted, will and should these services be included? (Those who argue that they are part of medicine will have a hard time saying no.) Failure to do so will make this procedure available only to the well-to-do, on a fee-for-service basis. Would that be a fair alternative? Perhaps; but it is unlikely to be tolerated. Indeed, the principle of equality—equal access to equal levels of medical care—is the leading principle in the pressure for medical reform. One can be certain that efforts will be forthcoming to make this procedure available equally to all, independent of ability to pay, under Medicaid or national health insurance or in some other way. (I have recently learned that a Boston-based group concerned with infertility has obtained private funding to pay for artificial insemination for women on welfare!)

Much as I sympathize with the plight of infertile couples, I do not believe that they are entitled to the provision of a child at the public expense, especially at this cost, especially by a procedure that also involves so many moral difficulties. Given the many vexing dilemmas that will surely be spawned by laboratory-assisted reproduction, the federal government should not be misled by compassion to embark on this imprudent course.

In considering the federal funding of such research for its other anticipated technological benefits, independent of its clinical use in baby-making, we face a more difficult matter. In brief, as is the case with all basic research, one simply cannot predict what kinds of techniques and uses this research will yield. But here, also, I think good sense would at present say that before one undertakes *human in vitro* fertilization to seek new methods of birth control—e.g., by developing antibodies to the human egg that would physically interfere with its fertilization—one should make adequate attempts to do this in animals. One simply can't get large enough numbers of human eggs to do this pioneering research well—at least not without subjecting countless women to additional risks not for their immediate benefit. Why not test this conceit first in the mouse or rabbit? Only if the results were very promising—and judged also to be relatively safe in practice—should one consider trying such things in humans. Likewise, the developmental research can and should be first carried out in animals, especially in primates. Though *in vitro* fertilization has yet to be achieved in monkeys, embryo transfer of *in vivo* fertilized eggs has been accomplished, thus permitting the relevant research to proceed. Purely *on scientific grounds,* the federal government ought not *now* to be investing funds in this research for its promised technological benefits—benefits which, in the absence of pilot studies in animals, must be regarded as mere wishful thoughts in the imaginings of scientists.

There remains the first justification, research for the sake of knowledge: knowledge about cell cleavage, cell-cell and cell-environment interactions, and cell differentiation; knowledge of gene action and of gene regulation; knowledge of the effects and mechanisms of action of various chemical and physical agents on growth and development; knowledge of the basic processes of fertilization and implantation. This is all knowledge worth having, and though much can be learned using animal sources—and these sources have barely begun to be sufficiently exploited—the investigation of these matters in man would, sooner or later, require the use of human-embryonic material. Here, again, there are questions of research priority about which there is room for disagreement, among scientists and laymen alike. But these questions of research priority, while not irrelevant to the decision at hand, are not the questions that the Ethics Advisory Board was constituted to answer.

It was constituted to consider whether such research is consistent with the ethical standards of our community. The question turns in large part on the status of the early embryo. If, as I have argued, the early embryo is deserving of respect because of what it is, now and potentially, it is difficult to justify submitting it to invasive experiments, and especially difficult to justify *creating it solely* for the purpose of experimentation. But even if this argument fails to sway the Board, another one should. For their decision, I remind you, is not whether *in vitro* fertilization should be permitted in the United States, but whether *our* tax dollars should encourage and foster it. One cannot, therefore, ignore the deeply held convictions of a sizable portion of our population—it may even be a majority on this issue—that regards the human embryo as protectable humanity, not to be experimented upon except for its own benefit. Never mind if these beliefs have a religious foundation—as if that should ever be a reason for dismissing them! The presence, sincerity, and depth of these beliefs, and the grave importance of their subject, are what must concern us. The holders of these beliefs have been very much alienated by the numerous court decisions and legislative enactments regarding abortion and research on fetuses. Many who, by and large, share their opinions about the humanity of prenatal life have with heavy heart gone along with the liberalization of abortion, out of deference to the wishes, desires, interests, or putative rights of pregnant women. But will they go along here with what they can only regard as gratuitous and willful assaults on human life, or at least on potential and salvageable human life, and on human dignity? We can ill afford to alienate them further, and it would be unstatesmanlike, to say the least, to do so, especially in a matter so little important to the national health and one so full of potential dangers.

Technological progress can be but one measure of our national health. Far more important are the affection and esteem in which our citizenry holds its laws and institutions. No amount of relieved infertility is worth the further disaffection and civil contention that the lifting of the moratorium on federal funding is likely to produce. People opposed to abortion and people grudgingly willing to permit women to obtain elective abortion, at their own expense, will not tolerate having their tax money spent on scientific research requiring what they regard as at best cruelty, at worst murder. A prudent Ethics Advisory Board and a prudent and wise Secretary of Health, Education, and Welfare should take this matter most seriously, and refuse to lift the moratorium—at least until they are persuaded that public opinion will overwhelmingly support them. Imprudence in this matter may be the worst sin of all.

## AN AFTERWORD

This has been for me a long and difficult exposition. Many of the arguments are hard to make. It is hard to get confident people to face unpleasant prospects. It is hard to get many people to take seriously such "soft" matters as lineage, identity, respect, and self-respect when they are in tension with such "hard" matters as a cure for infertility or new methods of contraception. It is hard to talk about the meaning of sexuality and embodiment in a culture that treats sex increasingly as sport and that has trivialized the significance of gender, marriage, and procreation. It is hard to oppose federal funding of baby-making in a society which increasingly demands that the federal government supply all demands, and which—contrary to so much evidence of waste, incompetence, and corruption—continues to believe that only Uncle Sam can do it. And, finally, it is hard to speak about restraint in a culture that seems to venerate very little above man's own attempt to master all. Here, I am afraid, is the biggest question and the one we perhaps can no longer ask or deal with: the question about the reasonableness of the desire to become masters and possessors of nature, human nature included.

Here we approach the deepest meaning of *in vitro* fertilization. Those who have likened it to artificial insemination are only partly correct. With *in vitro* fertilization, the human embryo emerges for the first time from the natural darkness and privacy of its own mother's womb, where it is hidden away in mystery, into the bright light and utter publicity of the scientist's laboratory, where it will be treated with unswerving rationality, before the clever and shameless eye of the mind and beneath the obedient and equally clever touch of the hand. What does it mean to hold the beginning of human life before your eyes, in your hands—even for five days (for the meaning does not depend on duration)? Perhaps the meaning is contained in the following story.

Long ago there was a man of great intellect and great courage. He was a remarkable man, a giant, able to answer questions that no other human being could answer, willing boldly to face any challenge or problem. He was a confident man, a masterful man. He saved his city from disaster and ruled it as a father rules his children, revered by all. But something was wrong in his city. A plague had fallen on generation; infertility afflicted plants, animals, and human beings. The man confidently promised to uncover the cause of the plague and to cure the infertility. Resolutely, dauntlessly, he put his sharp mind to work to solve the problem, to bring the dark things to light. No secrets, no reticences, a full public inquiry. He raged against the representatives of caution, moderation, prudence, and piety, who urged him to curtail his inquiry; he accused them of trying to usurp his rightfully earned power, of trying  to replace human and masterful control with submissive reverence. The story ends in tragedy: He solved the problem, but, in making visible and public the dark and intimate details of his origins, he ruined his life and that of his family. In the end, too late, he learns about the price of presumption, of overconfidence, of the overweening desire to master and control one's fate. In symbolic rejection of his desire to look into everything, he punishes his eyes with self-inflicted blindness.

Sophocles seems to suggest that such a man is always in principle—albeit unwittingly—a patricide, a regicide, and a practitioner of incest. We men of modern science may have something to learn from our forebear, Oedipus. It appears that Oedipus, being the kind of man an Oedipus is (the chorus calls him a paradigm of man), had no choice but to learn through suffering. Is it really true that we too have no other choice?

## NOTES

1. In the British procedures, several eggs are taken from each woman and fertilized, to increase the chance of success, but only one embryo is transferred for implantation. In Dr. Soupart's proposed experiments, as the embryos will be produced only for the purpose of research and not for transfer, all of them will be discarded or destroyed.
2. A perhaps justifiable exception would be the case of a universal plague on childbirth, say because of some epidemic that fatally attacks all fetuses *in utero* at age 5 months. Faced with the prospect of the end of the race, might we not condone the deliberate institution of pregnancies to provide fetuses for research, in the hope of finding a diagnosis and remedy for this catastrophic blight?
3. Peter Gwynne, "Was the Birth of Louise Brown Only a Happy Accident?" *Science Digest*, October 1978 (emphasis added).
4. For the supporting analysis of the concept of "viability," see my article "Determining Death and Viability in Fetuses and Abortuses," prepared for the National Commission for the Protection of Human Subjects of Biomedical and Behavioral Research, published in U.S. Department of

Health, Education, and Welfare, *Appendix: Research on the Fetus*, HEW Pub. No. (OS) 76–128 (Washington, DC, 1975).

5. Some people have suggested that the embryo be regarded like a vital organ, salvaged from a newly dead corpse, usable for transplantation or research, and that its donation by egg and sperm donors be governed by the Uniform Anatomical Gift Act, which legitimates premortem consent for organ donation upon death. But though this acknowledges that embryos are not things, it is mistaken in treating embryos as mere organs, thereby overlooking that they are early stages of a *complete, whole* human being. The Uniform Anatomical Gift Act does not apply to, nor should it be stretched to cover, donation of gonads, gametes (male sperm or female eggs), or—especially—zygotes and embryos.

6. There is a good chance that the problem of surplus embryos may be avoidable, for purely technical reasons. Some researchers believe that the uterine receptivity to the transferred embryo might be reduced during the particular menstrual cycle in which the ova are obtained, because of the effects of the hormones given to induce superovulation. They propose that the harvested *eggs* be frozen, and then defrosted one at a time each month for fertilization, culture, and transfer, until pregnancy is achieved. By refusing to fertilize all the eggs at once—i.e., not placing all one's eggs in one uterine cycle—there will not be surplus *embryos*, but at most only surplus eggs. This change in the procedure would make the demise of unimplanted embryos *exactly* analogous to the "natural" embryonic loss in ordinary reproduction.

7. The literature on intervention in reproduction is both confused and confusing on the crucial matter of the meanings of "nature" or "the natural," and their significance for the ethical issues. It may be as much a mistake to claim that "the natural" has *no* moral force as to suggest that the natural way is best, because natural. Though shallow and slippery thought about nature, and its relation to "good," is a likely source of these confusions, the nature of nature may itself be elusive, making it difficult for even careful thought to capture what is natural.

8. An unmarried woman in Dearborn, Michigan, offered to bear a child for her married friend, infertile because of a hysterectomy. She was impregnated by artificial insemination using semen produced by her friend's husband, his wife performing the injection. The threesome lived together all during the pregnancy. The child was delivered at birth by the biological-and-gestational-mother to the wife-and rearing-mother. The first (pregnancy) mother reports no feelings of attachment to the child she carried and bore. Everyone is reportedly delighted with the event. The trio has publicized its accomplishment and is reported to be considering selling rights to the story for a TV show, a book, and a movie. Their attorney has been swamped with letters requesting similar surrogate "mothers." (*American Medical News*, July 28, 1978, pp. 11–12.)

9. There are today numerous suits pending, throughout the United States, because of artificial insemination with donor semen (AID). Following

divorce, the ex-husbands are refusing child support for AID children, claiming, minimally, no paternity, or maximally that the child was the fruit of an adulterous union. In fact, a few states still treat AID as adultery. The importance of anonymity is revealed in the following bizarre case. A woman wanted to have a child, but abhorred the thought of marriage or of sexual relations with men. She learned a do-it-yourself technique of artificial insemination, and persuaded a male acquaintance to donate his semen. Now some 10 years after this virgin birth, the case has gone to court. The semen donor is suing for visitation privileges, to see his son.

10. To those who point out that the bond between sexuality and procreation has already been effectively and permanently cleaved by "the pill," and that this is therefore an idle worry in the case of *in vitro* fertilization, it must be said that the pill provides only sex without babies. Now the other shoe drops: babies without sex.

11. *Science 202*, no. 5 (October 6, 1978).

12. Some of these questions are addressed, albeit too briefly and polemically, in the latter part of my 1972 "Making Babies" article, to which the reader is referred. It has been pointed out to me by an astute colleague that the tone of the present article is less passionate and more accommodating than the first, which change he regards as an ironic demonstration of the inexorable way in which we get used to, and accept, our technological nightmares. I myself share his concern. I cannot decide whether the decline of my passion is to be welcomed; that is, whether it is due to greater understanding bred of more thought and experience, or to greater callousness and the contempt of familiarity bred from *too much* thought and experience. It does seem to me now that many of the fundamental beliefs and institutions that might be challenged by laboratory growth of human embryos and by laboratory-assisted reproduction are already severely challenged in perhaps more potent and important ways. Here, too, we see the creeping effect of the aggregated powers of modernity and the corrosive power of the familiar. Adaptiveness is our glory and our curse: as Raskolnikov put it, "Man gets used to everything, the beast!"

13. See "Making Babies—the New Biology and the 'Old' Morality," pp. 19–20. See also my "Regarding the End of Medicine and the Pursuit of Health," *The Public Interest*, Number 40, Summer 1975, especially pp. 11–18, and 33–35.

14. Consider the following contributions of federally-supported programs to rationalizing our sexual and reproductive practices. First, we have federally-supported programs of sex education in elementary schools, so that the children will know what can happen to them (and what they can make happen). Next, in high school, Uncle Sam provides for teenage contraception, to prevent the consequences of unavoidable sexual activity. Freed of a major deterrent to unrestricted sexual activity, our teenagers indulge, but not without consequences: They get gonorrhea, which some of them will have treated, again at the taxpayers' expense, through Medicaid. But for some the treatment comes too late to prevent scarring and oviduct

obstruction: federally supported *in vitro* fertilization research and services come to the rescue, to overcome their infertility. Uncle Sam will, of course, also provide Aid to Dependent Children, if the mother is or goes on welfare. How wonderful it is to be infinitely resourceful!

15. There has been much objection, largely from the scientific community, to the phrase "test-tube baby." More than one commentator has deplored the exploitation of its "flesh-creeping" connotations. They point out that a flat petri dish is used, not a test-tube—as if that mattered—and that the embryo spends but a few days in the dish. But they don't ask why the term "test-tube baby" remains the popular designation, and whether it does not embody more of the deeper truth than a more accurate, laboratory appellation. If the decisive difference is between "in the womb" or "in the lab," the popular designation conveys it. (See 'Afterword', below.) And it is right on target, and puts us on notice, if the justification for the present laboratory procedures tacitly also *justifies* future extensions, including full ectogenesis—say, if that were the only way a wombless woman could have a child of her own, without renting a human womb from a surrogate bearer.

16. This figure is calculated from estimates that between 10 and 15 percent of all couples are involuntarily infertile, and that in more than half of these cases the cause is in the female. Blocked oviducts account for perhaps 20 percent of the causes of female infertility. Perhaps 50 percent of these women might be helped to have a child by means of reconstructive surgery on the oviducts; the remainder could conceive *only* with the aid of laboratory fertilization and embryo transfer. These estimates do not include additional candidates with uterine disease (who could "conceive" only by embryo transfer to surrogate gestators), nor those with ovarian dysfunction who would need egg donation as well, nor that growing population of women who have had tubal ligations and who could later turn to *in vitro* fertilization. It is also worth noting that not all the infertile couples are childless; indeed, a surprising number are seeking to enlarge an existing family.

SELECTION 9

# Ending Reproductive Roulette

## Joseph Fletcher

*In this selection Joseph Fletcher advances his characteristic themes: that being human-
istic and religious is not the same as being fatalistic and antiscience, that the best way
to champion the dignity of humans is to give them choice and control over reproduction, and that the dangers of new forms of assisted reproduction are often exaggerated.*

We often tell our children that in defending any opinion or policy they ought
to know what the objections are—and, what is more, they should be able to
state those objections to the objector's satisfaction. It behooves us, then, to take
a good close look at the reservations, criticisms, reactions, and complaints
commonly raised against the new reproductive medicine. . . .

### RESPECT FOR LIFE

A common doubt has to do with respect for human life. If we exercise a radical control over the sources of life will it not result in a kind of arrogant and
contemptuous attitude? This is really a part of the wedge argument. Does it
not cheapen life, the objection goes, to tailor it genetically, to start and stop it
at will? Do we not degrade human life if we conceive it in laboratories or culti-
vate it in glass containers rather than in the human body? Is it not disrespectful of life to "manufacture" people by laboratory fertilization, for example, or
by intervening in the gene structure and heredity of people? Will it not end,
the objectors wonder with foreboding, in a world where sex is abolished and
reproduction is carried on by cloning?

*Source: The Ethics of Genetic Control: Ending Reproductive Roulette* (Garden City, N.Y.: Doubleday,
1974). Reprinted by permission of the estate of Joseph Fletcher. For biographical information on
Joseph Fletcher, see the introduction to Selection 3.

**118**

It is hard to take hold of a doubt like this one because it is so unobjective, so untied to any specific course of reasoning. The vitalist idea that life as such is sacrosanct, the highest good and somehow both sacred and untouchable, is obviously not tenable in actual practice. If we held to it consistently there would be no ethical basis for heroism or martyrdom or even of killing in self-defense. Like all such absolutes and universals it is constantly contradicted by those who preach it, even though some of them preach it with utter sincerity. For example, vitalists are very apt at the same time to defend capital punishment and military killing, along with "justifiable homicide" in a myriad of situations.

If their first concern was for *persons,* living people with minds and personalities, their moral inconsistencies would perhaps not be so obvious, but to hold as they do that *life* as such, and at any stage of development and quality, is untouchable runs into too many reasonable exceptions to stand up as a moral rule. An ideal, yes; a rule, no.

As an ideal, respect for life would be challenged by very few, if by anybody. Even Schopenhauer with all his pessimism urged only quietism, not suicide. But ideals are subject to all sorts of exceptions and qualifications on a tradeoff or tit-for-tat basis. The problem arises when we are confronted with a choice between having a defective baby or an abortion; between remaining ignorant of how to take care of fetuses or gaining the required knowledge by starting and stopping ("killing") conceptuses; between choosing childlessness or resorting to artificial reproduction; between accepting the exhaustion of the environment or having population control; between having an increasingly polluted gene pool and exerting genetic control; between voluntary or compulsory pregnancy. And so on. . . . .

Doubts based on "respect for life" remind us of the constant tension between a sanctity-of-life ethics and a quality-of-life ethics—two moral or value positions which are not only different but sometimes actually opposed to each other. This issue will surface time after time in what follows.

The respect-for-life objection is often tied psychologically to the feeling that mastery of life will kill its mystery and that the mystery of life is essential to respect for it. This attitude in turn reinforces the "stop meddling" attitude which favors blissful ignorance. If it were to dominate it would stifle or at least hobble not only biology but the chemistry on which biology is built.

## THE PROPER WAY TO PROPAGATE

There is a strong sentiment that it is somehow unnatural and "bad" to go outside of the coitus-gestation mode of reproduction. We might call this the proper-way-to-propagate thesis. More likely than not it arises from a strong sense of human romance and of the dynamic force of interpersonal relations. It may also come from a deep experience of the mutual commitment of a husband and wife in their lovemaking and babymaking, the historic and familiar nexus of the family.

After all, the phrase "in the family way" means far more than just being pregnant. It means a whole bundle of human ties and creative satisfactions. Will the new modes of reproduction undermine romantic and family love, even though they are hardly likely ever to be anything more than second choice to the natural mode? Could they not actually strengthen marriage in some situations? One objector [Leon Kass] asks if we want to eliminate "biological kinship"—although it should be obvious that it would be impossible to do so as long as we reproduce, whether we do it naturally or artificially.[1] What he really is asking is whether we are willing to eliminate sexual intercourse, and the answer should be obvious: "No. But we might be willing to reproduce another way in some situations."

Some psychologists and sociologists (and even some religiously oriented observers) believe it is a mistake ethically and humanly to equate being faithful in marriage with making it a sexual monopoly. Few of us any more look upon a husband or wife as property. Insemination or enovulation from a third-party donor is not an "invasion of monogamous marriage rights" if a couple agree in choosing it. If they understand their relationship morally and personally, rather than physically and sexually, the problem disappears. In the same vein, basing integrity and fidelity on personal relationship, we would regard an adopted child or one conceived by artificial insemination as being fully and truly one's child, whereas a battered or neglected child would *not* be its genetic parents' child even though they brought it into the world by coitus gestation.

The last sentence in one attack is "Have we enough sense to turn back?"—to which it might be answered, "No, not if we lack the sense to go ahead." People who feel as the objector does are apt to want a moratorium on reproductive science and medical research, or even to try to police or suppress them. There is a thin line somewhere at which the effort to politically control biological control will become the very dictatorship which the advocates of suppression are afraid of.

As Plato remarked (*Republic* 1.333), the same doctor who can keep us from disease would also be clever at producing it by stealth. The issue is whether human beings are to be trusted to use reproductive technology humanely. The critic we have just been reporting declares straightforwardly that noncoital reproduction is both dehumanizing and depersonalizing. This charge is of the *a priori* kind; it simply asserts that artificial modes are *as such* immoral. But he also tries to reinforce his condemnation by claiming that artificial modes are subject to abuse, and this is argument of a different kind; it appeals to consequences which allegedly will or might follow from the practice.

Of the two kinds of moral argument, pragmatic reasoning based on consequences is more rational and discussable. Bland *a priori* assertions of opinion we cannot either verify or falsify. How can we possibly check out the dire predictions of abuse and misuse on which the don't-trust-human-beings objection is based? On the record human beings have used their knowledge for *both* good and evil, and it is sensible to suppose that this "double effect" will happen also with the new reproductive medicine.

The "parade of horrors" strategy, however, is an ax that cuts two ways. After all, it was the "good old natural way" that the Third Reich officials turned to in their racist program, when they established the Ordenburgen where Aryan youth were sent to make babies—babies that met the phenotypic selection standards of the Nazi blood-and-soil mystique. Furthermore, the Nazis' pseudoscientific experiments with genetics and the cruelties perpetrated by some of their doctors were neither genetic nor eugenic anyway; they were aimed at ethnic politics and genocide.[2] The remedy lies in a more humane politics, not in the paralysis of biology and medicine.

Tyranny will always use whatever means lie at hand—it certainly has never waited for artificial insemination and enovulation, nor for ectogenesis and cloning. New modes are subject to tyrannous use just as the old ones are. Most things are vulnerable to misuse, just as marriage itself is; in the language of the traditional religious ceremony, marriage ought not to be "entered into unadvisedly or lightly." In any case, however, the fear of tyranny is a big element among the Doubting Thomases and we must try to appreciate it.

Another version of the fear of risk is the claim that misuse of artificial modes will be *unintentional* but none the less objectionable. This appeal to ignorance of the future as a reason for remaining ignorant in the present is an age-old weapon in the armory of reactionaries. They say, for example, that we cannot be sure that eradicating genetic diseases will be a good thing; if we succeed it might have unforeseeable and far worse end results. This is hypothetically possible, to be sure, but only in the same way that it is dangerous to be alive. The danger *if we do not eradicate genetic diseases* is far more real and evident.

Our champion [Leon Kass] follows up his attack by saying that the real danger comes not from the evil-doers but the do-gooders. He is more afraid of "the well-wishers of mankind, for folly is much harder to detect than wickedness"—he concludes that the dangerous people are the ones who want to prevent the birth of defective babies and who talk about the quality of life.[3] There, in a few cruel words, the issue stands stark naked.

Another general doubt appears in the claim that human traits and qualities are far too polygenic to be controlled by genetic means. This is a you-cannot-do-the-good-you-want argument. It is certainly true that much more needs to be known, and it may be true that not very much beyond control of single gene traits will ever be possible. The answer is not in yet, but not *wanting* it answered at all is merely self-crippling.

Almost diametrically opposed to this in logic is the objection that genetics will give *complete* control—turning people into robots or prefabricated automatons who will act out their designers' plans to the letter. This is a you-cannot-avoid-the-evil-you-do-not-want argument. Another form of this objection is based on our need for genetic variety, which is provided by sexual combination. Even the single-cell paramecia have to "merge" with one another after a series of asexual reproductions, before they can resume their solo system. The fear is that selective genetic control might end us up in a fixed and invariable gene pool, producing only a few interchangeable types. This notion is probably inspired by Aldous Huxley's clever picture of fixed human types: alpha personalities, betas, gammas, deltas, and epsilons.

Some doubters doubt that genetic engineering will work, while others have no doubt that it will work but they still doubt that it can serve humane purposes. The objection based on you *can* do it but shouldn't is worth a little closer look. Especially in certain religious circles it has been argued at great length (1) that individuality is of very great moral value; (2) that genetic controls—especially cloning—will prefabricate people right down to the minute details into preprogrammed creatures, just carbon or Xerox copies; and (3) that to practice designed or purposive reproduction wipes out individuality, which, to be authentic, must be the result of sexual chance. In this kind of reasoning reproductive control is therefore morally wrong. In its simplest form it is a syllogism: Individuality is essential to humanity, genetic control destroys individuality, *ergo* genetic control is inhumane. Now nobody wants to be a rubber stamp; objection along this line may appear to carry some weight in the eyes of the unwary who accept its presupposition that engineering *personalities* can be done genetically. The presupposition is false. . . .

## DO NO HARM

Still others have a fear of doing harm to people by these new birth technologies, especially while they are in their experimental or earlier stages. An old saying in medical ethics is *sed nil nocere* or *primum, non nocere*. These are the Latin words of a couple of versions of the Hippocratic oath (there are many other versions). It means that doctors cannot always help their patients but at least they ought not to do them any harm.

Some moralists include embryos among the "people" who might be hurt. They claim that we endanger actual human beings when we risk injuring an embryo during an *in vitro* fertilization or a subsequent implantation. They therefore oppose work like Shettles's and the English team Edwards and Steptoe's. Obstetricians, however, point out that some of the accidents feared can already be detected and such embryos aborted, that more will be discoverable as they progress, and that in any case there are no more congenital mishaps (if as many) in these artificial modes than in natural fertilizations and pregnancies. The English obstetrician R. F. R. Gardner, a professed Christian, calls it a "trivialization" to claim that spontaneously aborted conceptuses and *in vitro* conceptuses are human beings or persons or souls.[4]

Wise and humane as the principle of *non nocere* is, it cannot be a strict or universal rule. Surgery is an obvious exception to it. Medicine does its prescribing and treating with an unavoidable margin of uncertainty and risk, and there are innumerable treatments which hurt as well as help, on a tradeoff or "proportionate good" basis. This being so, medical ethics has always safeguarded the ideal of not doing harm with two further limiting principles. One is that any risks and injuries involved ought to be for the sick person's benefit, nobody else's; the other (its reverse) is that innocent third parties, people other than the patient, ought not to be victimized for the patient's sake.

It is pretty plain that an ethical code based on these general principles is going to run into practical difficulties. For example, it is almost impossible to carry out a scientifically sound clinical trial if you stick completely to the benefit principle; some of the patients involved will get a placebo or make-believe treatment, some will be given the outmoded treatment, still others will get the drug or treatment believed to be better. If such "double blind" tests are carried out widely enough to be valid there are bound to be some who suffer, either positively or negatively, for the sake of others. Even if "informed consent" is had from the patients participating, based on both knowledge of the risks and willingness to undergo them, there is still lack of benefit for some.

Several of Dr. Steptoe's patients are volunteers who know quite well that the attempt to do egg transfers (from the wife or from donors of the egg and/or sperm) may fail in their own case, but they do it because it might help others. The voluntary principle obtains in all artificial inseminations and egg transfers and it will, presumably, be an ethical requirement also in artificial gestation and nuclear transplants. Even so, even when people undergo it willingly, some critics object to running any risk of their being hurt.

An even more extreme version of the do-no-harm doctrine insists that zygotes and embryos (not just patients) may be harmed and that it is therefore immoral to do either research or therapy involving any risk of harm—known or unknown and no matter how unintentional. A critic of this type says, "We cannot morally *get to know* how to perfect" artificial inseminations and implantations "unless the *possibility* of such damage can definitely be excluded" from *in vitro* procedures. This would bring it all to a dead stop. Extensive animal studies should be done first, of course, but at some point *they* must be confirmed by human trials—as in all medical research.

Explaining that if embryos are damaged they can be discarded does not get around this argument's roadblock. Its major premise is that an embryo is a patient, a person, and that to discard a defective embryo is murder. The other side of the coin is that we cannot eliminate the possibility of damaged or defective natural or *in vivo* fertilizations either. Natural processes often damage the conceptus, so that the logic of the objection is to challenge both kinds of reproduction—the natural as well as the artificial.

Some objectors [such as Paul Ramsey] are prepared to go a lot further than this. They object on the ground that the embryos involved cannot give and have therefore not given their consent. Consent, they contend, is ethically required from every subject in investigative medicine. Not just from existing persons or patients, be it noted, but even from nonexisting or only potential persons. *In vitro* fertilizations, whether for experimental or therapeutic purposes, are ruled out because an embryo is obviously incapable of giving either willing or informed consent to anything.[5]

The assumption here, the main bone of contention in the abortion debate, is that embryos are persons. One religious moralist has argued that since "the unmade child" or "possible future human being" obviously cannot consent "he" (it) is not a volunteer and "before his beginning he is in no need of a physician to learn how not to harm him."[6]

A cohort puts it in slightly changed language. It is wrong, he asserts, ever to use children in medical experiments, but this condemnation applies "with even greater force" to experiments on "a hypothetical child (whose conception is as yet only intellectual)." This language has a somewhat Through-the-Looking-Glass unreality about it, basically because these moralists have saddled themselves with the claim that prenatal life is as human as anybody's and are trying to argue consistently with it. The absurdity of their objection is appreciated simply by remembering that babies produced in the coital-gestational or natural way could not have given *their* consent either. Which leaves us where?

Consistently enough the do-no-harm objection is also raised against amniocentesis, fetological therapy, egg transfers, artificial gestation, cloning—against all "manipulation" of reproduction. There is to be sure a marginal risk of injury in all of these things, just as there is in every other kind of medical treatment. But this is not a very weighty line of objection to artificial methods of reproduction, for the simple reason that a similar margin of risk is equally true of raw nature's way of making babies. Errors certainly occur in both sexual and asexual forms of reproduction when they take place in nature and without rational controls. Risk and error are always given factors; they exist in the very finiteness of things. And the point about artificial control is precisely that *it tends to reduce risk and error,* and is intended to do so.

Many of these protests are hardly more than mood expressions, feelings tied for the most part to traditional customs and values. They are *a priori,* not pragmatic; they are not conclusions based on a balance of good and evil consequences. Yet they are none the less influential.


## NOTES

1. L. Kass, "New Beginnings in Life," *The New Genetics and the Future of Man,* ed. Michael Hamilton (Grand Rapids: W. B. Eerdmans, 1972), pp. 53–63.
2. K. Ludmerer, *Genetics and American Society* (Baltimore: Johns Hopkins University Press, 1972), pp. 116–17.
3. L. Kass, "New Beginnings," p. 39.
4. R. F. R. Gardner, *Abortion: The Personal Dilemma* (London: Paternoster Press, 1972), p. 124.
5. P. Ramsey, "Shall We 'Reproduce'?" *Journal of the American Medical Association* 220 (1972), p. 1347.
6. Ibid., p. 1348. Observe the androcentric use of male or masculine pronouns.

## PART FOUR

# Assisted Reproduction: Surrogate Motherhood

# The Case against Surrogate Parenting

## Herbert T. Krimmel

*One controversial method of assisted reproduction, surrogate motherhood, first aroused widespread public debate in the mid-1980s in connection with the famous "Baby M" case. In the following selection Herbert Krimmel argues that it is unethical, for either altruistic or commercial reasons, for one woman to gestate a child that she intends to give to another woman to raise.*

*Herbert T. Krimmel, JD, is a professor of law at Southwestern University School of Law, Los Angeles. He specializes in jurisprudence and reproductive issues in bioethics.*

Is it ethical for someone to create a human life with the intention of giving it up? This seems to be the primary question for both surrogate mother arrangements and artificial insemination by donor (AID), since in both situations a person who is providing germinal material does so only upon the assurance that someone else will assume full responsibility for the child he or she helps to create.

### THE ETHICAL ISSUE

In analyzing the ethics of surrogate mother arrangements, it is helpful to begin by examining the roles the surrogate mother performs. First, she acts as a procreator in providing an ovum to be fertilized. Second, after her ovum has been fertilized by the sperm of the man who wishes to parent the child, she acts as host to the fetus, providing nurture and protection while the newly conceived individual develops.

*Source:* Hastings Center Report V 13, no. 5 (October 1983), pp. 35–39. Reprinted by permission of the author and publisher.

I see no insurmountable moral objections to the functions the mother performs in this second role as host. Her actions are analogous to those of a foster mother or of a wet-nurse who cares for a child when the natural mother cannot or does not do so. Using a surrogate mother as a host for the fetus when the biological mother cannot bear the child is no more morally objectionable than employing others to help educate, train, or otherwise care for a child. Except in extremes, where the parent relinquishes or delegates responsibilities for a child for trivial reasons, the practice would not seem to raise a serious moral issue.

I would argue, however, that the first role that the surrogate mother performs—providing germinal material to be fertilized—does pose a major ethical problem. The surrogate mother provides her ovum, and enters into a surrogate mother arrangement, with the clear understanding that she is to avoid responsibility for the life she creates. Surrogate mother arrangements are designed to separate in the mind of the surrogate mother the decision to create a child from the decision to have and raise that child. The cause of this dissociation is some other benefit she will receive, most often money.[1] In other words, her desire to create a child is born of some motive other than the desire to be a parent. This separation of the decision to create a child from the decision to parent it is ethically suspect. The child is conceived not because he is wanted by his biological mother, but because he can be useful to someone else. He is conceived in order to be given away.

At their deepest level, surrogate mother arrangements involve a change in motive for creating children: from a desire to have them for their own sake, to a desire to have them because they can provide some other benefit. The surrogate mother creates a child with the intention to abdicate parental responsibilities. Can we view this as ethical? My answer is no. I will explain why by analyzing various situations in which surrogate mother arrangements might be used.

## WHY MOTIVE MATTERS

Let's begin with the single parent. A single woman might use AID, or a single man might use a surrogate mother arrangement, if she or he wanted a child but did not want to be burdened with a spouse.[2] Either practice would intentionally deprive the child of a mother or a father. This, I assert, is fundamentally unfair to the child.

Those who disagree might point to divorce or to the death of a parent as situations in which a child is deprived of one parent and must rely solely or primarily upon the other. The comparison, however, is inapt. After divorce or the death of a parent, a child may find herself with a single parent as a result of circumstances that were unfortunate, unintended, and undesired. But when surrogate mother arrangements are used by a single parent, depriving the child of a second parent is one of the intended and desired effects. It is one thing to ask how to make the best of a bad situation when it is thrust upon a person. It is different altogether to ask whether one may intentionally set out to achieve the same result. The morality of identical results (for example, killings) will oftentimes differ depending upon whether the situation is invited by, or involuntarily thrust upon, the actor. Legal distinctions following and based upon this ethical distinction are abundant. The law of self-defense provides a notable example.[3]

Since a woman can get pregnant if she wishes whether or not she is married, and since there is little that society can do to prevent women from creating children even if their intention is to deprive the children of a father, why should we be so concerned about single men's using surrogate mother arrangements if they too want a child but not a spouse? To say that women can intentionally plan to be unwed mothers is not to condone the practice. Besides, society will hold the father liable in a paternity action if he can be found and identified, which indicates some social concern that people should not be able to abdicate the responsibilities that they incur in generating children. Otherwise, why do we condemn the proverbial sailor with a pregnant girlfriend in every port?

In many surrogate mother arrangements, of course, the surrogate mother will not be transferring custody of the child to a single man, but to a couple: the child's biological father and a stepmother, his wife. What are the ethics of surrogate mother arrangements when the child is taken into a two-parent family? Again, surrogate mother arrangements and AID pose similar ethical questions: The surrogate mother transfers her parental responsibilities to the wife of the biological father, while with AID the sperm donor relinquishes his interest in the child to the husband of the biological mother. In both cases the child is created with the intention of transferring the responsibility for its care to a new set of parents. The surrogate mother situation is more dramatic than AID since the transfer occurs after the child is born, while in the case of AID the transfer takes place at the time of the insemination. Nevertheless, the ethical point is the same: creating children for the purpose of transferring them. For a surrogate mother the question remains: Is it ethical to create a child for the purpose of transferring it to the wife of the biological father?

At first blush this looks to be little different from the typical adoption, for what is an adoption other than a transfer of responsibility from one set of parents to another? The analogy is misleading, however, for two reasons. First, it is difficult to imagine anyone's conceiving children for the purpose of putting them up for adoption. And, if such a bizarre event were to occur, I doubt that we would look upon it with moral approval. Most adoptions arise either because an undesired conception is brought to term, or because the parents wanted to have the child but find that they are unable to provide for it because of some unfortunate circumstances that develop after conception.

Second, even if surrogate mother arrangements were to be classified as a type of adoption, not all offerings of children for adoption are necessarily moral. For example, would it be moral for parents to offer their three-year-old for adoption because they are bored with the child? Would it be moral for a couple to offer for adoption their newborn female baby because they wanted a boy?

## HISTORICAL PARALLELS

Proponents of surrogate mother arrangements refer to biblical passages such as Genesis 16, which deals with Abram's having children by his handmaid, Hagar, and Deuteronomy 25:5–6, which deals with the duty of a man to raise up children to his dead brother by his sister-in-law. However, it is quite clear that when Abram conceived Ishmael by Hagar, he had done so only after his wife, Sarai, had given Hagar to him as a second *wife* (Genesis 16:3). Similarly, Deuteronomy 25:5–6 deals with a situation where the woman becomes a wife. In both cases the so-called surrogate mother is not a surrogate at all, but an extension (albeit polygamous) of the family unit. In the biblical tradition, the second wife in no way relinquishes control or responsibility for the children she creates: therefore, analogies between such biblical passages and present-day proposed surrogate mother arrangements are incorrect.

If the proponents of surrogate mother arrangements wish to take biblical authorities as analogies, they might well look to the end of the story of Hagar and Ishmael: how they were driven out by Sarah after Sarah gave birth to Isaac (Genesis 21). The family animosity of thousands of years ago is with us today as the sons of Ishmael (the Arabs) and the sons of Isaac (the Jews) still have some difficulties getting along.

Therefore, even though surrogate mother arrangements may in some superficial ways be likened to adoption, one must still ask whether it is ethical to separate the decision to create children from the desire to have them. I would answer no. The procreator should desire the child for its own sake, and not as a means to attaining some other end. Even though one of the ends may be stated altruistically as an attempt to bring happiness to an infertile couple, the child is still being used by the surrogate. She creates it not because she desires it, but because she desires something from it.

To sanction the use and treatment of human beings as means to the achievement of other goals instead of as ends in themselves is to accept an ethic with a tragic past and to establish a precedent with a dangerous future. Already the press has reported the decision of one couple to conceive a child for the purpose of using it as a bone marrow donor for its sibling.[4] And the bioethics literature contains articles seriously considering whether we should clone human beings to serve as an inventory of spare parts for organ transplants[5] and articles that foresee the use of comatose human beings as self-replenishing blood banks and manufacturing plants for human hormones.[6] How far our society is willing to proceed down this road is uncertain, but it is clear that the first step to all these practices is the acceptance of the same principle that the Nazis attempted to use to justify their medical experiments at the Nuremberg war-crimes trials: that human beings may be used as means to the achievement of other goals, and need not be treated as ends in themselves.[7]

But why, it might be asked, is it so terrible if the surrogate mother does not desire the child for its own sake, when under the proposed surrogate mother arrangements there will be a couple eagerly desiring to have the child and to be its parents? That this argument may not be entirely accurate will be illustrated in the following section, but the basic reply is that creating a child without desiring it fundamentally changes the way we look at children—instead of viewing them as unique individual personalities to be desired in their own right, we may come to view them as commodities or items of manufacture to be desired because of their utility. A recent newspaper account describes the business of an agency that matches surrogate mothers with barren couples as follows: "Its first product is due for delivery today. Twelve others are on the way and an additional 20 have been ordered. The 'company' is Surrogate Mothering Ltd., and the 'product' is babies."[8]

The dangers of this view are best illustrated by examining what might go wrong in a surrogate mother arrangement and, most important, by viewing how the various parties to the contract may react to the disappointment.

## WHAT MIGHT GO WRONG

Ninety-nine percent of the surrogate mother arrangements may work out just fine: the child will be born normal, and the adopting parents (that is, the biological father and his wife) will want it. But what happens when, unforeseeably, the child is born deformed? Since many defects cannot be discovered prenatally by amniocentesis or other means, the situation is bound to arise.[9] Similarly, consider what would happen if the biological father were to die before the birth of the child. Or if the "child" turns out to be twins or triplets. Each of these instances poses an inevitable situation where the adopting parents may be unhappy with the prospect of rearing the child or children. Although legislation can mandate that the adopting parents take the child or children in whatever condition they come or whatever the situation, provided the surrogate mother has abided by all the contractual provisions of the surrogate mother arrangement, the important point for our discussion is the attitude that the surrogate mother or the adopting parent might have. Consider the example of the deformed child.

When I participated in the Surrogate Parent Foundation's inaugural symposium in November 1981, I was struck by the attitude of both the surrogate mothers and the adopting parents to these problems. The adopting parents worried, "Do we have to take such a child?" and the surrogate mothers said in response, "Well, we don't want to be stuck with it." Clearly, both groups were anxious not to be responsible for the "undesirable child" born of the surrogate mother arrangement. What does this portend?

It is human nature that when one pays money, one expects value. Things that one pays for have a way of being seen as commodities. Unavoidable in surrogate mother arrangements are questions such as "Did I get a good one?" We see similar behavior with respect to the adoption of children: comparatively speaking, there is no shortage of black, Mexican-American, mentally retarded, or older children seeking homes; the shortage is in attractive, intelligent-looking Caucasian babies.[10] Similarly, surrogate mother arrangements involve more than just the desire to have a child. The desire is for a certain type of child.

But, it may be objected, don't all parents voice these same concerns in the normal course of having children? Not exactly. No one doubts or minimizes the pain and disappointment parents feel when they learn that their child has been born with some genetic or congenital birth defect. But this is different from the surrogate mother situation, where neither the surrogate mother nor the adopting parents may feel responsible, and both sides may feel that they have a legitimate excuse not to assume responsibility for the child. The surrogate mother might blame the biological father for having "defective sperm," as the adopting parents might blame the surrogate mother for a "defective ovum" or for improper care of the fetus during pregnancy. The adopting parents desire a normal child, not *this* child in any condition, and the surrogate mother doesn't want it in any event. So both sides will feel threatened by the birth of an "undesirable child." Like bruised fruit in the produce bin of a supermarket, this child is likely to become an object of avoidance.

Certainly, in the natural course of having children a mother may doubt whether she wants a child if the father has died before its birth; parents may shy away from a defective infant or be distressed at the thought of multiple births. Nevertheless, I believe they are more likely to accept these contingencies as a matter of fate. I do not think this is the case with surrogate mother arrangements. After all, in the surrogate mother arrangement the adopting parents can blame someone outside the marital relationship. The surrogate mother has been hosting this child all along, and she is delivering it. It certainly *looks* far more like a commodity than the child that arrives in the natural course within the family unit.

## A DANGEROUS AGENDA

Another social problem, which arises out of the first, is the fear that surrogate mother arrangements will fall prey to eugenic concerns.[11] Surrogate mother contracts typically have clauses requiring genetic tests of the fetus and stating that the surrogate mother must have an abortion (or keep the child herself) if the child does not pass these tests.[12]

In the last decade we have witnessed a renaissance of interest in eugenics. This, coupled with advances in biomedical technology, has created a host of abuses and new moral problems. For example, genetic counseling clinics now face a dilemma: amniocentesis, the same procedure that identifies whether a fetus suffers from certain genetic defects, also discloses the sex of a fetus. Genetic counseling clinics have reported that even when the fetus is normal, a disproportionate number of mothers abort female children.[13] Aborting normal fetuses simply because the prospective parents desire children of a certain sex is one result of viewing children as commodities. The recent scandal at the Repository for Germinal Choice, the so-called Nobel Sperm Bank, provides another chilling example. Their first "customer" was, unbeknownst to the staff, a woman who "had lost custody of two other children because they were abused in an effort to 'make them smart.' "[14] Of course, these and similar evils may occur whether or not surrogate mother arrangements are allowed by law. But to the extent that they promote the view of children as commodities, these arrangements contribute to these problems. There is nothing wrong with striving for betterment, as long as it does not result in intolerance to that which is not perfect. But I fear that the latter attitude will become prevalent.

Sanctioning surrogate mother arrangements can also exert pressures upon the family structure. First, as was noted earlier, there is nothing technically to prevent the use of surrogate mother arrangements by single males desiring to become parents. Indeed, single females can already do this with AID or even without it. But even if legislation were to limit the use of the surrogate mother arrangement to infertile couples, other pressures would occur, namely the intrusion of a third adult into the marital community.[15] I do not think that society is ready to accept either single parenting or quasi-adulterous arrangements as normal.

Another stress on the family structure arises within the family of the surrogate mother. When the child is surrendered to the adopting parents it is removed not only from the surrogate mother but also from her family. They too have interests to be considered. Do not the siblings of that child have an interest in the fact that their little baby brother has been "given" away?[16] One woman, the mother of a medical student who had often donated sperm for artificial insemination, expressed her feelings to me eloquently. She asked, "I wonder how many grandchildren I have that I have never seen and never been able to hold or cuddle."

Intrafamily tensions can also be expected to result in the family of the adopting parents because of the asymmetry of relationship the adopting parents will have toward the child. The adopting mother has no biological relationship to the child, whereas the adopting father is also the child's biological father. Won't this unequal biological claim on the child be used as a wedge in childrearing arguments? Can't we imagine the father saying, "Well, he is my son, not yours"? What if the couple eventually gets divorced? Should custody in a subsequent divorce between the adopting mother and the biological father be treated simply as a normal child custody dispute? Or should the biological relationship between father and child weigh more heavily? These questions do not arise in typical adoption situations since both parents are equally unrelated biologically to the child. Indeed, in adoption there is symmetry. The surrogate mother situation is more analogous to second marriage, where the children of one party by a prior marriage are adopted by the new spouse. Since asymmetry in second-marriage situations causes problems, we can anticipate similar difficulties arising from surrogate mother arrangements.

There is also the worry that the offspring of a surrogate mother arrangement will be deprived of important information about his or her heritage. This also happens with adopted children or children conceived by AID[17], who lack information about their biological parents, which could be important to them medically. Another less popularly recognized problem is the danger of half-sibling marriages,[18] where the child of the surrogate mother unwittingly falls in love with a half sister or brother. The only way to avoid these problems is to dispense with the confidentiality of parental records; however, the natural parents may not always want their identity disclosed.

The legalization of surrogate mother arrangements may also put undue pressure upon poor women to use their bodies in this way to support themselves and their families. Analogous problems have arisen in the past with the use of paid blood donors.[19] And occasionally the press reports someone desperate enough to offer to sell an eye or some other organ.[20] I believe that certain things should be viewed as too important to be sold as commodities, and I hope that we have advanced from the time when parents raised children for profitable labor, or found themselves forced to sell their children.

While many of the social dilemmas I have outlined here have their analogies in other present-day occurrences such as divorced families or in adoption, every addition is hurtful. Legalizing surrogate mother arrangements will increase the frequency of these problems and put more stress on our society's shared moral values.[21]

## A TALE FOR OUR TIME

An infertile couple might prefer to raise a child with a biological relationship to the husband, rather than to raise an adopted child who has no biological relationship to either the husband or the wife. But does the marginal increase in joy that they might therefore experience outweigh the potential pain that they, or the child conceived in such arrangements, or others might suffer? Does their preference outweigh the social costs and problems that the legalization of surrogate mothering might well engender? I honestly do not know. I don't even know on what hypothetical scale such interests could be weighed and balanced. But even if we could weigh such interests, and even if personal preference outweighed the costs, I still would not be able to say that we could justify achieving those ends by these means; that ethically it would be permissible for a person to create a child, not because she desired it, but because it could be useful to her.

Edmond Cahn has termed this ignoring of means in the attainment of ends the "Pompey syndrome":

> I have taken the name from young Sextus Pompey, who appears in Shakespeare's *Antony and Cleopatra* in an incident drawn directly from Plutarch. Pompey, whose navy has won control of the seas around Italy, comes to negotiate peace with the Roman triumvirs Mark Antony, Octavius Caesar, and Lepidus, and they meet in a roistering party on Pompey's ship. As they carouse, one of Pompey's lieutenants draws him aside and whispers that he can become lord of all the world if he will only grant the lieutenant leave to cut first the mooring cable and then the throats of the triumvirs. Pompey pauses, then replies in these words:

Ah, this thou shouldst have done,
And not have spoke on't!
In me 'tis villainy;
In thee't had been good service.
Thou must know 'tis not my profit that does lend mine honour;
Mine honour, it. Repent that e'er thy tongue
Hath so betrayed thine act; being done unknown,
I should have found it afterwards well done,
But must condemn it now. Desist, and drink.

Here we have the most pervasive of moral syndromes, the one most characteristic of so-called respectable men in a civilized society. To possess the end and yet not be responsible for the means, to grasp the fruit while disavowing the tree, to escape being told the cost until someone else has paid it irrevocably: this is the Pompey syndrome and the chief hypocrisy of our time.[22]

## NOTES

1. See Philip J. Parker, "Motivation of Surrogate Mothers: Initial Findings," *American Journal of Psychiatry* 140, no. 1 (January 1983), pp. 117–18; see also Doe v. Kelley, Circuit Court of Wayne County Michigan (1980), reported in 1980 Rep. on Human Reproduction and Law II-A-1.
2. See, e.g., C.M. v. C.C., 152 N.J. Supp. 160, 377 A.2d 821 (1977); "Why She Went to 'Nobel Sperm Bank' for Child," *Los Angeles Herald Examiner*, August 6, 1982, p. A9; "Womb for Rent," *Los Angeles Herald Examiner*, September 21, 1981, p. A3.
3. See also Richard McCormick, "Reproductive Technologies: Ethical Issues," in *Encyclopedia of Bioethics,* ed. Walter Reich, vol. 4 (New York: Free Press, 1978), pp. 1454, 1459; Robert Snowden and G. D. Mitchell, *The Artificial Family* (London: George Allen & Unwin, 1981), p. 71.
4. *Los Angeles Times,* April 17, 1979, p. I2.
5. See, e.g., Alexander Peters, "The Brave New World: Can the Law Bring Order within Traditional Concepts of Due Process?" *Suffolk Law Review* 4 (1970), pp. 901–2; Roderic Gorney, "The New Biology and the Future of Man," *UCLA Law Review* 15 (1968), p. 302; J. G. Castel, "Legal Implications of Biomedical Science and Technology in the Twenty-first Century," *Canadian Bar Review* 51 (1973), p. 127.
6. See Harry Nelson, "Maintaining Dead to Serve as Blood Makers Proposed Logical, Sociologist Says," *Los Angeles Times,* February 26, 1974, p. II-1; Hans Jonas, "Against the Stream: Comments on the Definition and Redefinition of Death," in *Philosophical Essays: From Ancient Creed to Technological Man* (Chicago: University of Chicago Press, 1974), pp. 132–40.
7. See Leo Alexander, "Medical Science under Dictatorship," *New England Journal of Medicine* 241, no. 2 (1949), p. 39; United States v. Brandt, Trial of

the Major War Criminals, International Military Tribunal, Nuremberg, 14 November 1945–1 October 1946.

8. Bob Dvorchak, "Surrogate Mothers: Pregnant Idea Now a Pregnant Business," *Los Angeles Herald Examiner,* December 27, 1983, p. A1.

9. "Surrogate's Baby Born with Deformities Rejected by All," *Los Angeles Times,* January 22, 1983, p. 1–17; "Man Who Hired Surrogate Did Not Father Ailing Baby," *Los Angeles Herald Examiner,* February 3, 1983, p. A6.

10. See, e.g., *Adoption in America: Hearing before the Subcommittee on Aging, Family, and Human Services of the Senate Committee on Labor and Human Resources,* 97th Cong., 1st sess. (1981), p. 3 (comments of Senator Jeremiah Denton) and 16–17 (statement of Warren Master, Acting Commissioner of Administration for Children, Youth, and Families, US Department of Health and Human Services).

11. Cf. "Discussion: Moral, Social and Ethical Issues," in *Law and Ethics of A.I.D. and Embryo Transfer* (1973) (comments of Himmelweit), reprinted in Michael Shapiro and Roy Spece, *Bioethics and Law* (St. Paul: West Publishing, 1981), p. 548.

12. See, e.g., Lane (*Newsday*), "Womb for Rent," *Tucson Citizen,* June 7, 1980, p. 3; Susan Lewis, "Baby Bartering? Surrogate Mothers Pose Issues for Lawyers, Courts," *Los Angeles Daily Journal,* April 20, 1981. See also Elaine Markoutsas, "Women Who Have Babies for Other Women," *Good Housekeeping* 96 (April 1981), p. 104.

13. See Morton A. Stenchever, "An Abuse of Prenatal Diagnosis," *JAMA* 221 (1972), p. 408; Charles Westoff and Ronald R. Rindfus, "Sex Preselection in the United States: Some Implications," *Science* 184 (1974), pp. 633, 636. See also Phyllis Battelle, "Is It a Boy or a Girl?" *Los Angeles Herald Examiner,* October 8, 1981, p. A17.

14. "2 Children Taken from Sperm Bank Mother," *Los Angeles Times,* July 14, 1981, p. I3; "The Sperm-Bank Scandal," *Newsweek* 24 (July 26, 1982).

15. See Helmut Thielicke, *The Ethics of Sex,* trans. John W. Doberstein (New York: Harper & Row, 1964).

16. According to one newspaper account, when a surrogate mother informed her nine-year-old daughter that the new baby would be given away, the daughter replied: "Oh, good. If it's a girl we can keep it and give Jeffrey [her two-year-old half brother] away"; "Womb for Rent," *Los Angeles Herald Examiner,* September 21, 1981, p. A3.

17. See, e.g., Lorraine Dusky, "Brave New Babies?" *Newsweek* 30 (December 6, 1982); also testimony of Suzanne Rubin before the California Assembly Committee on Judiciary, Surrogate Parenting Contracts, Assembly Publication no. 962 (November 19, 1982), pp. 72–75.

18. This has posed an increasing problem for children conceived through AID. See, e.g., Martin Curie-Cohen, et al., "Current Practice of Artificial Insemination by Donor in the United States," *New England Journal of Medicine* 300 (1979), pp. 585–89.

19. See, e.g., Richard M. Titmuss, *The Gift Relationship: From Human Blood to Social Policy* (New York: Random House, 1971).

20. See, e.g., "Man Desperate for Funds: Eye for Sale at $35,000," *Los Angeles Times*, February 1, 1975, p. II–1; "100 Answer Man's Ad for New Kidney," *Los Angeles Times*, September 12, 1974, p. I4.
21. See generally Guido Calabresi, "Reflections on Medical Experimentation in Humans," *Daedalus* 98 (1969), pp. 387–93; see also Michael Shapiro and Roy Spece, "On Being 'Unprincipled on Principle': The Limits of Decision Making 'On the Merits,' " in *Bioethics and Law*, pp. 67–71.
22. Edmond Cahn, "Drug Experiments and the Public Conscience," in *Drugs in Our Society*, ed. Paul Talalay (Baltimore: Johns Hopkins Press, 1964), pp. 255, 258–61.

SELECTION 11

# Surrogate Mothers: Not So Novel after All

## John A. Robertson

*During the "Baby M" case, one female judge in a New Jersey family court expressed dismay that so much fuss was being made. Having seen thousands of custody disputes among divorcing parents and disputing relatives, her view was that disputes in surrogacy cases simply come with the territory. No really novel moral question was being raised, she thought.*

*In the following pages John Robertson expresses sympathy with this view. He thinks that the dangers of this arrangement are exaggerated by critics and that all parties might benefit from surrogate gestation, even commercial surrogacy, if adequate safeguards were enforced. (Compare his views on this arrangement with his very conservative views on letting impaired infants die in Selection 17.)*

*John Robertson, JD, is the Thomas Watt Gregory Professor at the University of Texas Law School, Austin, and a fellow of the Hastings Center. He is the leading legal theorist in reproductive bioethics. His books include* The Rights of the Terminally Ill *and* Children of Choice: Freedom and the New Reproductive Technologies.

All reproduction is collaborative, for no man or woman reproduces alone. Yet the provision of sperm, egg, or uterus through artificial insemination, embryo transfer, and surrogate mothering makes reproduction collaborative in another way. A third person provides a genetic or gestational factor not present in ordinary paired reproduction. As these practices grow, we must confront the ethical issues raised and their implications for public policy.

Collaborative reproduction allows some persons who otherwise might remain childless to produce healthy children. However, its deliberate separation of genetic, gestational, and social parentage is troublesome. The offspring and

*Source: Hastings Center Report* 13, no. 5 (October 1983), pp. 28–34. Reprinted by permission of the author and publisher.

The author gratefully acknowledges the comments of Rebecca Dresser, Mark Frankel, Juga Markovits, Philip Parker, Bruce Russell, John Sampson, and Ted Schneyer on earlier drafts.

## HOW SURROGATE MOTHERING WORKS

For a fee of $5,000–10,000 a broker (usually a lawyer) will put an infertile couple (or, less often, a single man) in contact with women whom he has recruited and screened who are willing to serve as surrogates. If the parties strike a deal, they will sign a contract in which the surrogate agrees to be artificially inseminated (usually by a physician) with the husband's sperm, to bear the child, and then at or soon after birth to relinquish all parental rights and transfer physical custody of the child to the couple for adoption by the wife. Typically the contract has provisions dealing with prenatal screening, abortion, and other aspects of the surrogate's conduct during pregnancy, as well as her consent to relinquish the child at birth. The husband and wife agree to pay medical expenses related to the pregnancy, to take custody of the child, and to place approximately $10,000 in escrow to be paid to the surrogate when the child is transferred. The lawyer will also prepare papers establishing the husband's paternity, terminating the surrogate's rights, and legalizing the adoption.

participants may be harmed, and there is a risk of confusing family lineage and personal identity. In addition, the techniques intentionally manipulate a natural process that many persons want free of technical intervention. Yet many well-accepted practices, including adoption, artificial insemination by donor (AID), and blended families (families where children of different marriages are raised together) intentionally separate biologic and social parenting and have become an accepted thread in the social fabric. Should all collaborative techniques be similarly treated? When, if ever, are they ethical? Should the law prohibit, encourage, or regulate them, or should the practice be left to private actors? Surrogate motherhood—the controversial practice by which a woman agrees to bear a child conceived by artificial insemination and to relinquish it at birth to others for rearing—illustrates the legal and ethical issues arising in collaborative reproduction generally.

## AN ALTERNATIVE TO AGENCY ADOPTIONS

Infertile couples who are seeking surrogates hire attorneys and sign contracts with women recruited through newspaper ads. The practice at present probably involves at most a few hundred persons. But repeated attention on *Sixty Minutes* and the *Phil Donahue Show* and in the popular press is likely to engender more demand, for thousands of infertile couples might find surrogate mothers the answer to their reproductive needs. What began as an enterprise involving a few lawyers and doctors in Michigan, Kentucky, and California is now a national phenomenon. There are surrogate mother centers in Maryland, Arizona, and several other states, and even a surrogate mother newsletter.

Surrogate mother arrangements occur within a tradition of family law that gives the gestational mother (and her spouse, if any) rearing rights and obligations. (However, the presumption that the husband is the father can be challenged, and a husband's obligations to his wife's child by AID will usually require his consent.)[1] Although no state has legislation directly on the subject of surrogate motherhood, independently arranged adoptions are lawful in most states. It is no crime to agree to bear a child for another and then relinquish it for adoption. However, paying the mother a fee for adoption beyond medical expenses is a crime in some states, and in others will prevent the adoption from being approved.[2] Whether termination and transfer of parenting rights will be legally recognized depends on the state. Some states, like Hawaii and Florida, ask few questions and approve independent adoptions very quickly. Others, like Michigan and Kentucky, won't allow surrogate mothers to terminate and assign rearing rights to another if a fee has been paid, or even allow a paternity determination in favor of the sperm donor. The enforceability of surrogate contracts has also not been tested, and it is safe to assume that some jurisdictions will not enforce them. Legislation clarifying many of these questions has been proposed in several states, but has not yet been enacted.

Even this brief discussion highlights an important fact about surrogate motherhood and other collaborative reproductive techniques. They operate as an alternative to the nonmarket, agency system of allocating children for adoption, which has contributed to long queues for distributing healthy white babies. This form of independent adoption is controlled by the parties, planned before conception, involves a genetic link with one parent, and enables both the father and mother of the adopted child to be selected in advance.

Understood in these terms, the term "surrogate mother," which means substitute mother, is a misnomer. The natural mother, who contributes egg and uterus, is not so much a substitute mother as a substitute spouse who carries a child for a man whose wife is infertile. Indeed, it is the adoptive mother who is the surrogate mother for the child, since she parents a child borne by another. What, if anything, is wrong with this arrangement? Let us look more closely at its benefits and harms before discussing public policy.

## ALL THE PARTIES CAN BENEFIT

Reproduction through surrogate mothering is a deviation from our cultural norms of reproduction, and to many persons it seems immoral or wrong. But surrogate mothering may be a good for the parties involved.

Surrogate contracts meet the desire of a husband and wife to rear a healthy child and, more particularly, a child with one partner's genes. The need could arise because the wife has an autosomal dominant or sex-linked genetic disorder, such as hemophilia. More likely, she is infertile and the couple feels a strong need to have children. For many infertile couples the inability to conceive is a major personal problem causing marital conflict and filling both partners with anguish and self-doubt. It may also involve multiple medical workups and possibly even surgery. If the husband and wife have sought to adopt a child, they may have been told either that they do not qualify or to join the queue of couples waiting several years for agency adoptions (the wait has grown longer due to birth control, abortion, and the greater willingness of unwed mothers to keep their children).[3] For couples exhausted and frustrated by these efforts, the surrogate arrangement seems a godsend. While the intense desire to have a child often appears selfish, we must not lose sight of the deep-seated psychosocial and biological roots of the desire to generate children.[4]

The arrangement may also benefit the surrogate. Usually women undergo pregnancy and childbirth because they want to rear children. But some women want to have the experience of bearing and birthing a child without the obligation to rear. Philip Parker, a Michigan psychiatrist who has interviewed over 275 surrogate applicants, finds that the decision to be a surrogate springs from several motives.[5] Most women willing to be surrogates have already had children, and many are married. They choose the surrogate role primarily because the fee provides a better economic opportunity than alternative occupations, but also because they enjoy being pregnant and the respect and attention that it draws. The surrogate experience may also be a way to master, through reliving, guilt they feel from past pregnancies that ended in abortion or adoption. Some surrogates may also feel pleased, as organ donors do, that they have given the "gift of life" to another couple.[6]

The child born of a surrogate arrangement also benefits. Indeed, but for the surrogate contract, this child would not have been born at all. Unlike the ordinary agency or independent adoption, where a child is already conceived or brought to term, the conception of this child occurs solely as a result of the surrogate agreement. Thus even if the child does suffer identity problems, as adopted children often do because they are not able to know their mothers, this child has benefited, or at least has not been wronged, for without the surrogate arrangement, she would not have been born at all.[7]

## BUT PROBLEMS EXIST TOO

Surrogate mothering is also troublesome. Many people think that it is wrong for a woman to conceive and bear a child that she does not intend to raise, particularly if she receives a fee for her services. There are potential costs to the surrogate and her family, the adoptive couple, the child, and even society at large from satisfying the generative needs of infertile couples in this way.

The couple must be willing to spend about $20,000–25,000, depending on lawyers' fees and the supply of and demand for surrogate mothers. (While this price tag makes the surrogate contract a consumption item for the middle classes, it is not unjust to poor couples, for it does not leave them worse off than they were.) The couple must also be prepared to experience, along with the adjustment and demands of becoming parents, the stress and anxiety of participating in a novel social relationship that many still consider immoral or deviant. What do they tell their friends or family? What do they tell the child? Will the child have contact with the mother? What is the couple's relationship with the surrogate and her family during the pregnancy and after? Without established patterns for handling these questions, the parties may experience confusion, frustration, and embarrassment.

A major source of uncertainty and stress is likely to be the surrogate herself. In most cases she will be a stranger, and may never even meet the couple. The lack of a preexisting relation between the couple and surrogate and the possibility that they live far apart enhance the possibility of mistrust. Is the surrogate taking care of herself? Is she having sex with others during her fertile period? Will she contact the child afterwards? What if she demands more money to relinquish the child? To allay these anxieties, the couple could try to establish a relationship of trust with the surrogate, yet such a relationship creates reciprocal rights and duties and might create demands for an undesired relationship after the birth. Even good lawyering that specifies every contingency in the contract is unlikely to allay uncertainty and anxiety about the surrogate's trustworthiness.

The surrogate may also find the experience less satisfying than she envisioned. Conceiving the child may require insemination efforts over several months at inconvenient locations. The pregnancy and birth may entail more pain, unpleasant side effects, and disruption that she expected. The couple may be more intrusive or more aloof than she wishes. As the pregnancy advances and the birth nears, the surrogate may find it increasingly difficult to remain detached by thinking of the child as "theirs" rather than "hers." Relinquishing the baby after birth may be considerably more disheartening and disappointing than she anticipated. Even if informed of this possibility in advance, she may be distressed for several weeks with feelings of loss, depression, and sleep disturbance.[8] She may feel angry at the couple for cutting off all contact with her once the baby is delivered, and guilty at giving up her child. Finally, she will have to face the loss of all contact with "her" child. As the reality of her situation dawns, she may regret not having bargained harder for access to "her" baby.

As with the couple, the surrogate's experience will vary with the expectations, needs, and personalities of the parties, the course of the pregnancy, and an advance understanding of the problems that can arise. The surrogate should have a lawyer to protect her interests. Often, however, the couple's lawyer will end up advising the surrogate. Although he has recruited the surrogate, he is paid by and represents the couple. By disclosing his conflicting interest, he satisfies legal ethics, but he may not serve the interests of the surrogate as well as independent counsel.

## HARMS TO THE CHILD

Unlike embryo transfer, gene therapy, and other manipulative techniques (some of which are collaborative), surrogate arrangements do not pose the risk of physical harm to the offspring. But there is the risk of psychosocial harm. Surrogate mothering, like adoption and artificial insemination by donor (AID), deliberately separates genetic and gestational from social parentage. The mother who begets, bears, and births does not parent. This separation can pose a problem for the child who discovers it. Like adopted and AID children, the child may be strongly motivated to learn the absent parent's identity and to establish a relationship, in this case with the mother and her family. Inability to make that connection, especially inability to learn who the mother is, may affect the child's self-esteem, create feelings of rootlessness, and leave the child thinking that he had been rejected due to some personal fault.[9] While this is a serious concern, the situation is tolerated when it arises with AID and adoptive children. Intentional conception for adoption—the essence of surrogate mothering—poses no different issue.

The child can also be harmed if the adoptive husband and wife are not fit parents. After all, a willingness to spend substantial money to fulfill a desire to rear children is no guarantee of good parenting. But then neither is reproduction by paired mates who wish intensely to have a child. The nonbiologic parent may resent or reject the child, but the same possibility exists with adoption, AID, or ordinary reproduction.

There is also the fear, articulated by such commentators as Leon Kass and Paul Ramsey,[10] that collaborative reproduction confuses the lineage of children and destroys the meaning of family as we know it. In surrogate mothering, as with ovum or womb donors, the genetic and gestational mother does not rear the child, though the biologic father does. What implications does this hold for the family and the child's lineage?

The separation of the child from the genetic or biologic parent in surrogate mothering is hardly unique. It arises with adoption, but surrogate arrangements are more closely akin to AID or blended families, where at least one parent has a blood tie to the child and the child will know at least one genetic parent. He may, as adopted children often do, have intense desires to learn his biologic mother's identity and seek contact with her and her family. Failure to connect with biologic roots may cause suffering. But the fact that adoption through surrogate mother contracts is planned before conception does not increase the chance of identity confusion, lowered self-esteem, or the blurring of lineage that occurs with adoption or AID.

The greatest chance of confusing family lines arises if the child and couple establish relations with the surrogate and the surrogate's family. If that unlikely event occurs, questions about the child's relations with the surrogate's spouse, parents, and other children can arise. But these issues are not unique. Indeed, they are increasingly common with the growth of blended families. Surrogate mothering in a few instances may lead to a new variation on blended families, but its threat to the family is trivial compared to the rapid changes in family structure now occurring for social, economic, and demographic reasons.

In many cases surrogate motherhood and other forms of collaborative reproduction may shore up, rather than undermine, the traditional family by enabling couples who would otherwise be childless to have children. The practice of employing others to assist in child rearing—including wet-nurses, neonatal ICU nurses, daycare workers, and babysitters—is widely accepted. We also tolerate assistance in the form of sperm sales and donation of egg and gestation (adoption). Surrogate mothering is another method of assisting people to undertake child rearing, and thus serves the purposes of the marital union. It is hard to see how its planned nature obstructs that contribution.

## USING BIRTH FOR SELFISH ENDS

A basic fear about the new reproductive technologies is that they manipulate a natural physiologic process involved in the creation of human life. When one considers the potential power that resides in our ability to manipulate the genes of embryos, the charges of playing God or arrogantly tampering with nature and the resulting dark Huxleyian vision of genetically engineered babies decanted from bottles are not surprising. While *Brave New World* is the standard text for this fear, the 1982 film *Bladerunner* also evokes it. Trycorp., a genetic engineering corporation, manufactures "replicants," who resemble human beings in most respects, including their ability to remember their childhoods, but who are programmed to die in four years. In portraying the replicants' struggle for a long life and full human status, the film raises a host of ethical issues relevant to gene manipulation, from the meaning of personhood to the duties we have in "fabricating" people to make them as whole and healthy as possible.

Such fears, however, are not a sufficient reason to stop splicing genes or relieving infertility through external fertilization.[11] In any event they have no application to surrogate mothering, which does not alter genes or even manipulate the embryo. The only technological aid is a syringe to inseminate and a thermometer to determine when ovulation occurs. Although embryo manipulation would occur if the surrogate received the fertilized egg of another woman, the qualms about surrogate mothering stem less from its potential for technical manipulation, and more from its attitude toward the body and mother-child relations. Mothers bear and give up children for adoption rather frequently when the conception is unplanned. But here the mother conceives the child for that purpose, deliberately using her body for a fee to serve the needs of others. It is the cold willingness to use her body as a baby-making machine and deny the mother-child gestational bond that bothers. (Ironically, the natural bond may turn out to be deeper and stronger than the surrogate imagined.)

Since the transfer of rearing duties from the natural gestational mother to others is widely accepted, the unwillingness of the surrogate mother to rear her child cannot in itself be wrong. As long as she transfers rearing responsibility to capable parents, she is not acting irresponsibly. Still, some persons assert that it is wrong to use the reproductive process for ends other than the good of the child.[12] But the mere presence of selfish motives does not render reproduction immoral, as long as it is carried out in a way that respects the child's interests. Otherwise most pregnancies and births would be immoral, for people have children to serve individual ends as well as the good of the child. In terms of instrumentalism, surrogate mothering cannot be distinguished from most other reproductive situations, whether AID, adoption, or simply planning a child to experience the pleasures of parenthood.

In this vein the problems that can arise when a defective child is born are cited as proof of the immorality of surrogate mothering. The fear is that neither the contracting couple nor the surrogate will want the defective child. In one recent case a dispute arose when none of the parties wanted to take a child born with microcephaly, a condition related to mental retardation.[13] The contracting man claimed on the basis of blood typing that the baby was not his, and thus he was not obligated under the contract to take it or to pay the surrogate's fee. It turned out that surrogate had borne her husband's child, for she had unwittingly become pregnant by him before being artificially inseminated by the contracting man. The surrogate and her husband eventually assumed responsibility for the child.

An excessively instrumental and callous approach to reproduction when a less than perfect baby is born is not unique to surrogate mothering. Similar reactions can occur whenever married couples have a defective child, as the Baby Doe controversy, which involved the passive euthanasia of a child with Down syndrome, indicates. All surrogate mothering is not wrong because in some instances a handicapped child will be rejected. Nor is it clear that this reaction is more likely in surrogate mothering than in conventional births, for it reflects common attitudes toward handicapped newborns as much as alienation in the surrogate arrangement.

As with most situations, "how" something is done is more important than the mere fact of doing it. The morality of surrogate mothering thus depends on how the duties and responsibilities of the role are carried out, rather than on the mere fact that a couple produces a child with the aid of a collaborator. Depending on the circumstances, a surrogate mother can be praised as a benefactor to a suffering couple (the money is hardly adequate compensation) or condemned as a callous user of offspring to further her selfish ends. The view that one takes of her actions will also influence the role one wants the law to play.

## WHAT SHOULD THE STATE'S ROLE BE?

What stance should public policy and the law take toward surrogate mothering? As with all collaborative reproduction, a range of choices exists, from prohibition and regulation to active encouragement.

However, there may be constitutional limits to the state's power to restrict collaborative reproduction. The right not to procreate, through contraception and abortion, is now firmly established.[14] A likely implication of these cases, supported by rulings in other cases, is that married persons (and possibly single persons) have a right to bear, beget, birth, and parent children by natural coital means using such technological aids (microsurgery and *in vitro* fertilization, for example) as are medically available. It should follow that married persons also have a right to engage in noncoital, collaborative reproduction, at least where natural reproduction is not possible. The right of a couple to raise a child should not depend on their luck in the natural lottery, if they can obtain the missing factor of reproduction from others.[15]

If a married couple's right to procreative autonomy includes the right to contract with consenting collaborators, then the state will have a heavy burden of justification for infringing that right. The risks to surrogate, couple, and child do not seem sufficiently compelling to meet this burden, for they are no different from the harms of adoption and AID. Nor will it suffice to point to a communal feeling that such uses of the body are—aside from the consequences—immoral. Moral distaste alone does not justify interference with a fundamental right.

Although surrogate mothering is not now criminal, this discussion is not purely hypothetical. The ban in Michigan and several other states on paying fees for adoption beyond medical expenses has the same effect as an outright prohibition, for few surrogates will volunteer for altruistic reasons alone. A ban on fees is not necessary to protect the surrogate mother from coercion or exploitation, or to protect the child from abuse, the two objectives behind passage of those laws. Unlike the pregnant unmarried woman who "sells" her child, the surrogate has made a considered, knowing choice, often with the assistance of counsel, before becoming pregnant. She may of course choose to be a surrogate for financial reasons, but offering money to do unpleasant tasks is not in itself coercive.

Nor does the child's welfare support a ban on fees, for the risk is no greater than in natural paired reproduction that the parents will be unfit or abuse the child. The specter of slavery, which some opposed to surrogate mothering have raised, is unwarranted. It is quibbling to question whether the couple is "buying" a child or the mother's personal services. Quite clearly, the couple is buying the right to rear a child by paying the mother to beget and bear one for that very purpose. But the purchasers do not buy the right to treat the child or surrogate as a commodity or property. Child abuse and neglect laws still apply, with criminal and civil sanctions available for mistreatment.

The main concern with fees rests on moral and aesthetic grounds. An affront to moral sensibility arises over paying money for a traditionally noncommercial, intimate function. Even though blood and sperm are sold, and miners, professional athletes, and petrochemical workers sell some of their health and vitality, some persons think it wrong for women to bear children for money, in much the same way that paying money for sex or body organs is considered wrong. Every society excludes some exchanges from the marketplace on moral grounds. But the state's power to block exchanges that interfere with the exercise of a fundamental right is limited. Since blocking this exchange stops infertile couples from reproducing and rearing the husband's child, a harm greater than moral distaste is necessary to justify it.

Although the state cannot block collaborative reproductive exchanges on moral grounds, it need not subsidize or encourage surrogate contracts. One could argue that allowing the parties to a surrogate contract to use the courts to terminate parental rights, certify paternity, and legalize adoption is a subsidy and therefore not required of the state. Similarly, a state's refusal to enforce surrogate contracts as a matter of public policy could be taken as a refusal to subsidize rather than as interference with the right to reproduce. But given the state's monopoly of those functions and the impact its denial will have on the ability of infertile couples to find reproductive collaborators, it is more plausible to view the refusal to certify and effectuate surrogate contracts as an infringement of the right to procreate. Denying an adoption because it was agreed upon in advance for a fee interferes with the couple's procreative autonomy as much as any criminal penalty for paying a fee to or contracting with a collaborator. (The crucial distinction between interfering with and not encouraging the exercise of a right has been overlooked by the Michigan and Kentucky courts that have held constitutional the refusal to allow adoptions or paternity determinations where a fee has been paid to the surrogate mother. This error makes these cases highly questionable precedents.)[16]

A conclusion that surrogate contracts must be *enforced,* however, does not require that they be specifically carried out in all instances. As long as damage remedies remain, there is no constitutional right to specific performance. For example, a court need not enjoin the surrogate who changes her mind about abortion or relinquishing the child once it is born. A surrogate who wants to breach the contract by abortion should pay damages, but not be ordered to continue the pregnancy, because of the difficulty in enforcing or monitoring the order. (Whether damages are a practical alternative in such cases will depend on the surrogate's economic situation, or whether bonding or insurance to assure her contractual obligation is possible.) On the other hand, a court could reasonably order the surrogate after birth to relinquish the child. Whether such an order should issue will depend on whether the surrogate's interest in keeping the child is deemed greater than the couple's interest in rearing (assuming that both are fit parents). A commitment to freedom of contract and the rights of parties to arrange collaborative reproduction would favor the adoptive couple, while sympathy for the gestational bond between mother and child would favor the mother. If the mother prevailed, the couple should still have other remedies, including visitation rights for the father, restitution of the surrogate's fee and other expenses, and perhaps money damages as well.

The constitutional status of a married couple's procreative choice shields collaborative arrangements from interference on moral grounds alone, but not from all regulation. While the parties may assign the rearing rights according to contract, the state need not leave the entire transaction to the vagaries of the private sector. Regulation to minimize harm and to assure knowing choices would be permissible, as long as the regulation is reasonably related to promoting these goals.

For example, the state could set minimum standards for surrogate brokers, set age and health qualifications for surrogates, and structure the transaction to assure voluntary, knowing choices. The state could also define and allocate responsibilities among the parties to protect the best interests of the offspring—for example, refusing to protect the surrogate's anonymity, requiring that the contracting couple assume responsibility for a defective child, or even transferring custody to another if threats to the child's welfare justify such a move.

## NOT WHAT WE DO—BUT HOW WE DO IT

The central issue with surrogate mothering, as with other collaborative reproduction, is not the deliberate separation of biologic and social parentage, but
how the separation is effected and the resulting relationship with the third
party. If the third party's involvement in the reproduction is discrete and limited, collaborative reproduction is easily tolerated. Thus few people question
the anonymous sperm donor's lack of rights and duties toward the offspring,
except in the case where the mother and donor have expressly agreed that he
would have some access to the rearing of a child.[17] The donor's claim—and
possibly the child's need to connect—is less strong in such cases. Egg dona-
tions, though involving more risk and burden for the donor, should be similarly treated, for they are also discrete and limited.

Collaborative reproduction involving gestational contributors poses more
difficult problems, because the nine-month gestational period creates a unique
and powerful bond for both donor and offspring that seems to justify a claim
in its own right. Yet in adoption we allow those claims to be nullified by the
gestational mother's choice. Surrogate motherhood presents the same issue.
The difference is that it is planned before conception, but that hardly seems to
matter once the child is born and the mother wishes to fulfill her commitment.
The issue of whether the mother should be held to a promise on which others
have relied is distinct from the question of whether mothers can relinquish
children deliberately conceived for others outside the agency-controlled adoption process.

Surrogate mothering casts particular light on one other collaborative technique that may soon be widely available—the transfer of the externally (or in-
ternally) fertilized egg of one woman to another woman who gestates and
births it.[18] The third party in this situation is a gestational surrogate for a genetic and rearing mother who is unable or unwilling to bear and birth her
child. At first glance the gestational mother's claim to the child seems less compelling than the claim of the surrogate mother, because the child is not genetically hers. Yet concerns will arise, as with surrogate mothers, over the severing
or denial of the gestational bond, the degree to which the contract should be
honored, and the gestational mother's relationship (if any) with the child.

The moral issues surrounding surrogate mothering also cast light on the
problems with manipulative techniques such as genetic alteration of the embryo and nonuterine gestation of the fertilized egg. Since those techniques will
be used primarily for paired reproduction, the main concerns will be the
safety of the offspring and the morality of genetic manipulation. However,
when manipulation and collaborative reproduction are combined, the relationship of the offspring to the third party contributor will come into question.

Surrogate mothering for a fee is neither the evil nor the panacea that many
have thought. It is barely distinguishable from the many current practices that
separate biologic and social parentage and that seek parenthood for personal
satisfaction. The differences do not appear to be great enough to justify

prohibition, active discouragement, or, for that matter, encouragement. Like many human endeavors, in the final analysis what matters is not *whether* but *how* it is done. In that respect public scrutiny, through regulation of the process of drawing up the contract rather than its specific terms, could help to assure that it is done well.

## NOTES

1. People v. Sorenson, 68 Cal. 2d 280, 437 P.2d 495; Walter Wadlington, "Artificial Insemination: The Dangers of a Poorly Kept Secret," *Northwestern Law Review* 64 (1970), p. 777.
2. See, e.g., Michigan Statutes Annotated, 27.3178 (555.54)(555.69) (1980).
3. William Landes and Eleanor Posner, "The Economics of the Baby Shortage," *Journal of Legal Studies* 7 (1978), p. 323.
4. See Erik Erikson, *The Life Cycle Completed* (New York: W. W. Norton, 1980), pp. 122–24.
5. Philip Parker, "Surrogate Mother's Motivations: Initial Findings," *American Journal of Psychiatry* 140, no. 1 (January 1983), pp. 117–18; idem, "The Psychology of Surrogate Motherhood: A Preliminary Report of a Longitudinal Pilot Study" (manuscript). See also Dava Sobel, "Surrogate Mothers: Why Women Volunteer," *New York Times*, June 25, 1981, p. 18.
6. Mark Frankel, "Surrogate Motherhood: An Ethical Perspective," paper presented at Wayne State University Symposium on Surrogate Motherhood, November 20, 1982, pp. 1–2.
7. See John Robertson, "In Vitro Conception and Harm to the Unborn," *Hastings Center Report* 8 (October 1978), pp. 13–14; Michael Bayles, "Harm to the Unconceived," *Philosophy and Public Affairs* 5 (1976), p. 295.
8. A small, uncontrolled study found these effects to last some four to six weeks; statement of Nancy Reame, RN, at Wayne State University Symposium on Surrogate Motherhood, November 20, 1982.
9. Betty Jane Lifton, *Twice Born: Memoirs of an Adopted Daughter* (New York: Penguin, 1977); L. Dusky, "Brave New Babies," *Newsweek*, December 6, 1982, p. 30.
10. Leon Kass, "Making Babies—the New Biology and the Old Morality," *Public Interest* 26 (1972), p. 18; " 'Making Babies' Revisited," *Public Interest* 54 (1979), p. 32; Paul Ramsey, *Fabricated Man: The Ethics of Genetic Control* (New Haven: Yale University Press, 1970).
11. President's Commission for the Study of Ethical Problems in Medicine and Biomedical and Behavioral Research, *Splicing Life: The Social and Ethical Issues of Genetic Engineering with Human Beings* (Washington, DC, 1982), pp. 53–60.
12. Herbert Krimmel, testimony before the California Assembly Committee on Judiciary, *Surrogate Parenting Contracts*, Assembly Publication no. 962 (November 14, 1982), pp. 89–96.

13. *New York Times,* January 28, 1983, p. 18.

14. Griswold v. Connecticut, 381 U.S. 479 (1964); Eisenstadt v. Baird, 405 U.S. 438 (1972); Roe v. Wade, 410 U.S. 113 (1973); Planned Parenthood v. Danforth, 428 U.S. 52 (1976); Bellotti v. Baird, 443 U.S. 622 (1979); Carey v. Population Services International, 431 U.S. 678 (1977).

15. Although this article does not address the right of single persons to contract with others for reproductive purposes, it should be noted that the right of married persons to engage in collaborative reproduction does not entail a similar right for unmarried persons. For a more detailed exposition of the arguments for the reproductive rights of married and single persons, see John Robertson, "Procreative Liberty and the Control of Conception, Pregnancy and Childbirth," *Virginia Law Review* 69 (April 1983), pp. 418–20.

16. See Doe v. Kelley, 106 Mich. App. 164, 307 N.W.2d 438 (1981); Syrkowski v. Appleyard, 9 Family Law Rptr. 2348 (April 5, 1983); In re Baby Girl, 9 Family Law Reptr. 2348 (March 8, 1983).

17. See C.M. v. C.C., 152 N.J. 160, 377 A.2d 821 (man who provided sperm for artificial insemination held to have visitation rights because of express agreement with the mother).

18. See Richard D. Lyons, "2 Women Become Pregnant With Transferred Embryos," *New York Times,* July 22, 1983, pp. A1, B7.

## PART FIVE

# Abortion

# A Defense of Abortion

## Judith Jarvis Thomson

*The following 1971 article on abortion by Judith Jarvis Thomson is widely regarded as a watershed event in 20th-century ethics in America. Published during the era of the Vietnam War, the patients' rights movement, and the hippie counterculture, it showed the value of using analysis on topics in everyday morality. Suddenly it seemed that philosophers had something important to say about contemporary moral issues. Following Thomson's lead, they started writing and publishing articles on euthanasia, contraception, genetics, population policy, and psychosurgery. Symbolically, Thomson's article was published in the first issue of a new journal dedicated to the idea that two fields could illuminate each other:* Philosophy and Public Affairs. *Thomson's essay presents a limited defense of the right of a woman to have an abortion. At the time it was written, abortion was still illegal in most states; the* Roe v. Wade *decision by the U.S. Supreme Court was two years away.*

*First-time readers of Thomson's article today are frequently disappointed because they had hoped for a more general discussion of abortion. Yet Thomson's central idea—that an innocent person can have a right to life and still, in some situations, be permissibly killed—was, and still is, a brilliant one. The ideal way to read the essay today is as a classic piece of conceptual analysis.*

*Judith Jarvis Thomson, PhD, is professor of philosophy at the Massachusetts Institute of Technology.*

Most opposition to abortion relies on the premise that the fetus is a human being, a person, from the moment of conception. The premise is argued for, but, as I think, not well. Take, for example, the most common argument. We are asked to notice that the development of a human being from conception through birth into childhood is continuous; then it is said that to draw a line,

*Source: Philosophy and Public Affairs* 1, no. 1 (1971), pp. 47–66. Reprinted by permission of the author and publisher. The author is indebted to James Thomson for discussion, criticism, and many helpful suggestions.

to choose a point in this development and say "before this point the thing is not a person, after this point it is a person" is to make an arbitrary choice, a choice for which in the nature of things no good reason can be given. It is concluded that the fetus is, or anyway that we had better say it is, a person from the moment of conception. But this conclusion does not follow. Similar things might be said about the development of an acorn into an oak tree, and it does not follow that acorns are oak trees, or that we had better say they are. Arguments of this form are sometimes called "slippery slope arguments"—the phrase is perhaps self-explanatory—and it is dismaying that opponents of abortion rely on them so heavily and uncritically.

I am inclined to agree, however, that the prospects for "drawing a line" in the development of the fetus look dim. I am inclined to think also that we shall probably have to agree that the fetus has already become a human person well before birth. Indeed, it comes as a surprise when one first learns how early in its life it begins to acquire human characteristics. By the tenth week, for example, it already has a face, arms and legs, fingers and toes; it has internal organs, and brain activity is detectable.[1] On the other hand, I think that the premise is false, that the fetus is not a person from the moment of conception. A newly fertilized ovum, a newly implanted clump of cells, is no more a person than an acorn is an oak tree. But I shall not discuss any of this. For it seems to me to be of great interest to ask what happens if, for the sake of argument, we allow the premise. How, precisely, are we supposed to get from there to the conclusion that abortion is morally impermissible? Opponents of abortion commonly spend most of their time establishing that the fetus is a person, and hardly any time explaining the step from there to the impermissibility of abortion. Perhaps they think the step too simple and obvious to require much comment. Or perhaps instead they are simply being economical in argument. Many of those who defend abortion rely on the premise that the fetus is not a person, but only a bit of tissue that will become a person at birth; and why pay out more arguments than you have to? Whatever the explanation, I suggest that the step they take is neither easy nor obvious, that it calls for closer examination than it is commonly given, and that when we do give it this closer examination we shall feel inclined to reject it.

I propose, then, that we grant that the fetus is a person from the moment of conception. How does the argument go from here? Something like this, I take it. Every person has a right to life. So the fetus has a right to life. No doubt the mother has a right to decide what shall happen in and to her body; everyone would grant that. But surely a person's right to life is stronger and more stringent than the mother's right to decide what happens in and to her body, and so outweighs it. So the fetus may not be killed; an abortion may not be performed.

It sounds plausible. But now let me ask you to imagine this. You wake up in the morning and find yourself back to back in bed with an unconscious violinist. A famous unconscious violinist. He has been found to have a fatal kidney ailment, and the Society of Music Lovers has canvassed all the available medical records and found that you alone have the right blood type to help.

They have therefore kidnapped you, and last night the violinist's circulatory system was plugged into yours, so that your kidneys can be used to extract poisons from his blood as well as your own. The director of the hospital now tells you, "Look, we're sorry the Society of Music Lovers did this to you—we would never have permitted it if we had known. But still, they did it, and the violinist now is plugged into you. To unplug you would be to kill him. But never mind, it's only for nine months. By then he will have recovered from his ailment, and can safely be unplugged from you." Is it morally incumbent on you to accede to this situation? No doubt it would be very nice of you if you did, a great kindness. But do you *have* to accede to it? What if it were not nine months, but nine years? Or longer still? What if the director of the hospital says, "Tough luck, I agree, but you've now got to stay in bed, with the violinist plugged into you, for the rest of your life. Because remember this. All persons have a right to life, and violinists are persons. Granted you have a right to decide what happens in and to your body, but a person's right to life outweighs your right to decide what happens in and to your body. So you cannot ever be unplugged from him." I imagine you would regard this as outrageous, which suggests that something really is wrong with that plausible-sounding argument I mentioned a moment ago.

In this case, of course, you were kidnapped; you didn't volunteer for the operation that plugged the violinist into your kidneys. Can those who oppose abortion on the ground I mentioned make an exception for a pregnancy due to rape? Certainly. They can say that persons have a right to life only if they didn't come into existence because of rape; or they can say that all persons have a right to life, but that some have less of a right to life than others, in particular, that those who came into existence because of rape have less. But these statements have a rather unpleasant sound. Surely the question of whether you have a right to life at all, or how much of it you have, shouldn't turn on the question of whether or not you are the product of a rape. And in fact the people who oppose abortion on the ground I mentioned do not make this distinction, and hence do not make an exception in case of rape.

Nor do they make an exception for a case in which the mother has to spend the nine months of her pregnancy in bed. They would agree that would be a great pity, and hard on the mother; but all the same, all persons have a right to life, the fetus is a person, and so on. I suspect, in fact, that they would not make an exception for a case in which, miraculously enough, the pregnancy went on for nine years, or even the rest of the mother's life.

Some won't even make an exception for a case in which continuation of the pregnancy is likely to shorten the mother's life; they regard abortion as impermissible even to save the mother's life. Such cases are nowadays very rare, and many opponents of abortion do not accept this extreme view. All the same, it is a good place to begin: a number of points of interest come out in respect to it.

1. Let us call the view that abortion is impermissible even to save the mother's life "the extreme view." I want to suggest first that it does not issue from the argument I mentioned earlier without the addition of some fairly

powerful premises. Suppose a woman has become pregnant, and now learns that she has a cardiac condition such that she will die if she carries the baby to term. What may be done for her? The fetus, being a person, has a right to life, but as the mother is a person too, so has she a right to life. Presumably they have an equal right to life. How is it supposed to come out that an abortion may not be performed? If mother and child have an equal right to life, shouldn't we perhaps flip a coin? Or should we add to the mother's right to life her right to decide what happens in and to her body, which everybody seems to be ready to grant—the sum of her rights now outweighing the fetus' right to life?

The most familiar argument here is the following. We are told that performing the abortion would be directly killing the child,[2] whereas doing nothing would not be killing the mother, but only letting her die. Moreover, in killing the child, one would be killing an innocent person, for the child has committed no crime, and is not aiming at his mother's death. And then there are a variety of ways in which this might be continued. (1) But as directly killing an innocent person is always and absolutely impermissible, an abortion may not be performed. Or, (2) as directly killing an innocent person is murder, and murder is always and absolutely impermissible, an abortion may not be performed.[3] Or, (3) as one's duty to refrain from directly killing an innocent person is more stringent than one's duty to keep a person from dying, an abortion may not be performed. Or, (4) if one's only options are directly killing an innocent person or letting a person die, one must prefer letting the person die, and thus an abortion may not be performed.[4]

Some people seem to have thought that these are not further premises which must be added if the conclusion is to be reached, but that they follow from the very fact that an innocent person has a right to life.[5] But this seems to me to be a mistake, and perhaps the simplest way to show this is to bring out that while we must certainly grant that innocent persons have a right to life, the theses in (1) through (4) are all false. Take (2), for example. If directly killing an innocent person is murder, and thus is impermissible, then the mother's directly killing the innocent person inside her is murder, and thus is impermissible. But it cannot seriously be thought to be murder if the mother performs an abortion on herself to save her life. It cannot seriously be said that she *must* refrain, that she *must* sit passively by and wait for her death. Let us look again at the case of you and the violinist. There you are, in bed with the violinist, and the director of the hospital says to you, "It's all most distressing, and I deeply sympathize, but you see this is putting an additional strain on your kidneys, and you'll be dead within the month. But you *have* to stay where you are all the same. Because unplugging you would be directly killing an innocent violinist, and that's murder, and that's impermissible." If anything in the world is true, it is that you do not commit murder, you do not do what is impermissible, if you reach around to your back and unplug yourself from that violinist to save your life.

The main focus of attention in writings on abortion has been on what a third party may or may not do in answer to a request from a woman for an abortion. This is in a way understandable. Things being as they are, there isn't much a woman can safely do to abort herself. So the question asked is what a third party may do, and what the mother may do, if it is mentioned at all, is deduced, almost as an afterthought, from what it is concluded that third parties may do. But it seems to me that to treat the matter in this way is to refuse to grant to the mother that very status of person which is so firmly insisted on for the fetus. For we cannot simply read off what a person may do from what a third party may do. Suppose you find yourself trapped in a tiny house with a growing child. I mean a very tiny house, and a rapidly growing child—you are already up against the wall of the house and in a few minutes you'll be crushed to death. The child on the other hand won't be crushed to death; if nothing is done to stop him from growing he'll be hurt, but in the end he'll simply burst open the house and walk out a free man. Now I could well understand it if a bystander were to say, "There's nothing we can do for you. We cannot choose between your life and his, we cannot be the ones to decide who is to live, we cannot intervene." But it cannot be concluded that you too can do nothing, that you cannot attack it to save your life. However innocent the child may be, you do not have to wait passively while it crushes you to death. Perhaps a pregnant woman is vaguely felt to have the status of house, to which we don't allow the right of self-defense. But if the woman houses the child, it should be remembered that she is a person who houses it.

I should perhaps stop to say explicitly that I am not claiming that people have a right to do anything whatever to save their lives. I think, rather, that there are drastic limits to the right of self-defense. If someone threatens you with death unless you torture someone else to death, I think you have not the right, even to save your life, to do so. But the case under consideration here is very different. In our case there are only two people involved, one whose life is threatened, and one who threatens it. Both are innocent: the one who is threatened is not threatened because of any fault, the one who threatens does not threaten because of any fault. For this reason we may feel that we bystanders cannot intervene. But the person threatened can.

In sum, a woman surely can defend her life against the threat to it posed by the unborn child, even if doing so involves its death. And this shows not merely that the theses in (1) through (4) are false; it shows also that the extreme view of abortion is false, and so we need not canvass any other possible ways of arriving at it from the argument I mentioned at the outset.

2. The extreme view could of course be weakened to say that while abortion is permissible to save the mother's life, it may not be performed by a third party, but only by the mother herself. But this cannot be right either. For what we have to keep in mind is that the mother and the unborn child are not like two tenants in a small house which has, by an unfortunate mistake, been rented to both: the mother *owns* the house. The fact that she does adds to the offensiveness of deducing that the mother can do nothing from the supposition that third parties can do nothing. But it does more than this: it casts a bright light on the supposition that third parties can do nothing. Certainly it lets us see that a third party who says "I cannot choose between you" is fooling

himself if he thinks this is impartiality. If Jones has found and fastened on a certain coat, which he needs to keep him from freezing, but which Smith also needs to keep him from freezing, then it is not impartiality that says "I cannot choose between you" when Smith owns the coat. Women have said again and again "This body is *my* body!" and they have reason to feel angry, reason to feel that it has been like shouting into the wind. Smith, after all, is hardly likely to bless us if we say to him, "Of course it's your coat, anybody would grant that it is. But no one may choose between you and Jones who is to have it."

We should really ask what it is that says "no one may choose" in the face of the fact that the body that houses the child is the mother's body. It may be simply a failure to appreciate this fact. But it may be something more interesting, namely the sense that one has a right to refuse to lay hands on people, even where it would be just and fair to do so, even where justice seems to require that somebody do so. Thus justice might call for somebody to get Smith's coat back from Jones, and yet you have a right to refuse to be the one to lay hands on Jones, a right to refuse to do physical violence to him. This, I think, must be granted. But then what should be said is not "no one may choose," but only "*I* cannot choose," and indeed not even this, but "*I* will not act," leaving it open that somebody else can or should, and in particular that anyone in a position of authority, with the job of securing people's rights, both can and should. So this is no difficulty. I have not been arguing that any given third party must accede to the mother's request that he perform an abortion to save her life, but only that he may.

I suppose that in some views of human life the mother's body is only on loan to her, the loan not being one which gives her any prior claim to it. One who held this view might well think it impartiality to say "I cannot choose." But I shall simply ignore this possibility. My own view is that if a human being has any just, prior claim to anything at all, he has a just, prior claim to his own body. And perhaps this needn't be argued for here anyway, since, as I mentioned, the arguments against abortion we are looking at do grant that the woman has a right to decide what happens in and to her body.

But although they do grant it, I have tried to show that they do not take seriously what is done in granting it. I suggest the same thing will reappear even more clearly when we turn away from cases in which the mother's life is at stake, and attend, as I propose we now do, to the vastly more common cases in which a woman wants an abortion for some less weighty reason than preserving her own life.

3. Where the mother's life is not at stake, the argument I mentioned at the outset seems to have a much stronger pull. "Everyone has a right to life, so the unborn person has a right to life." And isn't the child's right to life weightier than anything other than the mother's own right to life, which she might put forward as ground for an abortion?

This argument treats the right to life as if it were unproblematic. It is not, and this seems to me to be precisely the source of the mistake.

For we should now, at long last, ask what it comes to, to have a right to life. In some views having a right to life includes having a right to be given at least the bare minimum one needs for continued life. But suppose that what in fact *is* the bare minimum a man needs for continued life is something he has no right at all to be given? If I am sick unto death, and the only thing that will save my life is the touch of Henry Fonda's cool hand on my fevered brow, then all the same, I have no right to be given the touch of Henry Fonda's cool hand on my fevered brow. It would be frightfully nice of him to fly in from the West Coast to provide it. It would be less nice, though no doubt well meant, if my friends flew out to the West Coast and carried Henry Fonda back with them. But I have no right at all against anybody that he should do this for me. Or again, to return to the story I told earlier, the fact that for continued life that violinist needs the continued use of your kidneys does not establish that he has a right to be given the continued use of your kidneys. He certainly has no right against you that *you* should give him continued use of your kidneys. For nobody has any right to use your kidneys unless you give him such a right; and nobody has the right against you that you shall give such a right; and nobody has the right against you that you shall give him this right—if you do allow him to go on using your kidneys, this is a kindness on your part, and not something he can claim from you as his due. Nor has he any right against anybody else that *they* should give him continued use of your kidneys. Certainly he had no right against the Society of Music Lovers that they should plug him into you in the first place. And if you now start to unplug yourself, having learned that you will otherwise have to spend nine years in bed with him, there is nobody in the world who must try to prevent you, in order to see to it that he is given something he has a right to be given.

Some people are rather stricter about the right to life. In their view, it does not include the right to be given anything, but amounts to, and only to, the right not to be killed by anybody. But here a related difficulty arises. If everybody is to refrain from killing that violinist, then everybody must refrain from doing a great many different sorts of things. Everybody must refrain from slitting his throat, everybody must refrain from shooting him—and everybody must refrain from unplugging you from him. But does he have a right against everybody that they shall refrain from unplugging you from him? To refrain from doing this is to allow him to continue to use your kidneys. It could be argued that he has a right against us that *we* should allow him to continue to use your kidneys. That is, while he had no right against us that we should give him the use of your kidneys, it might be argued that he anyway has a right against us that we shall not now intervene and deprive him of the use of your kidneys. I shall come back to third-party interventions later. But certainly the violinist has no right against you that *you* shall allow him to continue to use your kidneys. As I said, if you do allow him to use them, it is a kindness on your part, and not something you owe him.

The difficulty I point to here is not peculiar to the right to life. It reappears in connection with all the other natural rights; and it is something which an adequate account of rights must deal with. For present purposes it is enough just to draw attention to it. But I would stress that I am not arguing that people do not have a right to life—quite to the contrary, it seems to me that the primary control we must place on the acceptability of an account of rights is that it should turn out in that account to be a truth that all persons have a right to life. I am arguing only that having a right to life does not guarantee having either a right to be given the use of or a right to be allowed continued use of another person's body—even if one needs it for life itself. So the right to life will not serve the opponents of abortion in the very simple and clear way in which they seem to have thought it would.

4. There is another way to bring out the difficulty. In the most ordinary sort of case, to deprive someone of what he has a right to is to treat him unjustly. Suppose a boy and his small brother are jointly given a box of chocolates for Christmas. If the older boy takes the box and refuses to give his brother any of the chocolates, he is unjust to him, for the brother has been given a right to half of them. But suppose that, having learned that otherwise it means nine years in bed with that violinist, you unplug yourself from him. You surely are not being unjust to him, for you gave him no right to use your kidneys, and no one else can have given him any such right. But we have to notice that in unplugging yourself, you are killing him; and violinists, like everybody else, have a right to life, and thus in the view we were considering just now, the right not to be killed. So here you do what he supposedly has a right you shall not do, but you do not act unjustly to him in doing it.

The emendation which may be made at this point is this: the right to life consists not in the right not to be killed, but rather in the right not to be killed unjustly. This runs a risk of circularity, but never mind: it would enable us to square the fact that the violinist has a right to life with the fact that you do not act unjustly toward him in unplugging yourself, thereby killing him. For if you do not kill him unjustly, you do not violate his right to life, and so it is no wonder you do him no injustice.

But if this emendation is accepted, the gap in the argument against abortion stares us plainly in the face: it is by no means enough to show that the fetus is a person, and to remind us that all persons have a right to life—we need to be shown also that killing the fetus violates its right to life, i.e., that abortion is unjust killing. And is it?

I suppose we may take it as a datum that in a case of pregnancy due to rape the mother has not given the unborn person a right to the use of her body for food and shelter. Indeed, in what pregnancy could it be supposed that the mother has given the unborn person such a right? It is not as if there were unborn persons drifting about the world, to whom a woman who wants a child says "I invite you in."

But it might be argued that there are other ways one can have acquired a right to the use of another person's body than by having been invited to use it by that person. Suppose a woman voluntarily indulges in intercourse, knowing of the chance it will issue in pregnancy, and then she does become pregnant; is she not in part responsible for the presence, in fact the very existence, of the unborn person inside her? No doubt she did not invite it in. But doesn't her partial responsibility for its being there itself give it a right to the use of her body?[6] If so, then her aborting it would be more like the boy's taking away the chocolates, and less like your unplugging yourself from the violinist—doing so would be depriving it of what it does have a right to, and thus would be doing it an injustice.

And then, too, it might be asked whether or not she can kill it even to save her own life: If she voluntarily called it into existence, how can she now kill it, even in self-defense?

The first thing to be said about this is that it is something new. Opponents of abortion have been so concerned to make out the independence of the fetus, in order to establish that it has a right to life, just as its mother does, that they have tended to overlook the possible support they might gain from making out that the fetus is *dependent* on the mother, in order to establish that she has a special kind of responsibility for it, a responsibility that gives it rights against her which are not possessed by any independent person—such as an ailing violinist who is a stranger to her.

On the other hand, this argument would give the unborn person a right to its mother's body only if her pregnancy resulted from a voluntary act, undertaken in full knowledge of the chance a pregnancy might result from it. It would leave out entirely the unborn person whose existence is due to rape. Pending the availability of some further argument, then, we would be left with the conclusion that unborn persons whose existence is due to rape have no right to the use of their mothers' bodies, and thus that aborting them is not depriving them of anything they have a right to and hence is not unjust killing.

And we should also notice that it is not at all plain that this argument really does go even as far as it purports to. For there are cases and cases, and the details make a difference. If the room is stuffy, and I therefore open a window to air it, and a burglar climbs in, it would be absurd to say, "Ah, now he can stay, she's given him a right to the use of her house—for she is partially responsible for his presence there, having voluntarily done what enabled him to get in, in full knowledge that there are such things as burglars, and that burglars burgle." It would be still more absurd to say this if I had had bars installed outside my windows, precisely to prevent burglars from getting in, and a burglar got in only because of a defect in the bars. It remains equally absurd if we imagine it is not a burglar who climbs in, but an innocent person who blunders or falls in. Again, suppose it were like this: people-seeds drift about in the air like pollen, and if you open your windows, one may drift in and take root in your carpets or upholstery. You don't want children, so you fix up your windows with fine mesh screens, the very best you can buy. As can happen, however, and on very, very rare occasions does happen, one of the screens is defective; and a seed drifts in and takes root. Does the person-plant who now develops have a right to the use of your house? Surely not—despite the fact that you voluntarily opened your windows, you knowingly kept carpets and upholstered furniture, and you knew that screens were sometimes defective. Someone may argue that you are responsible for its rooting, that it does have a right to your house, because after all you *could* have lived out your life with bare floors and furniture, or with sealed windows and doors. But this won't do—for by the same token anyone can avoid a pregnancy due to rape by having a hysterectomy, or anyway by never leaving home without a (reliable!) army.

It seems to me that the argument we are looking at can establish at most that there are *some* cases in which the unborn person has a right to the use of its mother's body, and therefore *some* cases in which abortion is unjust killing. There is room for much discussion and argument as to precisely which, if any. But I think we should sidestep this issue and leave it open, for at any rate the argument certainly does not establish that all abortion is unjust killing.

5. There is room for yet another argument here, however. We surely must all grant that there may be cases in which it would be morally indecent to detach a person from your body at the cost of his life. Suppose you learn that what the violinist needs is not nine years of your life, but only one hour: all you need do to save his life is to spend one hour in that bed with him. Suppose also that letting him use your kidneys for that one hour would not affect your health in the slightest. Admittedly you were kidnapped. Admittedly you did not give anyone permission to plug him into you. Nevertheless it seems to me plain you *ought* to allow him to use your kidneys for that hour—it would be indecent to refuse.

Again, suppose pregnancy lasted only an hour, and constituted no threat to life or health. And suppose that a woman becomes pregnant as a result of rape. Admittedly she did not voluntarily do anything to bring about the existence of a child. Admittedly she did nothing at all which would give the unborn person a right to the use of her body. All the same it might well be said, as in the newly emended violinist story, that she *ought* to allow it to remain for that hour—that it would be indecent in her to refuse.

Now some people are inclined to use the term "right" in such a way that it follows from the fact that you ought to allow a person to use your body for the hour he needs, that he has a right to use your body for the hour he needs, even though he has not been given that right by any person or act. They may say that it follows also that if you refuse, you act unjustly toward him. This use of the term is perhaps so common that it cannot be called wrong; nevertheless it seems to me to be an unfortunate loosening of what we would do better to keep a tight rein on. Suppose that box of chocolates I mentioned earlier had not been given to both boys jointly, but was given only to the older boy. There he sits, stolidly eating his way through the box, his small brother watching enviously. Here we are likely to say "You ought not to be so mean. You ought to give your brother some of those chocolates." My own view is that it just does not follow from the truth of this that the brother has any right to any of the chocolates. If the boy refuses to give his brother any, he is greedy, stingy, callous—but not unjust. I suppose that the people I have in mind will say it does follow that the brother has a right to some of the chocolates, and thus that the boy does act unjustly if he refuses to give his brother any. But the effect of saying this is to obscure what we should keep distinct, namely the difference between the boy's refusal in this case and the boy's refusal in the earlier case, in which the box was given to both boys jointly, and in which the small brother thus had what was from any point of view clear title to half.

A further objection to so using the term "right" that from the fact that A ought to do a thing for B, it follows that B has a right against A that A do it for him, is that it is going to make the question of whether or not a man has a right to a thing turn on how easy it is to provide him with it; and this seems not merely unfortunate, but morally unacceptable. Take the case of Henry Fonda again. I said earlier that I had no right to the touch of his cool hand on my fevered brow, even though I needed it to save my life. I said it would be frightfully nice of him to fly in from the West Coast to provide me with it, but that I had no right against him that he should do so. But suppose he isn't on the West Coast. Suppose he has only to walk across the room, place a hand briefly on my brow—and lo, my life is saved. Then surely he ought to do it, it would be indecent to refuse. Is it to be said "Ah, well, it follows that in this case she has a right to the touch of his hand on her brow, and so it would be an injustice in him to refuse"? So that I have a right to it when it is easy for him to provide it, though no right when it's hard? It's rather a shocking idea that anyone's rights should fade away and disappear as it gets harder and harder to accord them to him.

So my own view is that even though you ought to let the violinist use your kidneys for the one hour he needs, we should not conclude that he has a right to do so—we should say that if you refuse, you are, like the boy who owns all the chocolates and will give none away, self-centered and callous, indecent in fact, but not unjust. And similarly, that even supposing a case in which a woman pregnant due to rape ought to allow the unborn person to use her body for the hours he needs, we should not conclude that he has a right to do so; we should conclude that she is self-centered, callous, indecent, but not unjust, if she refuses. The complaints are no less grave; they are just different. However, there is no need to insist on this point. If anyone does wish to deduce "he has a right" from "you ought," then all the same he must surely grant that there are cases in which it is not morally required of you that you allow that violinist to use your kidneys, and in which he does not have a right to use them, and in which you do not do him an injustice if you refuse. And so also for mother and unborn child. Except in such cases as the unborn person has a right to demand it—and we were leaving open the possibility that there may be such cases— nobody is morally *required* to make large sacrifices, of health, of all other interests and concerns, of all other duties and commitments, for nine years, or even for nine months, in order to keep another person alive.

6. We have in fact to distinguish between two kinds of Samaritan: the Good Samaritan and what we might call the Minimally Decent Samaritan. The story of the Good Samaritan, you will remember, goes like this (Luke 10:30–35):

> A certain man went down from Jerusalem to Jerico, and fell among thieves, which stripped him of his raiment, and wounded him, and departed, leaving him half dead.

> And by chance there came down a certain priest that way; and when he saw him, he passed by on the other side.

And likewise a Levite, when he was at the place, came and looked on him, and passed by on the other side.

But a certain Samaritan, as he journeyed, came where he was; and when he saw him he had compassion on him.

And went to him, and bound up his wounds, pouring in oil and wine, and set him on his own beast, and brought him to an inn, and took care of him.

And on the morrow, when he departed, he took out two pence, and gave them to the host, and said unto him, "Take care of him; and whatsoever thou spendest more, when I come again, I will repay thee."

The Good Samaritan went out of his way, at some cost to himself, to help one in need of it. We are not told what the options were, that is, whether or not the priest and the Levite could have helped by doing less than the Good Samaritan did, but assuming they could have, then the fact they did nothing at all shows they were not even Minimally Decent Samaritans, not because they were not Samaritans, but because they were not even minimally decent.

These things are a matter of degree, of course, but there is a difference, and it comes out perhaps most clearly in the story of Kitty Genovese, who, as you will remember, was murdered while thirty-eight people watched or listened, and did nothing at all to help her. A Good Samaritan would have rushed out to give direct assistance against the murderer. Or perhaps we had better allow that it would have been a Splendid Samaritan who did this, on the ground that it would have involved a risk of death for himself. But the thirty-eight not only did not do this, they did not even trouble to pick up a phone to call the police. Minimally Decent Samaritanism would call for doing at least that, and their not having done it was monstrous.

After telling the story of the Good Samaritan, Jesus said "Go, and do thou likewise." Perhaps he meant that we are morally required to act as the Good Samaritan did. Perhaps he was urging people to do more than is morally required of them. At all events it seems plain that it was not morally required of any of the thirty-eight that he rush out to give direct assistance at the risk of his own life, and that it is not morally required of anyone that he give long stretches of his life—nine years or nine months—to sustaining the life of a person who has no special right (we were leaving open the possibility of this) to demand it.

Indeed, with one rather striking class of exceptions, no one in any country in the world is *legally* required to do anywhere near as much as this for anyone else. The class of exceptions is obvious. My main concern here is not the state of the law in respect to abortion, but it is worth drawing attention to the fact that in no state in this country is any man compelled by law to be even a Minimally Decent Samaritan to any person; there is no law under which charges could be brought against the thirty-eight who stood by while Kitty Genovese died. By contrast, in most states in this country women are compelled by law to be not merely Minimally Decent Samaritans, but Good Samaritans to unborn persons inside them. This doesn't by itself settle anything one way or the other, because it may well be argued that there should be laws in this country—as there are in many European countries—compelling at least Minimally Decent Samaritanism.[7] But it does show that there is a gross injustice in the existing state of the law. And it shows also that the groups currently working against liberalization of abortion laws, in fact working toward having it declared unconstitutional for a state to permit abortion, had better start working for the adoption of Good Samaritan laws generally, or earn the charge that they are acting in bad faith.

I should think, myself, that Minimally Decent Samaritan laws would be one thing, Good Samaritan laws quite another, and in fact highly improper. But we are not here concerned with the law. What we should ask is not whether anybody should be compelled by law to be a Good Samaritan, but whether we must accede to a situation in which somebody is being compelled—by nature, perhaps—to be a Good Samaritan. We have, in other words, to look now at third-party interventions. I have been arguing that no person is morally required to make large sacrifices to sustain the life of another who has no right to demand them, and this even where the sacrifices do not include life itself; we are not morally required to be Good Samaritans or anyway Very Good Samaritans to one another. But what if a man cannot extricate himself from such a situation? What if he appeals to us to extricate him? It seems to me plain that there are cases in which we can, cases in which a Good Samaritan would extricate him. There you are, you were kidnapped, and nine years in bed with that violinist lie ahead of you. You have your own life to lead. You are sorry, but you simply cannot see giving up so much of your life to the sustaining of his. You cannot extricate yourself, and ask us to do so. I should have thought that—in light of his having no right to the use of your body—it was obvious that we do not have to accede to your being forced to give up so much. We can do what you ask. There is no injustice to the violinist in our doing so.

7. Following the lead of the opponents of abortion, I have throughout been speaking of the fetus merely as a person, and what I have been asking is whether or not the argument we began with, which proceeds only from the fetus' being a person, really does establish its conclusion. I have argued that it does not.

But of course there are arguments and arguments, and it may be said that I have simply fastened on the wrong one. It may be said that what is important is not merely the fact that the fetus is a person, but that it is a person for whom the woman has a special kind of responsibility issuing from the fact that she is its mother. And it might be argued that all my analogies are therefore irrelevant—for you do not have that special kind of responsibility for that violinist, Henry Fonda does not have that special kind of responsibility for me. And our attention might be drawn to the fact that men and women both *are* compelled by law to provide support for their children.

I have in effect dealt (briefly) with this argument in section 4 above; but a (still briefer) recapitulation now may be in order. Surely we do not have any such "special responsibility" for a person unless we have assumed it, explicitly or implicitly. If a set of parents do not try to prevent pregnancy, do not obtain an abortion, and then at the time of birth of the child do not put it out for adoption, but rather take it home with them, then they have assumed responsibility for it, they have given it rights, and they cannot *now* withdraw support from it at the cost of its life because they now find it difficult to go on providing for it. But if they have taken all reasonable precautions against having a child, they do not simply by virtue of their biological relationship to the child who comes into existence have a special responsibility for it. They may wish to assume responsibility for it, or they may not wish to. And I am suggesting that if assuming responsibility for it would require large sacrifices, then they may refuse. A good Samaritan would not refuse—or anyway, a Splendid Samaritan, if the sacrifices that had to be made were enormous. But then so would a Good Samaritan assume responsibility for that violinist; so would Henry Fonda, if he is a Good Samaritan, fly in from the West Coast and assume responsibility for me.

8. My argument will be found unsatisfactory on two counts by many of those who want to regard abortion as morally permissible. First, while I do argue that abortion is not impermissible, I do not argue that it is always permissible. There may well be cases in which carrying the child to term requires only Minimally Decent Samaritanism of the mother, and this is a standard we must not fall below. I am inclined to think it a merit of my account precisely that it does *not* give a general yes or a general no. It allows for and supports our sense that, for example, a sick and desperately frightened fourteen-year-old schoolgirl, pregnant due to rape, may *of course* choose abortion, and that any law which rules this out is an insane law. And it also allows for and supports our sense that in other cases resort to abortion is even positively indecent. It would be indecent in the woman to request an abortion, and indecent in a doctor to perform it, if she is in her seventh month, and wants the abortion just to avoid the nuisance of postponing a trip abroad. The very fact that the arguments I have been drawing attention to treat all cases of abortion, or even all cases of abortion in which the mother's life is not at stake, as morally on a par ought to have made them suspect at the outset.

Secondly, while I am arguing for the permissibility of abortion in some cases, I am not arguing for the right to secure the death of the unborn child. It is easy to confuse these two things in that up to a certain point in the life of the fetus it is not able to survive outside the mother's body; hence removing it from her body guarantees its death. But they are importantly different. I have argued that you are not morally required to spend nine months in bed, sustaining the life of that violinist; but to say this is by no means to say that if, when you unplug yourself, there is a miracle and he survives, you then have a right to turn round and slit his throat. You may detach yourself even if this costs him his life; you have no right to be guaranteed his death, by some other means, if unplugging yourself does not kill him. There are some people who will feel dissatisfied by this feature of my argument. A woman may be utterly devastated by the thought of a child, a bit of herself, put out for adoption and never seen or heard of again. She may therefore want not merely that the child be detached from her, but more, that it die. Some opponents of abortion are inclined to regard this as beneath contempt—thereby showing insensitivity to what is surely a powerful source of despair. All the same, I agree that the desire for the child's death is not one which anybody may gratify, should it turn out to be possible to detach the child alive.

At this place, however, it should be remembered that we have only been pretending throughout that the fetus is a human being from the moment of conception. A very early abortion is surely not the killing of a person, and so is not dealt with by anything I have said here.

## NOTES

1. Daniel Callahan, *Abortion: Law, Choice, and Morality* (New York, 1970), p. 373. This book gives a fascinating survey of the available information on abortion. The Jewish tradition is surveyed in David M. Feldman, *Birth Control in Jewish Law* (New York, 1968), part 5; and the Catholic tradition in John T. Noonan Jr., "An Almost Absolute Value in History," in *The Morality of Abortion,* ed. John T. Noonan Jr. (Cambridge Mass., 1970).
2. The term "direct" in the arguments I refer to is a technical one. Roughly, what is meant by "direct killing" is either killing as an end in itself or killing as a means to some end, for example, the end of saving someone else's life. See note 5 below for an example of its use.
3. Cf. *Encyclical Letter of Pope Pius XI on Christian Marriage* (Boston, n.d.), p. 32: "however much we may pity the mother whose health and even life is gravely imperiled in the performance of the duty allotted to her by nature, nevertheless what could ever be a sufficient reason for excusing in any way the direct murder of the innocent? This is precisely what we are dealing with here." Noonan ("An Almost Absolute Value," p. 43) reads this as follows: "What cause can ever avail to excuse in any way the direct killing of the innocent? For it is a question of that."
4. The thesis in (4) is in an interesting way weaker than those in (1), (2), and (3): they rule out abortion even in cases in which both mother *and* child will die if the abortion is not performed. By contrast, one who held the view expressed in (4) could consistently say that one needn't prefer letting two persons die to killing one.

5. Cf. the following passage from Pope Pius XII, *Address to the Italian Catholic Society of Midwives:* "The baby in the maternal breast has the right to life immediately from God.—Hence there is no man, no human authority, no science, no medical, eugenic, social, economic or moral 'indication' which can establish or grant a valid juridical ground for a direct deliberate disposition of an innocent human life, that is a disposition which looks to its destruction either as an end or as a means to another end perhaps in itself not illicit.—The baby, still not born, is a man in the same degree and for the same reason as the mother" (quoted in Noonon, "An Almost Absolute Value," p. 45).
6. The need for a discussion of this argument was brought home to me by members of the Society for Ethical and Legal Philosophy, to whom this paper was originally presented.
7. For a discussion of the difficulties involved and a survey of the European experience with such laws, see James M. Ratcliffe, ed., *The Good Samaritan and the Law* (New York, 1966).

# On the Moral and Legal Status of Abortion

## Mary Anne Warren

*In January 1973, the same year and month as the U.S. Supreme Court's landmark* Roe v. Wade *decision on abortion, philosopher Mary Anne Warren published the following famous article on abortion. She begins by discussing some points made by Judith Jarvis Thomson (see Selection 12) and then defends what can be called the "cognitive criterion of personhood," laid out and defended by Joseph Fletcher in 1972.*

*In many ways, Warren gives the general defense of abortion that students sought unsuccessfully in Thomson's earlier article. She argues that the qualities that are most important for personhood are consciousness, reasoning, agency, communication, and a self-concept: a being that lacks* all *these qualities cannot be a person.*

*Mary Anne Warren is professor of philosophy at San Francisco State University. She is the author of many articles on ethical issues and reproductive rights.*

We will be concerned with both the moral status of abortion, which for our purposes we may define as the act which a woman performs in voluntarily terminating, or allowing another person to terminate, her pregnancy, and the legal status which is appropriate for this act. I will argue that, while it is not possible to produce a satisfactory defense of a woman's right to obtain an abortion without showing that a fetus is not a human being, in the morally relevant sense of that term, we ought not to conclude that the difficulties involved in determining whether or not a fetus is human make it impossible to produce any satisfactory solution to the problem of the moral status of abortion. For it is possible to show that, on the basis of intuitions which we may expect even the opponents of abortion to share, a fetus is not a person, and hence not the sort of entity to which it is proper to ascribe full moral rights.

Source: *The Monist* 57, no. 1 (January 1973), pp. 43–61. Reprinted by permission of the publisher. The author is grateful to Herbert Gold, Gene Glass, Anne Lauterbach, Judith Thomson, Mary Mothersill, and Timothy Binkley for reading and criticizing an earlier version of this article.

Of course, while some philosophers would deny the possibility of any such proof,[1] others will deny that there is any need for it, since the moral permissibility of abortion appears to them to be too obvious to require proof. But the inadequacy of this attitude should be evident from the fact that both the friends and the foes of abortion consider their position to be morally self-evident. Because proabortionists have never adequately come to grips with the conceptual issues surrounding abortion, most, if not all, of the arguments which they advance in opposition to laws restricting access to abortion fail to refute or even weaken the traditional antiabortion argument, i.e., that a fetus is a human being, and therefore abortion is murder.

These arguments are typically of one of two sorts. Either they point to the terrible side effects of the restrictive laws, e.g., the deaths due to illegal abortions, and the fact that it is poor women who suffer the most as a result of these laws, or else they state that to deny a woman access to abortion is to deprive her of her right to control her own body. Unfortunately, however, the fact that restricting access to abortion has tragic side effects does not, in itself, show that the restrictions are unjustified, since murder is wrong regardless of the consequences of prohibiting it; and the appeal to the right to control one's body, which is generally construed as a property right, is at best a rather feeble argument for the permissibility of abortion. Mere ownership does not give me the right to kill innocent people whom I find on my property, and indeed I am apt to be held responsible if such people injure themselves while on my property. It is equally unclear that I have any moral right to expel an innocent person from my property when I know that doing so will result in his death.

Furthermore, it is probably inappropriate to describe a woman's body as her property, since it seems natural to hold that a person is something distinct from her property, but not from her body. Even those who would object to the identification of a person with his body, or with the conjunction of his body and his mind, must admit that it would be very odd to describe, say, breaking a leg as damaging one's property, and much more appropriate to describe it as injuring one*self.* Thus it is probably a mistake to argue that the right to obtain an abortion is in any way derived from the right to own and regulate property.

But however we wish to construe the right to abortion, we cannot hope to convince those who consider abortion a form of murder of the existence of any such right unless we are able to produce a clear and convincing refutation of the traditional antiabortion argument, and this has not, to my knowledge, been done. With respect to the two most vital issues which that argument involves, i.e., the humanity of the fetus and its implication for the moral status of abortion, confusion has prevailed on both sides of the dispute.

Thus, both proabortionists and antiabortionists have tended to abstract the question of whether abortion is wrong to that of whether it is wrong to destroy a fetus, just as though the rights of another person were not necessarily involved. This mistaken abstraction has led to the almost universal assumption that if a fetus is a human being, with a right to life, then it follows immediately that abortion is wrong (except perhaps when necessary to save the woman's life), and that it ought to be prohibited. It has also been generally assumed that unless the question about the status of the fetus is answered, the moral status of abortion cannot possibly be determined.

Two recent papers, one by B. A. Brody and one by Judith Thomson, have attempted to settle the question of whether abortion ought to be prohibited apart from the question of whether or not the fetus is human.[2] Brody examines the possibility that the following two statements are compatible: (1) that abortion is the taking of innocent human life, and therefore wrong; and (2) that nevertheless it ought not to be prohibited by law, at least under the present circumstances.[3] Not surprisingly, Brody finds it impossible to reconcile these two statements, since, as he rightly argues, none of the unfortunate side effects of the prohibition of abortion is bad enough to justify legalizing the *wrongful* taking of human life. He is mistaken, however, in concluding that the incompatibility of (1) and (2), in itself, shows that "the legal problem about abortion cannot be resolved independently of the status of the fetus problem."[4]

What Brody fails to realize is that (1) embodies the questionable assumption that if a fetus is a human being, then of course abortion is morally wrong, and that an attack on *this* assumption is more promising, as a way of reconciling the humanity of the fetus with the claim that laws prohibiting abortion are unjustified, than is an attack on the assumption that if abortion is the wrongful killing of innocent human beings then it ought to be prohibited. He thus overlooks the possibility that a fetus may have a right to life and abortion still be morally permissible, in that the right of a woman to terminate an unwanted pregnancy might override the right of the fetus to be kept alive. This immorality of abortion is no more demonstrated by the humanity of the fetus, in itself, than the immorality of killing in self-defense is demonstrated by the fact that the assailant is a human being. Neither is it demonstrated by the *innocence* of the fetus, since there may be situations in which the killing of innocent human beings is justified.

It is perhaps not surprising that Brody fails to spot this assumption, since it has been accepted with little or no argument by nearly everyone who has written on the morality of abortion. John Noonan is correct in saying that "the fundamental question in the long history of abortion is, How do you determine the humanity of a being?"[5] He summarizes his own antiabortion argument, which is a version of the official position of the Catholic church, as follows: "it is wrong to kill humans, however poor, weak, defenseless, and lacking in opportunity to develop their potential they may be. It is therefore morally wrong to kill Biafrans. Similarly, it is morally wrong to kill embryos."[6]

Noonan bases his claim that fetuses are human upon what he calls the theologians' criterion of humanity: that whoever is conceived of human beings is human. But although he argues at length for the appropriateness of this criterion, he never questions the assumption that if a fetus is human then abortion is wrong for exactly the same reason that murder is wrong.

Judith Thomson is, in fact, the only writer I am aware of who has seriously questioned this assumption; she has argued that, even if we grant the antiabortionist his claim that a fetus is a human being, with the same right to life as any other human being, we can still demonstrate that, in at least some and perhaps most cases, a woman is under no moral obligation to complete an unwanted pregnancy. Her argument is worth examining, since if it holds up it may enable us to establish the moral permissibility of abortion without becoming involved in problems about what entitles an entity to be considered human, and accorded full moral rights. To be able to do this would be a great gain in the power and simplicity of the proabortion position, since, although I will argue that these problems can be solved at least as decisively as can any other moral problem, we should certainly be pleased to be able to avoid having to solve them as part of the justification of abortion.

On the other hand, even if Thomson's argument does not hold up, her insight, i.e., that it requires argument to show that if fetuses are human then abortion is properly classified as murder, is an extremely valuable one. The assumption she attacks is particularly invidious, for it amounts to the decision that it is appropriate, in deciding the moral status of abortion, to leave the rights of the pregnant woman out of consideration entirely, except possibly when her life is threatened. Obviously, this will not do; determining what moral rights, if any, a fetus possesses is only the first step in determining the moral status of abortion. Step two, which is at least equally essential, is finding a just solution to the conflict between whatever rights the fetus may have, and the rights of the woman who is unwillingly pregnant. While the historical error has been to pay far too little attention to the second step, Ms. Thomson's suggestion is that if we look at the second step first we may find that a woman has a right to obtain an abortion *regardless* of what rights the fetus has.

Our own inquiry will also have two stages. In Section I, we will consider whether or not it is possible to establish that abortion is morally permissible even on the assumption that a fetus is an entity with a full-fledged right to life. I will argue that in fact this cannot be established, at least not with the conclusiveness which is essential to our hopes of convincing those who are skeptical about the morality of abortion, and that we therefore cannot avoid dealing with the question of whether or not a fetus really does have the same right to life as a (more fully developed) human being.

In Section II, I will propose an answer to this question, namely, that a fetus cannot be considered a member of the moral community, the set of beings with full and equal moral rights, for the simple reason that it is not a person, and that it is personhood, and not genetic humanity, i.e., humanity as defined by Noonan, which is the basis for a membership in this community. I will argue that a fetus, whatever its stage of development, satisfies none of the basic criteria of personhood, and is not even enough *like* a person to be accorded even some of the same rights on the basis of this resemblance. Nor, as we will see, is a fetus' *potential* personhood a threat to the morality of abortion, since, whatever the rights of potential people may be, they are invariably overridden in any conflict with the moral rights of actual people.

# I

We turn now to Professor Thomson's case for the claim that even if a fetus has full moral rights, abortion is still morally permissible, at least sometimes, and for some reasons other than to save the woman's life. Her argument is based upon a clever, but I think faulty, analogy. She asked us to picture ourselves waking up one day, in bed with a famous violinist. Imagine that you have been kidnapped, and your bloodstream hooked up to that of the violinist, who happens to have an ailment which will certainly kill him unless he is permitted to share your kidneys for a period of nine months. No one else can save him, since you alone have the right type of blood. He will be unconscious all that time, and you will have to stay in bed with him, but after the nine months are over he may be unplugged, completely cured, that is, provided that you have cooperated.

Now then, she continues, what are your obligations in this situation? The antiabortionist, if he is consistent, will have to say that you are obligated to stay in bed with the violinist: for all people have a right to life, and violinists are people, and therefore it would be murder for you to disconnect yourself from him and let him die. But this is outrageous, and so there must be something wrong with the same argument when it is applied to abortion. It would certainly be commendable of you to agree to save the violinist, but it is absurd to suggest that your refusal to do so would be murder. His right to life does not obligate you to do whatever is required to keep him alive; nor does it justify anyone else in forcing you to do so. A law which required you to stay in bed with the violinist would clearly be an unjust law, since it is no proper function of the law to force unwilling people to make huge sacrifices for the sake of other people toward whom they have no such prior obligation.

Thomson concludes that, if this analogy is an apt one, then we can grant the antiabortionist his claim that a fetus is a human being, and still hold that it is at least sometimes the case that a pregnant woman has the right to refuse to be a Good Samaritan towards the fetus, i.e., to obtain an abortion. For there is a great gap between the claim that $x$ has a right to life, and the claim that $y$ is obligated to do whatever is necessary to keep $x$ alive, let alone that he ought to be forced to do so. It is $y$'s duty to keep $x$ alive only if he has somehow contracted a *special* obligation to do so; and a woman who is unwillingly pregnant, e.g., who was raped, has done nothing which obligates her to make the enormous sacrifice which is necessary to preserve the conceptus.

This argument is initially quite plausible, and in the extreme case of pregnancy due to rape it is probably conclusive. Difficulties arise, however, when we try to specify more exactly the range of cases in which abortion is clearly justifiable even on the assumption that the fetus is human. Professor Thomson considers it a virtue of her argument that it does not enable us to conclude that abortion is *always* permissible. It would, she says, be "indecent" for a woman in her seventh month to obtain an abortion just to avoid having to postpone a trip to Europe. On the other hand, her argument enables us to see that "a sick and desperately frightened schoolgirl pregnant due to rape may *of course* choose abortion, and that any law which rules this out is an insane law."[7] So far, so good; but what are we to say about the woman who becomes pregnant not though rape but as a result of her own carelessness, or because of contraceptive failure, or who gets pregnant intentionally and then changes her mind about wanting a child? With respect to such cases, the violinist analogy is of much less use to the defender of the woman's right to obtain an abortion.

Indeed, the choice of a pregnancy due to rape, as an example of a case in which abortion is permissible even if a fetus is considered a human being, is extremely significant; for it is only in the case of pregnancy due to rape that the woman's situation is adequately analogous to the violinist case for our intuitions about the latter to transfer convincingly. The crucial difference between a pregnancy due to rape and the normal case of an unwanted pregnancy is that in the normal case we cannot claim that the woman is in no way responsible for her predicament; she could have remained chaste, or taken her pills more faithfully, or abstained on dangerous days, and so on. If, on the other hand, you are kidnapped by strangers, and hooked up to a strange violinist, then you are free of any shred of responsibility for the situation, on the basis of which it would be argued that you are obligated to keep the violinist alive. Only when her pregnancy is due to rape is a woman clearly just as nonresponsible.[8]

Consequently, there is room for the antiabortionist to argue that in the normal case of unwanted pregnancy a woman has, by her own actions, assumed responsibility for the fetus. For if $x$ behaves in a way which he could have avoided, and which he knows involves, let us say, a 1 percent chance of bringing into existence a human being, with a right to life, and does so knowing that if this should happen then that human being will perish unless $x$ does certain things to keep him alive, then it is by no means clear that when it does happen $x$ is free of any obligation to what he knew in advance would be required to keep that human being alive.

The plausibility of such an argument is enough to show that the Thomson analogy can provide a clear and persuasive defense of a woman's right to obtain an abortion only with respect to those cases in which the woman is in no way responsible for her pregnancy, e.g., where it is due to rape. In all other cases, we would almost certainly conclude that it was necessary to look carefully at the particular circumstances in order to determine the extent of the woman's responsibility, and hence the extent of her obligation. This is an extremely unsatisfactory outcome, from the viewpoint of the opponents of restrictive abortion laws, most of whom are convinced that a woman has a right to obtain an abortion regardless of how and why she got pregnant.

Of course a supporter of the violinist analogy might point out that it is absurd to suggest that forgetting her pill one day might be sufficient to obligate a woman to complete an unwanted pregnancy. And indeed it *is* absurd to suggest this. As we will see, the moral right to obtain an abortion is not in the least dependent upon the extent to which the woman is responsible for her pregnancy. But unfortunately, once we allow the assumption that a fetus has full moral rights, we cannot avoid taking this absurd suggestion seriously.

Perhaps we can make this point more clear by altering the violinist story just enough to make it more analogous to a normal unwanted pregnancy and less to a pregnancy due to rape, and then seeing whether it is still obvious that you are not obligated to stay in bed with the fellow.

Suppose, then, that violinists are peculiarly prone to the sort of illness the only cure for which is the use of someone else's bloodstream for nine months, and that because of this there has been formed a society of music lovers who agree that whenever a violinist is stricken they will draw lots and the loser will, by some means, be made the one and only person capable of saving him. Now then, would you be obligated to cooperate in curing the violinist if you had voluntarily joined this society, knowing the possible consequences, and then your name had been drawn and you had been kidnapped? Admittedly, you did not promise ahead of time that you would, but you did deliberately place yourself in a position in which it might happen that a human life would be lost if you did not. Surely this is at least a prima facie reason for supposing that you have an obligation to stay in bed with the violinist. Suppose that you had gotten your name drawn deliberately; surely *that* would be quite a strong reason for thinking that you had such an obligation.

It might be suggested that there is one important disanalogy between the modified violinist case and the case of an unwanted pregnancy, which makes the woman's responsibility significantly less, namely, the fact that the fetus *comes into existence* as the result of the result of the woman's actions. This fact might give her a right to refuse to keep it alive, whereas she would not have had this right had it existed previously, independently, and then as a result of her actions become dependent upon her for its survival.

My own intuition, however, is that $x$ has no more right to bring into existence, either deliberately or as a foreseeable result of actions he could have avoided, a being with full moral rights ($y$), and then refuse to do what he knew beforehand would be required to keep that being alive, than he has to enter into an agreement with an existing person, whereby he may be called upon to save that person's life, and then refuse to do so when so called upon. Thus $x$'s responsibility for $y$'s existence does not seem to lessen his obligation to keep $y$ alive, if he is also responsible for $y$'s being in a situation in which only he can save him.

Whether or not this intuition is entirely correct, it brings us back once again to the conclusion that once we allow the assumption that a fetus has full moral rights it becomes an extremely complex and difficult question whether and when abortion is justifiable. Thus the Thomson analogy cannot help us produce a clear and persuasive proof of the moral permissibility of abortion. Nor will the opponents of the restrictive laws thank us for anything less; for their conviction (for the most part) is that abortion is obviously *not* a morally serious and extremely unfortunate, even though sometimes justified, act comparable to killing in self-defense or to letting the violinist die, but rather is closer to being a morally neutral act, like cutting one's hair.

The basis of this conviction, I believe, is the realization that a fetus is not a person, and thus does not have a full-fledged right to life. Perhaps the reason why this claim has been so inadequately defended is that it seems self-evident to those who accept it. And so it is, insofar as it follows from what I take to be perfectly obvious claims about the nature of personhood, and about the proper grounds for ascribing moral rights, claims which ought, indeed, to be obvious to both the friends and foes of abortion. Nevertheless, it is worth examining these claims, and showing how they demonstrate the moral innocuousness of abortion, since this apparently has not been adequately done before.

II

The question which we must answer in order to produce a satisfactory solution to the problem of the moral status of abortion is this: How are we to define the moral community, the set of beings with full and equal moral rights, such that we can decide whether a human fetus is a member of this community or not? What sort of entity, exactly, has the inalienable rights to life, liberty, and the pursuit of happiness? Jefferson attributed these rights to all *men*, and it may or may not be fair to suggest that he intended to attribute them *only* to men. Perhaps he ought have attributed them to all human beings. If so, then we arrive, first, at Noonan's problem of defining what makes a being human, and, second, at the equally vital question, which Noonan does not consider, namely, What reason is there for identifying the moral community with the set of all human beings, in whatever way we have chosen to define that term?

## On the Definition of "Human"

One reason why this vital second question is so frequently overlooked in the debate over the moral status of abortion is that the term "human" has two distinct, but not often distinguished, senses. This fact results in a slide of meaning, which serves to conceal the fallaciousness of the traditional argument that since (1) it is wrong to kill innocent human beings, and (2) fetuses are innocent human beings, then (3) it is wrong to kill fetuses. For if "human" is used in the same sense in both (1) and (2) then, whichever of the two senses is meant, one of these premises is question-begging. And if it is used in two different senses then of course the conclusion doesn't follow.

Thus, (1) is a self-evident moral truth,[9] and avoids begging the question about abortion, only if "human being" is used to mean something like "a full-fledged member of the moral community." (It may or may not also be meant to refer exclusively to members of the species *Homo sapiens*.) We may call this the *moral* sense of "human." It is not to be confused with what we will call the *genetic* sense, i.e., the sense in which *any* member of the species is a human being, and no member of any other species could be. If (1) is acceptable only if the moral sense is intended, (2) is non-question-begging only if what is intended is the genetic sense.

In "Deciding Who Is Human," Noonan argues for the classification of fetuses with human beings by pointing to the presence of the full genetic code, and the potential capacity for rational thought. It is clear that what he needs to show, for his version of the traditional argument to be valid, is that fetuses are human in the moral sense, the sense in which it is analytically true that all human beings have full moral rights. But, in the absence of any argument showing that whatever is genetically human is also morally human, and he gives none, nothing more than genetic humanity can be demonstrated by the presence of the human genetic code. And, as we will see, the *potential* capacity for rational thought can at most show that an entity has the potential for *becoming* human in the moral sense.

## Defining the Moral Community

Can it be established that genetic humanity is sufficient for moral humanity? I think that there are very good reasons for not defining the moral community in this way. I would like to suggest an alternative way of defining the moral community, which I will argue for only to the extent of explaining why it is, or should be, self-evident. The suggestion is simply that the moral community consists of all and *only* people, rather than all and only human beings;[10] and probably the best way of demonstrating its self-evidence is by considering the concept of personhood, to see what sorts of entity are and are not persons, and what the decision that a being is or is not a person implies about its moral rights.

What characteristics entitle an entity to be considered a person? This is obviously not the place to attempt a complete analysis of the concept of personhood, but we do not need such a fully adequate analysis just to determine whether and why a fetus is or isn't a person. All we need is a rough and approximate list of the most basic criteria of personhood, and some idea of which, or how many, of these an entity must satisfy in order to properly be considered a person.

In searching for such criteria, it is useful to look beyond the set of people with whom we are acquainted, and ask how we would decide whether a totally alien being was a person or not. (For we have no right to assume that genetic humanity is necessary for personhood.) Imagine a space traveler who lands on an unknown planet and encounters a race of beings utterly unlike any he has ever seen or heard of. If he wants to be sure of behaving morally toward these beings, he has somehow to decide whether they are people, and hence have full moral rights, or whether they are the sort of thing which he need not feel guilty about treating as, for example, a source of food.

How should he go about making this decision? If he has some anthropological background, he might look for such things as religion, art, and the manufacturing of tools, weapons, or shelters, since these factors have been used to distinguish our human from our prehuman ancestors, in what seems to be closer to the moral than the genetic sense of "human." And no doubt he would be right to consider the presence of such factors as good evidence that the alien beings were people, and morally human. It would, however, be overly anthropocentric of him to take the absence of these things as adequate evidence that they were not, since we can imagine people who have progressed beyond, or evolved without ever developing, these cultural characteristics.

I suggest that the traits which are most central to the concept of personhood, or humanity in the moral sense, are, very roughly, the following:

1. Consciousness (of objects and events external and/or internal to the being), and in particular the capacity to feel pain
2. Reasoning (the *developed* capacity to solve new and relatively complex problems)
3. Self-motivated activity (activity which is relatively independent of either genetic or direct external control)
4. The capacity to communicate, by whatever means, messages of an indefinite variety of types, that is, not just with an indefinite number of possible contents, but on indefinitely many possible topics
5. The presence of self-concepts and self-awareness, either individual or racial, or both

Admittedly, there are apt to be a great many problems involved in formulating precise definitions of these criteria, let alone in developing universally valid behavioral criteria for deciding when they apply. But I will assume that both we and our explorer know approximately what (1)–(5) mean, and that he is also able to determine whether or not they apply. How, then, should he use his findings to decide whether or not the alien beings are people? We needn't suppose that an entity must have *all* these attributes to be properly considered a person; (1) and (2) alone may well be sufficient for personhood, and quite probably (1)–(3) are sufficient. Neither do we need to insist that any one of these criteria is necessary for personhood, although once again (1) and (2) look like fairly good candidates for necessary conditions, as does (3), if "activity" is construed so as to include the activity of reasoning.

All we need to claim, to demonstrate that a fetus is not a person, is that any being which satisfies *none* of (1)–(5) is certainly not a person. I consider this claim to be so obvious that I think anyone who denied it, and claimed that a being which satisfied none of (1)–(5) was a person all the same, would thereby demonstrate that he had no notion at all of what a person is—perhaps because he had confused the concept of a person with that of genetic humanity. If the opponents of abortion were to deny the appropriateness of these five criteria, I do not know what further arguments would convince them. We would probably have to admit that our conceptual schemes were indeed irreconcilably different, and that our dispute could not be settled objectively.

I do not expect this to happen, however, since I think that the concept of a person is one which is very nearly universal (to people), and that it is common to both proabortionists and antiabortionists, even though neither group has fully realized the relevance of this concept to the resolution of their dispute. Furthermore, I think that on reflection even the antiabortionists ought to agree not only that (1)–(5) are central to the concept of personhood, but also that it is a part of this concept that all and only people have full moral rights. The concept of a person is in part a moral concept; once we have admitted that *x* is a person we have recognized, even if we have not agreed to respect *x*'s right to be treated as a member of the moral community. It is true that the claim that *x* is a *human being* is more commonly voiced as part of an appeal to treat *x* decently than is the claim that *x* is a person, but this is either because "human being" is here used in the sense which implies personhood, or because the genetic and moral senses of "human" have been confused.

Now if (1)–(5) are indeed the primary criteria of personhood, then it is clear that genetic humanity is neither necessary nor sufficient for establishing that an entity is a person. Some human beings are not people, and there may well be people who are not human beings. A man or woman whose consciousness has been permanently obliterated but who remains alive is a human being which is no longer a person; defective human beings, with no appreciable mental capacity, are not and presumably never will be people; and a fetus is a human being which is not yet a person, and which therefore cannot coherently be said to have full moral rights. Citizens of the next century should be prepared to recognize highly advanced, self-aware robots or computers, should such be developed, and intelligent inhabitants of other worlds, should such be found, as people in the fullest sense, and to respect their moral rights. But to ascribe full moral rights to an entity which is not a person is as absurd as to ascribe moral obligations and responsibilities to such an entity.

## Fetal Development and the Right to Life

Two problems arise in the application of these suggestions for the definition of the moral community to the determination of the precise moral status of a human fetus. Given that the paradigm example of a person is a normal adult being, then (1) How like this paradigm, in particular how far advanced since conception, does a human being need to be before it begins to have a right to life by virtue, not of being fully a person as of yet, but of being *like* a person? and (2) To what extent, if any, does the fact that a fetus has the *potential* for becoming a person endow it with some of the same rights? Each of these questions requires some comment.

In answering the first question, we need not attempt a detailed consideration of the moral rights of organisms which are not developed enough, aware enough, intelligent enough, etc., to be considered people, but which resemble people in some respects. It does seem reasonable to suggest that the more like a person, in the relevant respects, a being is, the stronger is the case for regarding it as having a right to life, and indeed the stronger its right to life is. Thus we ought to take seriously the suggestion that, insofar as "the human individual develops biologically in a continuous fashion . . . the rights of a human person might develop in the same way."[11] But we must keep in mind that the attributes which are relevant in determining whether or not an entity is enough like a person to be regarded as having some of the same moral rights are no different from those which are relevant to determining whether or not it is fully a person—i.e., are no different from (1)–(5)—and that being genetically human, or having recognizably human facial and other physical features, or detectable brain activity, or the capacity to survive outside the uterus, is simply not among these relevant attributes.

Thus it is clear that even though a seven- or eight-month fetus has features which make it apt to arouse in us almost the same powerful protective instinct as is commonly aroused by a small infant, nevertheless, it is not significantly more personlike than is a very small embryo. It is *somewhat* more personlike; it can apparently feel and respond to pain, and it may even have a rudimentary form of consciousness, insofar as its brain is quite active. Nevertheless, it seems safe to say that it is not fully conscious, in the way that an infant of a few months is, and that it cannot reason, or communicate messages of indefinitely many sorts, does not engage in self-motivated activity, and has no self-awareness. Thus, in the *relevant* respects, a fetus, even a fully developed one, is considerably less personlike than is the average mature mammal, indeed the average fish. And I think that a rational person must conclude that if the right to life of a fetus is to be based upon its resemblance to a person, then it cannot be said to have any more right to life than, let us say, a newborn guppy (which also seems to be capable of feeling pain), and that a right of that magnitude could never override a woman's right to obtain an abortion, at any stage of her pregnancy.

There may, of course, be other arguments in favor of placing legal limits upon the stage of pregnancy in which an abortion may be performed. Given the relative safety of the new techniques of artificially inducing labor during the third trimester, the danger to the woman's life or health is no longer such an argument. Neither is the fact that people tend to respond to the thought of abortion in the later stages of pregnancy with emotional revulsion, since mere emotional responses cannot take the place of moral reasoning in determining what ought to be permitted. Nor, finally, is the frequently heard argument that legalizing abortion, especially late in the pregnancy, may erode the level of re-spect for human life, leading, perhaps, to an increase in unjustified euthanasia and other crimes. For this threat, if it is a threat, can be better met by educating people to the kinds of moral distinctions which we are making here than by limiting access to abortion (which limitation may, in its disregard for the rights of women, be just as damaging to the level of respect for human rights).

Thus, since the fact that even a fully developed fetus is not personlike enough to have any significant right to life on the basis of its personlikeness shows that no legal restrictions upon the stage of pregnancy in which an abor-tion may be performed can be justified on the grounds that we should protect the rights of the older fetus, and since there is no other apparent justification for such restrictions, we may conclude that they are entirely unjustified. Whether or not it would be *indecent* (whatever that means) for a woman in her seventh month to obtain an abortion just to avoid having to postpone a trip to Europe, it would not, in itself, be *immoral,* and therefore it ought to be permitted.

## Potential Personhood and the Right to Life

We have seen that a fetus does not resemble a person in any way which can support the claim that it has even some of the same rights. But what about its *potential*, the fact that if nurtured and allowed to develop naturally it will very probably become a person? Doesn't that alone give it at least some right to life? It is hard to deny that the fact than an entity is a potential person is a strong prima facie reason for not destroying it; but we need not conclude from this that a potential person has a right to life, by virtue of that potential. It may be that our feeling that it is better, other things being equal, not to destroy a potential person is better explained by the fact that potential people are still (felt to be) an invaluable resource, not to be lightly squandered. Surely, if every speck of dust were a potential person, we would be much less apt to conclude that every potential person has a right to become actual.

Still, we do not need to insist that a potential person has no right to life whatever. There may well be something immoral, and not just imprudent, about wantonly destroying potential people, when doing so isn't necessary to protect anyone's rights. But even if a potential person does have some prima facie right to life, such a right could not possibly outweigh the right of a woman to obtain an abortion, since the rights of any actual person invariably outweigh those of any potential person, whenever the two conflict. Since this may not be immediately obvious in the case of a human fetus, let us look at another case.

Suppose that our space explorer falls into the hands of an alien culture, whose scientists decide to create a few hundred thousand or more human beings, by breaking his body into its component cells, and using these to create fully developed human beings, with, of course, his genetic code. We may imagine that each of these newly created men will have all of the original man's abilities, skills, knowledge, and so on, and also have an individual self-concept, in short that each of them will be a bona fide (though hardly unique) person. Imagine that the whole project will take only seconds, and that its chances of success are extremely high, and that our explorer knows all of this, and also knows that these people will be treated fairly. I maintain that in such a situation he would have every right to escape if he could, and thus to deprive all these potential people of their potential lives; for his right to life outweighs all of theirs together, in spite of the fact that they are all genetically human, all innocent, and all have a very high probability of becoming people very soon, if only he refrains from acting.

Indeed, I think he would have a right to escape even if it were not his life which the alien scientists planned to take, but only a year of his freedom or, indeed, only a day. Nor would he be obligated to stay if he had gotten captured (thus bringing all these people-potentials into existence) because of his own carelessness, or even if he had done so deliberately, knowing the consequences. Regardless of how he got captured, he is not morally obligated to remain in captivity for *any* period of time for the sake of permitting any number of potential people to come into actuality, so great is the margin by which one actual person's right to liberty outweighs whatever right to life even a hundred thousand potential people have. And it seems reasonable to conclude that the rights of a woman will outweigh by a similar margin whatever right to life a fetus may have by virtue of its potential personhood.

Thus, neither a fetus' resemblance to a person nor its potential for becoming a person provides any basis whatever for the claim that it has any significant right to life. Consequently, a woman's right to protect her health, happiness, freedom, and even her life,[12] by terminating an unwanted pregnancy, will always override whatever right to life it may be appropriate to ascribe to a fetus, even a fully developed one. And thus, in the absence of any overwhelming social need for every possible child, the laws which restrict the right to obtain an abortion, or limit the period of pregnancy during which an abortion may be performed, are a wholly unjustified violation of a woman's most basic moral and constitutional rights.

## NOTES

1. For example, Roger Wertheimer, who in "Understanding the Abortion Argument," *Philosophy and Public Affairs* 1, no. I (Fall 1971), pp. 67–95, argues that the problem of the moral status of abortion is insoluble, in that the dispute over the status of the fetus is not a question of fact at all, but only a question of how one responds to the facts.
2. B. A. Brody, "Abortion and the Law," *Journal of Philosophy* 68, no. 12 (June 17, 1971), pp. 357–69; Judith Thomson, "A Defense of Abortion," *Philosophy and Public Affairs* 1, no. 1 (Fall 1971), pp. 47–66.
3. I have abbreviated these statements somewhat, but not in a way which affects the argument.
4. Brody, "Abortion and the Law," p. 369.
5. John Noonan, "Abortion and the Catholic Church: A Summary History," *Natural Law Forum* 12 (1967), p. 125.
6. John Noonan, "Deciding Who Is Human," *Natural Law Forum* 13 (1968), p. 134.
7. Thomson, "A Defense of Abortion," p. 65.
8. We may safely ignore the fact that she might have avoided getting raped, e.g., by carrying a gun, since by similar means you might likewise have avoided getting kidnapped, and in neither case does the victim's failure to take all possible precautions against a highly unlikely event (as opposed to reasonable precautions against a rather likely event) mean that he is morally responsible for what happens.
9. Of course, the principle that it is (always) wrong to kill innocent human beings is in need of many other modifications, e.g., that it may be permissible to do so to save a greater number of other innocent human beings; but we may safely ignore these complications here.
10. From here on, we will use "human" to mean genetically human, since the moral sense seems closely connected to, and perhaps derived from, the assumption that genetic humanity is sufficient for membership in the moral community.
11. Thomas L. Hayes, "A Biological View," *Commonweal* 85 (March 17, 1967), pp. 677–78; quoted by Daniel Callahan in *Abortion, Law, Choice, and Morality* (London: Macmillan, 1970).
12. That is, insofar as the death rate, for the woman, is higher for childbirth than for early abortion.

# Why Abortion Is Immoral

## Don Marquis

*For many years the literature in philosophy and medical ethics lacked an attack on abortion from philosophically strong grounds. In 1989 Don Marquis filled this omission.*

*Marquis begins by asking: if we do not depend on metaphysical premises about God and an afterlife to explain why murder is wrong, how do we explain it? One promising answer is to argue that what is wrong about killing adult persons is that in doing so, the murderer deprives the victim of the rich set of experiences—in thinking, loving, and growing old—that the victim otherwise would have had. It is wrong to deprive people of such future experiences, and this deprivation explains why murder is wrong.*

*If this argument is valid, Marquis asks, then why is aborting a human fetus not wrong? For surely, doing so deprives a potential person of a rich set of future experiences. The philosophical challenge posed by Marquis is to explain why abortion is permissible but killing adults is not.*

*Don Marquis is professor of philosophy at the University of Kansas, Lawrence.*

The view that abortion is, with rare exceptions, seriously immoral has received little support in the recent philosophical literature. No doubt most philosophers affiliated with secular institutions of higher education believe that the anti-abortion position is either a symptom of irrational religious dogma or a conclusion generated by seriously confused philosophical argument. The purpose of this essay is to undermine this general belief. This essay sets out an argument that purports to show, as well as any argument in ethics can show, that abortion is, except possibly in rare cases, seriously immoral, that it is in the same moral category as killing an innocent adult human being.

*Source: Journal of Philosophy* 86, no. 4 (April 1989), pp. 183–202. Reprinted by permission of the author and publisher.

The argument is based on a major assumption. Many of the most insightful and careful writers on the ethics of abortion—such as Joel Feinberg, Michael Tooley, Mary Anne Warren, H. Tristram Engelhardt, Jr., L. W. Sumner, John T. Noonan, Jr., and Philip Devine—believe that whether or not abortion is morally permissible stands or falls on whether or not a fetus is the sort of being whose life it is seriously wrong to end.[1] The argument of this essay will assume, but not argue, that they are correct.

Also, this essay will neglect issues of great importance to a complete ethics of abortion. Some anti-abortionists will allow that certain abortions, such as abortion before implantation or abortion when the life of a woman is threatened by a pregnancy or abortion after rape, may be morally permissible. This essay will not explore the casuistry of these hard cases. The purpose of this essay is to develop a general argument for the claim that the overwhelming majority of deliberate abortions are seriously immoral.

# I

A sketch of standard anti-abortion and pro-choice arguments exhibits how those arguments possess certain symmetries that explain why partisans of those positions are so convinced of the correctness of their own positions, why they are not successful in convincing their opponents, and why, to others, this issue seems to be unresolvable. An analysis of the nature of this standoff suggests a strategy for surmounting it.

Consider the way a typical anti-abortionist argues. She will argue or assert that life is present from the moment of conception or that fetuses look like babies or that fetuses possess a characteristic such as a genetic code that is both necessary and sufficient for being human. Anti-abortionists seem to believe that (1) the truth of all of these claims is quite obvious, and (2) establishing any of these claims is sufficient to show that abortion is morally akin to murder.

A standard pro-choice strategy exhibits similarities. The pro-choicer will argue or assert that fetuses are not persons or that fetuses are not rational agents or that fetuses are not social beings. Pro-choicers seem to believe that (1) the truth of any of these claims is quite obvious, and (2) establishing any of these claims is sufficient to show that an abortion is not a wrongful killing.

In fact, both the pro-choice and the anti-abortion claims do seem to be true, although the "it looks like a baby" claim is more difficult to establish the earlier the pregnancy. We seem to have a standoff. How can it be resolved?

As everyone who has taken a bit of logic knows, if any of these arguments concerning abortion is a good argument, it requires not only some claim characterizing fetuses, but also some general moral principle that ties a characteristic of fetuses to having or not having the right to life or to some other moral characteristic that will generate the obligation or the lack of obligation not to end the life of a fetus. Accordingly, the arguments of the anti-abortionist and the pro-choicer need a bit of filling in to be regarded as adequate.

Note what each partisan will say. The anti-abortionist will claim that her position is supported by such generally accepted moral principles as "It is always prima facie seriously wrong to take a human life" or "It is always prima facie seriously wrong to end the life of a baby." Since these are generally accepted moral principles, her position is certainly not obviously wrong. The pro-choicer will claim that her position is supported by such plausible moral principles as "Being a person is what gives an individual intrinsic moral worth" or "It is only seriously prima facie wrong to take the life of a member of the human community." Since these are generally accepted moral principles, the pro-choice position is certainly not obviously wrong. Unfortunately, we have again arrived at a standoff.

Now, how might one deal with this standoff? The standard approach is to try to show how the moral principles of one's opponent lose their plausibility under analysis. It is easy to see how this is possible. On the one hand, the anti-abortionist will defend a moral principle concerning the wrongness of killing which tends to be broad in scope in order that even fetuses at an early stage of pregnancy will fall under it. The problem with broad principles is that they often embrace too much. In this particular instance, the principle "It is always prima facie wrong to take a human life" seems to entail that it is wrong to end the existence of a living human cancer-cell culture, on the grounds that the culture is both living and human. Therefore, it seems that the anti-abortionist's favored principle is too broad.

On the other hand, the pro-choicer wants to find a moral principle concerning the wrongness of killing which tends to be narrow in scope in order that fetuses will *not* fall under it. The problem with narrow principles is that they often do not embrace enough. Hence, the needed principles such as "It is prima facie seriously wrong to kill only persons" or "It is prima facie wrong to kill only rational agents" do not explain why it is wrong to kill infants or young children or the severely retarded or even perhaps the severely mentally ill. Therefore, we seem again to have a standoff. The anti-abortionist charges, not unreasonably, that pro-choice principles concerning killing are too narrow to be acceptable; the pro-choicer charges, not unreasonably, that anti-abortionist principles concerning killing are too broad to be acceptable.

Attempts by both sides to patch up the difficulties in their positions run into further difficulties. The anti-abortionist will try to remove the problem in her position by reformulating her principle concerning killing in terms of human beings. Now we end up with: "It is always prima facie seriously wrong to end the life of a human being." This principle has the advantage of avoiding the problem of the human cancer-cell culture counterexample. But this advantage is purchased at a high price. For although it is clear that a fetus is both human and alive, it is not at all clear that a fetus is a human *being*. There is at least something to be said for the view that something becomes a human being only after a process of development, and that therefore first trimester fetuses and perhaps all fetuses are not yet human beings. Hence, the anti-abortionist, by this move, has merely exchanged one problem for another.[2]

The pro-choicer fares no better. She may attempt to find reasons why killing infants, young children, and the severely retarded is wrong which are independent of her major principle that is supposed to explain the wrongness of taking human life, but which will not also make abortion immoral. This is no easy task. Appeals to social utility will seem satisfactory only to those who resolve not to think of the enormous difficulties with a utilitarian account of the wrongness of killing and the significant social costs of preserving the lives of the unproductive.[3] A pro-choice strategy that extends the definition of "person" to infants or even to young children seems just as arbitrary as an anti-abortion strategy that extends the definition of "human being" to fetuses. Again, we find symmetries in the two positions and we arrive at a standoff.

There are even further problems that reflect symmetries in the two positions. In addition to counterexample problems, or the arbitrary application problems that can be exchanged for them, the standard anti-abortionist principle "It is prima facie seriously wrong to kill a human being," or one of its variants, can be objected to on the grounds of ambiguity. If "human being" is taken to be a *biological* category, then the anti-abortionist is left with the problem of explaining why a merely biological category should make a moral difference. Why, it is asked, is it any more reasonable to base a moral conclusion on the number of chromosomes in one's cells than on the color of one's skin?[4] If "human being," on the other hand, is taken to be a *moral* category, then the claim that a fetus is a human being cannot be taken to be a premise in the anti-abortion argument, for it is precisely what needs to be established. Hence, either the anti-abortionist's main category is a morally irrelevant, merely biological category, or it is of no use to the anti-abortionist in establishing (noncircularly, of course) that abortion is wrong.

Although this problem with the anti-abortionist position is often noticed, it is less often noticed that the pro-choice position suffers from an analogous problem. The principle "Only persons have the right to life" also suffers from an ambiguity. The term "person" is typically defined in terms of psychological characteristics, although there will certainly be disagreement concerning which characteristics are most important. Supposing that this matter can be settled, the pro-choicer is left with the problem of explaining why *psychological* characteristics should make a *moral* difference. If the pro-choicer should attempt to deal with this problem by claiming that an explanation is not necessary, that in fact we do treat such a cluster of psychological properties as having moral significance, the sharp-witted anti-abortionist should have a ready response. We do treat being both living and human as having moral significance. If it is legitimate for the pro-choicer to demand that the anti-abortionist provide an explanation of the connection between the biological character of being a human being and the wrongness of being killed (even though people accept this connection), then it is legitimate for the anti-abortionist to demand that the pro-choicer provide an explanation of the connection between psychological criteria for being a person and the wrongness of being killed (even though that connection is accepted).[5]

Feinberg has attempted to meet this objection (he calls psychological personhood "commonsense personhood"):

> The characteristics that confer commonsense personhood are not arbitrary bases for rights and duties, such as race, sex, or species membership; rather they are traits that make sense out of rights and duties and without which those moral attributes would have no point or function. It is because people are conscious; have a sense of their personal identities; have plans, goals, and projects; experience emotions; are liable to pains, anxieties, and frustrations; can reason and bargain, and so on—it is because of these attributes that people have values and interests, desires and expectations of their own, including a stake in their own futures, and a personal well-being of a sort we cannot ascribe to unconscious or nonrational beings. Because of their developed capacities they can assume duties and responsibilities and can have and make claims on one another. Only because of their sense of self, their life plans, their value hierarchies, and their stakes in their own futures can they be ascribed fundamental rights. There is nothing arbitrary about these linkages.[6]

The plausible aspects of this attempt should not be taken to obscure its implausible features. There is a great deal to be said for the view that being a psychological person under some description is a necessary condition for having duties. One cannot have a duty unless one is capable of behaving morally, and a being's capability of behaving morally will require having a certain psychology. It is far from obvious, however, that having rights entails consciousness or rationality, as Feinberg suggests. We speak of the rights of the severely retarded or the severely mentally ill, yet some of these persons are not rational. We speak of the rights of the temporarily unconscious. The New Jersey Supreme Court based their decision in the Quinlan case on Karen Ann Quinlan's right to privacy, and she was known to be permanently unconscious at that time. Hence, Feinberg's claim that having rights entails being conscious is, on its face, obviously false.

Of course, it might not make sense to attribute rights to a being that would never in its natural history have certain psychological traits. This modest connection between psychological personhood and moral personhood will create a place for Karen Ann Quinlan and the temporarily unconscious. But then it makes a place for fetuses also. Hence, it does not serve Feinberg's pro-choice purposes. Accordingly, it seems that the pro-choicer will have as much difficulty bridging the gap between psychological personhood and personhood in the moral sense as the anti-abortionist has bridging the gap between being a biological human being and being a human being in the moral sense.

Furthermore, the pro-choicer cannot any more escape her problem by making person a purely moral category than the anti-abortionist could escape by the analogous move. For if person is a moral category, then the pro-choicer is left without the resources for establishing (noncircularly, of course) the claim that a fetus is not a person, which is an essential premise in her argument. Again, we have both a symmetry and a standoff between pro-choice and anti-abortion views.

Passions in the abortion debate run high. There are both plausibilities and difficulties with the standard positions. Accordingly, it is hardly surprising that partisans of either side embrace with fervor the moral generalizations that support the conclusions they preanalytically favor, and reject with disdain the moral generalizations of their opponents as being subject to inescapable difficulties. It is easy to believe that the counterexamples to one's own moral principles are merely temporary difficulties that will dissolve in the wake of further philosophical research, and that the counterexamples to the principles of one's opponents are as straightforward as the contradiction between *A* and *O* propositions in traditional logic. This might suggest to an impartial observer (if there are any) that the abortion issue is unresolvable.

There is a way out of this apparent dialectical quandary. The moral generalizations of both sides are not quite correct. The generalizations hold for the most part, for the usual cases. This suggests that they are all *accidental* generalizations, that the moral claims made by those on both sides of the dispute do not touch on the *essence* of the matter.

This use of the distinction between essence and accident is not meant to invoke obscure metaphysical categories. Rather, it is intended to reflect the rather atheoretical nature of the abortion discussion. If the generalization a partisan in the abortion dispute adopts were derived from the reason why ending the life of a human being is wrong, then there could not be exceptions to that generalization unless some special case obtains in which there are even more powerful countervailing reasons. Such generalizations would not be merely accidental generalizations; they would point to, or be based upon, the essence of the wrongness of killing, what it is that makes killing wrong. All this suggests that a necessary condition of resolving the abortion controversy is a more theoretical account of the wrongness of killing. After all, if we merely believe, but do not understand, why killing adult human beings such as ourselves is wrong, how could we conceivably show that abortion is either immoral or permissible?

## II

In order to develop such an account, we can start from the following unproblematic assumption concerning our own case: it is wrong to kill *us*. Why is it wrong? Some answers can be easily eliminated. It might be said that what makes killing us wrong is that a killing brutalizes the one who kills. But the brutalization consists of being inured to the performance of an act that is hideously immoral; hence, the brutalization does not explain the immorality. It might be said that what makes killing us wrong is the great loss others would experience as a result of our absence. Although such hubris is understandable, such an explanation does not account for the wrongness of killing hermits, or those whose lives are relatively independent and whose friends find it easy to make new friends.

A more obvious answer is better. What primarily makes killing wrong is neither its effect on the murderer nor its effect on the victim's friends and relatives, but its effect on the victim. The loss of one's life is one of the greatest losses one can suffer. The loss of one's life deprives one of all the experiences, activities, projects, and enjoyments that would otherwise have constituted one's future. Therefore, killing someone is wrong, primarily because the killing inflicts (one of) the greatest possible losses on the victim. To describe this as the loss of life can be misleading, however. The change in my biological state does not by itself make killing me wrong. The effect of the loss of my biological life is the loss to me of all those activities, projects, experiences, and enjoyments which would otherwise have constituted my future personal life. These activities, projects, experiences, and enjoyments are either valuable for their own sakes or are means to something else that is valuable for its own sake. Some parts of my future are not valued by me now, but will come to be valued by me as I grow older and as my values and capacities change. When I am killed, I am deprived both of what I now value which would have been part of my future personal life, but also of what I would come to value. Therefore, when I die, I am deprived of all of the value of my future. Inflicting this loss on me is ultimately what makes killing me wrong. This being the case, it would seem that what makes killing *any* adult human being prima facie seriously wrong is the loss of his or her future.[7]

How should this rudimentary theory of the wrongness of killing be evaluated? It cannot be faulted for deriving an "ought" from an "is," for it does not. The analysis assumes that killing me (or you, reader) is prima facie seriously wrong. The point of the analysis is to establish which natural property ultimately explains the wrongness of the killing, given that it is wrong. A natural property will ultimately explain the wrongness of killing, only if (1) the explanation fits with our intuitions about the matter and (2) there is no other natural property that provides the basis for a better explanation of the wrongness of killing. This analysis rests on the intuition that what makes killing a particular human or animal wrong is what it does to that particular human or animal. What makes killing wrong is some natural effect or other of the killing. Some would deny this. For instance, a divine-command theorist in ethics would deny it. Surely this denial is, however, one of those features of divine-command theory which renders it so implausible.

The claim that what makes killing wrong is the loss of the victim's future is directly supported by two considerations. In the first place, this theory explains why we regard killing as one of the worst of crimes. Killing is especially wrong, because it deprives the victim of more than perhaps any other crime. In the second place, people with AIDS or cancer who know they are dying believe, of course, that dying is a very bad thing for them. They believe that the loss of a future to them that they would otherwise have experienced is what makes their premature death a very bad thing for them. A better theory of the wrongness of killing would require a different natural property associated with killing which better fits with the attitudes of the dying. What could it be?

The view that what makes killing wrong is the loss to the victim of the value of the victim's future gains additional support when some of its implications are examined. In the first place, it is incompatible with the view that it is wrong to kill only beings who are biologically human. It is possible that there exists a different species from another planet whose members have a future like ours. Since having a future like that is what makes killing someone wrong, this theory entails that it would be wrong to kill members of such a species. Hence, this theory is opposed to the claim that only life that is biologically human has great moral worth, a claim which many anti-abortionists have seemed to adopt. This opposition, which this theory has in common with personhood theories, seems to be a merit of the theory.

In the second place, the claim that the loss of one's future is the wrong-making feature of one's being killed entails the possibility that the futures of some actual nonhuman mammals on our own planet are sufficiently like ours that it is seriously wrong to kill them also. Whether some animals do have the same right to life as human beings depends on adding to the account of the wrongness of killing some additional account of just what it is about my future or the futures of other adult human beings which makes it wrong to kill us. No such additional account will be offered in this essay. Undoubtedly, the provision of such an account would be a very difficult matter. Undoubtedly, any such account would be quite controversial. Hence, it surely should not reflect badly on this sketch of an elementary theory of the wrongness of killing that it is indeterminate with respect to some very difficult issues regarding animal rights.

In the third place, the claim that the loss of one's future is the wrong-making feature of one's being killed does not entail, as sanctity-of-human-life theories do, that active euthanasia is wrong. Persons who are severely and incurably ill, who face a future of pain and despair, and who wish to die will not have suffered a loss if they are killed. It is, strictly speaking, the value of a human's future which makes killing wrong in this theory. This being so, killing does not necessarily wrong some persons who are sick and dying. Of course, there may be other reasons for a prohibition of active euthanasia, but that is another matter. Sanctity-of-human-life theories seem to hold that active euthanasia is seriously wrong even in an individual case where there seems to be good reason for it independently of public policy considerations. This consequence is most implausible, and it is a plus for the claim that the loss of a future of value is what makes killing wrong that it does not share this consequence.

In the fourth place, the account of the wrongness of killing defended in this essay does straightforwardly entail that it is prima facie seriously wrong to kill children and infants, for we do presume that they have futures of value. Since we do believe that it is wrong to kill defenseless little babies, it is important that a theory of the wrongness of killing easily account for this. Personhood theories of the wrongness of killing, on the other hand, cannot straightforwardly account for the wrongness of killing infants and young children.[8] Hence, such theories must add special ad hoc accounts of the wrongness of killing the young. The plausibility of such ad hoc theories seems to be a function of how desperately one wants such theories to work. The claim that the primary wrong-making feature of a killing is the loss to the victim of the value of its future accounts for the wrongness of killing young children and infants directly; it makes the wrongness of such acts as obvious as we actually think it is. This is a further merit of this theory. Accordingly, it seems that this value of a future-like-ours theory of the wrongness of killing shares strengths of both sanctity-of-life and personhood accounts while avoiding weaknesses of both. In addition, it meshes with a central intuition concerning what makes killing wrong.

The claim that the primary wrong-making feature of a killing is the loss to the victim of the value of its future has obvious consequences for the ethics of abortion. The future of a standard fetus includes a set of experiences, projects, activities, and such which are identical with the futures of adult human beings and are identical with the futures of young children. Since the reason that is sufficient to explain why it is wrong to kill human beings after the time of birth is a reason that also applies to fetuses, it follows that abortion is prima facie seriously morally wrong.

This argument does not rely on the invalid inference that, since it is wrong to kill persons, it is wrong to kill potential persons also. The category that is morally central to this analysis is the category of having a valuable future like ours; it is not the category of personhood. The argument to the conclusion that abortion is prima facie seriously morally wrong proceeded independently of the notion of person or potential person or any equivalent. Someone may wish to start with this analysis in terms of the value of a human future, conclude that abortion is, except perhaps in rare circumstances, seriously morally wrong, infer that fetuses have the right to life, and then call fetuses "persons" as a result of their having the right to life. Clearly, in this case, the category of person is being used to state the *conclusion* of the analysis rather than to generate the *argument* of the analysis.

The structure of this anti-abortion argument can be both illuminated and defended by comparing it to what appears to be the best argument for the wrongness of the wanton infliction of pain on animals. This latter argument is based on the assumption that it is prima facie wrong to inflict pain on me (or you, reader). What is the natural property associated with the infliction of pain which makes such infliction wrong? The obvious answer seems to be that the infliction of pain causes suffering and that suffering is a misfortune. The suffering caused by the infliction of pain is what makes the wanton infliction of pain on me wrong. The wanton infliction of pain on other adult humans causes suffering. The wanton infliction of pain on animals causes suffering. Since causing suffering is what makes the wanton infliction of pain wrong and since the wanton infliction of pain on animals causes suffering, it follows that the wanton infliction of pain on animals is wrong.

This argument for the wrongness of the wanton infliction of pain on animals shares a number of structural features with the argument for the serious prima facie wrongness of abortion. Both arguments start with an obvious assumption concerning what it is wrong to do to me (or you, reader). Both then look for the characteristic or the consequence of the wrong action which makes the action wrong. Both recognize that the wrong-making feature of these immoral actions is a property of actions sometimes directed at individuals other than postnatal human beings. If the structure of the argument for the wrongness of the wanton infliction of pain on animals is sound, then the structure of the argument for the prima facie serious wrongness of abortion is also sound, for the structure of the two arguments is the same. The structure common to both is the key to the explanation of how the wrongness of abortion can be demonstrated without recourse to the category of person. In neither argument is that category crucial.

This defense of an argument for the wrongness of abortion in terms of a structurally similar argument for the wrongness of the wanton infliction of pain on animals succeeds only if the account regarding animals is the correct account. Is it? In the first place, it seems plausible. In the second place, its major competition is Kant's account. Kant believed that we do not have direct duties to animals at all, because they are not persons. Hence, Kant had to explain and justify the wrongness of inflicting pain on animals on the grounds that "he who is hard in his dealings with animals becomes hard also in his dealing with men."[9] The problem with Kant's account is that there seems to be no reason for accepting this latter claim unless Kant's account is rejected. If the alternative to Kant's account is accepted, then it is easy to understand why someone who is indifferent to inflicting pain on animals is also indifferent to inflicting pain on humans, for one is indifferent to what makes inflicting pain wrong in both cases. But if Kant's account is accepted, there is no intelligible reason why one who is hard in his dealings with animals (or crabgrass or stones) should also be hard in his dealings with men. After all, men are persons; animals are no more persons than crabgrass or stones. Persons are Kant's crucial moral category. Why, in short, should a Kantian accept the basic claim in Kant's argument?

Hence, Kant's argument for the wrongness of inflicting pain on animals rests on a claim that, in a world of Kantian moral agents, is demonstrably false. Therefore, the alternative analysis, being more plausible anyway, should be accepted. Since this alternative analysis has the same structure as the anti-abortion argument being defended here, we have further support for the argument for the immorality of abortion being defended in this essay.

Of course, this value of a future-like-ours argument, if sound, shows only that abortion is prima facie wrong, not that it is wrong in any and all circumstances. Since the loss of the future to a standard fetus, if killed, is, however, at least as great a loss as the loss of the future to a standard adult human being who is killed, abortion, like ordinary killing, could be justified only by the most compelling reasons. The loss of one's life is almost the greatest misfortune that can happen to one. Presumably abortion could be justified in some circumstances, only if the loss consequent on failing to abort would be at least as great. Accordingly, morally permissible abortions will be rare indeed unless, perhaps, they occur so early in pregnancy that a fetus is not yet definitely an individual. Hence, this argument should be taken as showing that abortion is presumptively very seriously wrong, where the presumption is very strong—as strong as the presumption that killing another adult human being is wrong.

## III

How complete an account of the wrongness of killing does the value of a future-like-ours account have to be in order that the wrongness of abortion is a consequence? This account does not have to be an account of the necessary conditions for the wrongness of killing. Some persons in nursing homes may lack valuable human futures, yet it may be wrong to kill them for other reasons. Furthermore, this account does not obviously have to be the sole reason killing is wrong where the victim did have a valuable future. This analysis claims only that, for any killing where the victim did have a valuable future like ours, having that future by itself is sufficient to create the strong presumption that the killing is seriously wrong.

One way to overturn the value of a future-like-ours argument would be to find some account of the wrongness of killing which is at least as intelligible and which has different implications for the ethics of abortion. Two rival accounts possess at least some degree of plausibility. One account is based on the obvious fact that people value the experience of living and wish for that valuable experience to continue. Therefore, it might be said, what makes killing wrong is the discontinuation of that experience for the victim. Let us call this the *discontinuation account*.[10] Another rival account is based upon the obvious fact that people strongly desire to continue to live. This suggests that what makes killing us so wrong is that it interferes with the fulfillment of a strong and fundamental desire, the fulfillment of which is necessary for the fulfillment of any other desires we might have. Let us call this the *desire account*.[11]

Consider first the desire account as a rival account of the ethics of killing which would provide the basis for rejecting the anti-abortion position. Such an account will have to be stronger than the value of a future-like-ours account of the wrongness of abortion if it is to do the job expected of it. To entail the wrongness of abortion, the value of a future-like-ours account has only to provide a sufficient, but not a necessary condition for the wrongness of killing. The desire account, on the other hand, must provide us also with a necessary condition for the wrongness of killing in order to generate a pro-choice conclusion on abortion. The reason for this is that presumably the argument from the desire account moves from the claim that what makes killing wrong is interference with a very strong desire to the claim that abortion is not wrong because the fetus lacks a strong desire to live. Obviously, this inference fails if someone's having the desire to live is not a necessary condition of its being wrong to kill that individual.

One problem with the desire account is that we do regard it as seriously wrong to kill persons who have little desire to live or who have no desire to

live or, indeed, have a desire not to live. We believe it is seriously wrong to kill
the unconscious, the sleeping, those who are tired of life, and those who are
suicidal. The value-of-a-human-future account renders standard morality intelligible in these cases; these cases appear to be incompatible with the desire
account.

The desire account is subject to a deeper difficulty. We desire life, because
we value the goods of this life. The goodness of life is not secondary to our desire for it. If this were not so, the pain of one's own premature death could be
done away with merely by an appropriate alteration in the configuration of
one's desires. This is absurd. Hence, it would seem that it is the loss of the
goods of one's future, not the interference with the fulfillment of a strong desire to live, which accounts ultimately for the wrongness of killing.

It is worth noting that, if the desire account is modified so that it does not
provide a necessary, but only a sufficient, condition for the wrongness of
killing, the desire account is compatible with the value of a future-like-ours account. The combined accounts will yield an anti-abortion ethic. This suggests
that one can retain what is intuitively plausible about the desire account without a challenge to the basic argument of this essay.

It is also worth noting that, if future desires have moral force in a modified desire account of the wrongness of killing, one can find support for an
anti-abortion ethic even in the absence of a value of a future-like-ours account.
If one decides that a morally relevant property, the possession of which is sufficient to make it wrong to kill some individual, is the desire at some future
time to live--one might decide to justify one's refusal to kill suicidal teenagers
on these grounds, for example—then, since typical fetuses will have the desire
in the future to live, it is wrong to kill typical fetuses. Accordingly, it does not
seem that a desire account of the wrongness of killing can provide a justification of a pro-choice ethic of abortion which is nearly as adequate as the value
of a human-future justification of an anti-abortion ethic.

The discontinuation account looks more promising as an account of the
wrongness of killing. It seems just as intelligible as the value of a future-like-
ours account, but it does not justify an anti-abortion position. Obviously, if it is
the continuation of one's activities, experiences, and projects, the loss of which
makes killing wrong, then it is not wrong to kill fetuses for that reason, for fetuses do not have experiences, activities, and projects to be continued or discontinued. Accordingly, the discontinuation account does not have the anti-
abortion consequences that the value of a future-like-ours account has. Yet it
seems as intelligible as the value of a future-like-ours account, for when we
think of what would be wrong with our being killed, it does seem as if it is the
discontinuation of what makes our lives worthwhile which makes killing us
wrong.

Is the discontinuation account just as good an account as the value of a
future-like-ours account? The discontinuation account will not be adequate at
all, if it does not refer to the *value* of the experience that may be discontinued.
One does not want the discontinuation account to make it wrong to kill a patient who begs for death and who is in severe pain that cannot be relieved

short of killing. (I leave open the question of whether it is wrong for other reasons.) Accordingly, the discontinuation account must be more than a bare discontinuation account. It must make some reference to the positive value of the patient's experiences. But, by the same token, the value of a future-like-ours account cannot be a bare future account either. Just having a future surely does not itself rule out killing the above patient. This account must make some reference to the value of the patient's future experiences and projects also. Hence, both accounts involve the value of experiences, projects, and activities. So far we still have symmetry between the accounts.

The symmetry fades, however, when we focus on the time period of the value of the experiences, etc., which has moral consequences. Although both accounts leave open the possibility that the patient in our example may be killed, this possibility is left open only in virtue of the utterly bleak future for the patient. It makes no difference whether the patient's immediate past contains intolerable pain, or consists in being in a coma (which we can imagine is a situation of indifference), or consists in a life of value. If the patient's future is a future of value, we want our account to make it wrong to kill the patient. If the patient's future is intolerable, whatever his or her immediate past, we want our account to allow killing the patient. Obviously, then, it is the value of that patient's future which is doing the work in rendering the morality of killing the patient intelligible.

This being the case, it seems clear that whether one has immediate past experiences or not does no work in the explanation of what makes killing wrong. The addition the discontinuation account makes to the value of a human future account is otiose. Its addition to the value-of-a-future account plays no role at all in rendering intelligible the wrongness of killing. Therefore, it can be discarded with the discontinuation account of which it is a part.

## IV

The analysis of the previous section suggests that alternative general accounts of the wrongness of killing are either inadequate or unsuccessful in getting around the anti-abortion consequences of the value of a future-like-ours argument. A different strategy for avoiding these anti-abortion consequences involves limiting the scope of the value of a future argument. More precisely, the strategy involves arguing that fetuses lack a property that is essential for the value-of-a-future argument (or for any anti-abortion argument) to apply to them.

One move of this sort is based upon the claim that a necessary condition of one's future being valuable is that one values it. Value implies a valuer. Given this, one might argue that, since fetuses cannot value their futures, their futures are not valuable to them. Hence, it does not seriously wrong them deliberately to end their lives.

This move fails, however, because of some ambiguities. Let us assume that something cannot be of value unless it is valued by someone. This does not entail that my life is of no value unless it is valued by me. I may think, in a

**196**

Part 5   Abortion

period of despair, that my future is of no worth whatsoever, but I may be wrong because others rightly see value—even great value—in it. Furthermore, my future can be valuable to me even if I do not value it. This is the case when a young person attempts suicide, but is rescued and goes on to significant human achievements. Such young people's futures are ultimately valuable to them, even though such futures do not seem to be valuable to them at the moment of attempted suicide. A fetus' future can be valuable to it in the same way. Accordingly, this attempt to limit the anti-abortion argument fails.

Another similar attempt to reject the anti-abortion position is based on Tooley's claim that an entity cannot possess the right to life unless it has the capacity to desire its continued existence. It follows that, since fetuses lack the conceptual capacity to desire to continue to live, they lack the right to life. Accordingly, Tooley concludes that abortion cannot be seriously prima facie wrong.[12]

What could be the evidence for Tooley's basic claim? Tooley once argued that individuals have a prima facie right to what they desire and that the lack of the capacity to desire something undercuts the basis of one's right to it.[13] This argument plainly will not succeed in the context of the analysis of this essay, however, since the point here is to establish the fetus' right to life on other grounds. Tooley's argument assumes that the right to life cannot be established in general on some basis other than the desire for life. This position was considered and rejected in the preceding section.

One might attempt to defend Tooley's basic claim on the grounds that, because a fetus cannot apprehend continued life as a benefit, its continued life cannot be a benefit or cannot be something it has a right to or cannot be something that is in its interest. This might be defended in terms of the general proposition that, if an individual is literally incapable of caring about or taking an interest in some $X$, then one does not have a right to $X$ or $X$ is not a benefit or $X$ is not something that is in one's interest.[14]

Each member of this family of claims seems to be open to objections. As John C. Stevens has pointed out, one may have a right to be treated with a certain medical procedure (because of a health insurance policy one has purchased), even though one cannot conceive of the nature of the procedure.[15] And, as Tooley himself has pointed out, persons who have been indoctrinated, or drugged, or rendered temporarily unconscious may be literally incapable of caring about or taking an interest in something that is in their interest or is something to which they have a right, or is something that benefits them. Hence, the Tooley claim that would restrict the scope of the value of a future-like-ours argument is undermined by counterexamples.[16]

Finally, Paul Bassen has argued that even though the prospects of an embryo might seem to be a basis for the wrongness of abortion, an embryo cannot be a victim and therefore cannot be wronged.[17] An embryo cannot be a victim, he says, because it lacks sentience. His central argument for this seems to be that even though plants and the permanently unconscious are alive, they clearly cannot be victims. What is the explanation of this? Bassen claims that the explanation is that their lives consist of mere metabolism, and mere metabolism is not enough to ground victimizability. Mentation is required.

The problem with this attempt to establish the absence of victimizability is that both plants and the permanently unconscious clearly lack what Bassen calls "prospects" or what I have called "a future life like ours." Hence, it is surely open to one to argue that the real reason we believe plants and the permanently unconscious cannot be victims is that killing them cannot deprive them of a future life like ours; the real reason is not their absence of present mentation.

Bassen recognizes that his view is subject to this difficulty, and he recognizes that the case of children seems to support this difficulty, for "much of what we do for children is based on prospects." He argues, however, that in the case of children and in other such cases, "potentiality comes into play only where victimizability has been secured on other grounds."[18]

Bassen's defense of his view is patently question-begging, since what is adequate to secure victimizability is exactly what is at issue. His examples do not support his own view against the thesis of this essay. Of course, embryos can be victims: when their lives are deliberately terminated, they are deprived of their futures of value, their prospects. This makes them victims, for it directly wrongs them.

The seeming plausibility of Bassen's view stems from the fact that paradigmatic cases of imagining someone as a victim involve empathy, and empathy requires mentation of the victim. The victims of flood, famine, rape, or child abuse are all persons with whom we can empathize. That empathy seems to be part of seeing them as victims.[19]

In spite of the strength of these examples, the attractive intuition that a situation in which there is victimization requires the possibility of empathy is subject to counterexamples. Consider a case that Bassen himself offers: "Posthumous obliteration of an author's work constitutes a misfortune for him only if he had wished his work to endure."[20] The conditions Bassen wishes to impose upon the possibility of being victimized here seem far too strong. Perhaps this author, due to his unrealistic standards of excellence and his low self-esteem, regarded his work as unworthy of survival, even though it possessed genuine literary merit. Destruction of such work would surely victimize its author. In such a case, empathy with the victim concerning the loss is clearly impossible.

Of course, Bassen does not make the possibility of empathy a necessary condition of victimizability; he requires only mentation. Hence, on Bassen's actual view, this author, as I have described him, can be a victim. The problem is that the basic intuition that renders Bassen's view plausible is missing in the author's case. In order to attempt to avoid counterexamples, Bassen has made his thesis too weak to be supported by the intuitions that suggested it.

Even so, the mentation requirement on victimizability is still subject to counterexamples. Suppose a severe accident renders me totally unconscious for a month, after which I recover. Surely killing me while I am unconscious victimizes me, even though I am incapable of mentation during that time. It follows that Bassen's thesis fails. Apparently, attempts to restrict the value of a future-like-ours argument so that fetuses do not fall within its scope do not succeed.

## V

In this essay, it has been argued that the correct ethic of the wrongness of killing can be extended to fetal life and used to show that there is a strong presumption that any abortion is morally impermissible. If the ethic of killing adopted here entails, however, that contraception is also seriously immoral, then there would appear to be a difficulty with the analysis of this essay.

But this analysis does not entail that contraception is wrong. Of course, contraception prevents the actualization of a possible future of value. Hence, it follows from the claim that futures of value should be maximized that contraception is prima facie immoral. This obligation to maximize does not exist, however; furthermore, nothing in the ethics of killing in this paper entails that it does. The ethics of killing in this essay would entail that contraception is wrong only if something were denied a human future of value by contraception. Nothing at all is denied such a future by contraception, however.

Candidates for a subject of harm by contraception fall into four categories: (1) some sperm or other, (2) some ovum or other, (3) a sperm and an ovum separately, and (4) a sperm and an ovum together. Assigning the harm to some sperm is utterly arbitrary, for no reason can be given for making a sperm the subject of harm rather than an ovum. Assigning the harm to some ovum is utterly arbitrary, for no reason can be given for making an ovum the subject of harm rather than a sperm. One might attempt to avoid these problems by insisting that contraception deprives both the sperm and the ovum separately of a valuable future like ours. On this alternative, too many futures are lost. Contraception was supposed to be wrong because it deprived us of one future of value, not two. One might attempt to avoid this problem by holding that contraception deprives the combination of sperm and ovum of a valuable future like ours. But here the definite article misleads. At the time of contraception, there are hundreds of millions of sperm, one (released) ovum, and millions of possible combinations of all of these. There is no actual combination at all. Is the subject of the loss to be a merely possible combination? Which one? This alternative does not yield an actual subject of harm either. Accordingly, the immorality of contraception is not entailed by the loss of a future-like-ours argument, simply because there is no nonarbitrarily identifiable subject of the loss in the case of contraception.

## VI

The purpose of this essay has been to set out an argument for the serious presumptive wrongness of abortion subject to the assumption that the moral permissibility of abortion stands or falls on the moral status of the fetus. Since a fetus possesses a property, the possession of which in adult human beings is sufficient to make killing an adult human being wrong, abortion is wrong. This way of dealing with the problem of abortion seems superior to other approaches to the ethics of abortion, because it rests on an ethics of killing which is close to self-evident, because the crucial morally relevant property clearly applies to fetuses, and because the argument avoids the usual equivocations on "human life," "human being," or "person." The argument rests neither on religious claims nor on papal dogma. It is not subject to the objection of "speciesism." Its soundness is compatible with the moral permissibility of euthanasia and contraception. It deals with our intuitions concerning young children.

Finally, this analysis can be viewed as resolving a standard problem—indeed, *the* standard problem—concerning the ethics of abortion. Clearly, it is wrong to kill adult human beings. Clearly, it is not wrong to end the life of some arbitrarily chosen single human cell. Fetuses seem to be like arbitrarily chosen human cells in some respects and like adult humans in other respects. The problem of the ethics of abortion is the problem of determining the fetal property that settles this moral controversy. The thesis of this essay is that the problem of the ethics of abortion, so understood, is solvable.

## NOTES

1. Joel Feinberg, "Abortion," in *Matters of Life and Death: New Introductory Essays in Moral Philosophy*, ed. Tom Regan (New York: Random House, 1986), pp. 256–93; Michael Tooley, "Abortion and Infanticide," *Philosophy and Public Affairs*, 11, no. 1 (1972), pp. 37–65, idem, *Abortion and Infanticide* (New York: Oxford University Press, 1984); Mary Anne Warren, "On the Moral and Legal Status of Abortion," *The Monist* 57, no. 1 (1973), pp. 43–61; H. Tristram Engelhardt Jr., "The Ontology of Abortion," *Ethics* 84, no. 3 (1974), pp. 217–34; L. W. Sumner, *Abortion and Moral Theory* (Princeton: Princeton University Press, 1981); John T. Noonan Jr., "An Almost Absolute Value in History," in *The Morality of Abortion: Legal and Historical Perspectives*, ed. Noonan (Cambridge: Harvard University Press, 1970); and Philip Devine, *The Ethics of Homicide* (Ithaca: Cornell University Press, 1978).
2. For interesting discussions of this issue, see Warren Quinn, "Abortion: Identity and Loss," *Philosophy and Public Affairs* 13, no. 1 (1984), pp. 24–54; and Lawrence C. Becker, "Human Being: The Boundaries of the Concept," *Philosophy and Public Affairs* 4, no. 4 (1975), pp. 334–59.
3. See, e.g., Don Marquis, "Ethics and the Elderly: Some Problems," in *Aging and the Elderly: Humanistic Perspectives in Gerontology*, ed. Stuart Spicker, Kathleen Woodward, and David Van Tassel (Atlantic Highlands, NJ: Humanities Press, 1978), pp. 341–55.
4. See Warren, "Moral and Legal Status"; and Tooley, "Abortion and Infanticide."

5. This seems to be the fatal flaw in Warren's treatment of this issue.

6. Feinberg, "Abortion," p. 270.

7. I have been most influenced on this matter by Jonathan Glover, *Causing Death and Saving Lives* (New York: Penguin, 1977), chap. 3; and Robert Young, "What Is So Wrong with Killing People?" *Philosophy* 54, no. 210 (1979), pp. 515–28.

8. Feinberg, Tooley, Warren, and Engelhardt have all dealt with this problem.

9. Immanuel Kant, "Duties to Animals and Spirits," in *Lectures on Ethics*, trans. Louis Infeld (New York: Harper, 1963), p. 239.

10. I am indebted to Jack Bricke for raising this objection.

11. Presumably a preference utilitarian would press such an objection. Tooley once suggested that his account has such a theoretical underpinning; "Abortion and Infanticide," pp. 44–45.

12. Tooley, "Abortion and Infanticide," pp. 46–47.

13. Ibid., pp. 44–45.

14. Donald VanDeVeer seems to think this is self-evident; see his "Whither Baby Doe?" in Regan, *Matters of Life and Death*, p. 233.

15. John C. Stevens, "Must the Bearer of a Right Have the Concept of That to Which He Has a Right?" *Ethics* 95, no. 1 (1984), pp. 68–74.

16. See Tooley, "Abortion and Infanticide," pp. 47–49.

17. Paul Bassen, "Present Sakes and Future Prospects: The Status of Early Abortion," *Philosophy and Public Affairs* 11, no. 4 (1982), pp. 322–26.

18. Ibid., p. 333.

19. Note carefully the reasons he gives on the bottom of ibid., p. 316.

20. Ibid., p. 318.

## PART SIX

# Imperiled Newborns

# Abortion and Infanticide

## Michael Tooley

*The following essay by Michael Tooley appeared in* Philosophy and Public Affairs *a year after Judith Thomson's famous article. This piece is notable for two distinct claims.*

*First, Tooley argues that one's position on abortion and infanticide should be consistent. For example, if one believes that a genetic impairment of the fetus justifies an abortion during the second trimester, then why shouldn't a similar impairment, discovered at birth, justify killing the newborn? Does visibility make so much difference that inconsistency can be allowed? With this point Tooley makes it clear that justifications about abortion could be linked in a "slippery slope" of justification to an expanding range of cases.*

*Second, Tooley distinguishes between humans and persons and proposes a criterion for when a person cannot be killed. To be a person, Tooley argues, is to be a subject who can desire his continued existence. (In this regard Tooley anticipates Don Marquis' objections to abortion in Selection 14.)*

*Michael Tooley is professor of philosophy at the University of Colorado at Boulder.*

This essay deals with the question of the morality of abortion and infanticide. The fundamental ethical objection traditionally advanced against these practices rests on the contention that human fetuses and infants have a right to life. It is this claim which will be the focus of attention here. The basic issue to be discussed, then, is what properties a thing must possess in order to have a serious right to life. My approach will be to set out and defend a basic moral principle specifying a condition an organism must satisfy if it is to have a serious right to life. It will be seen that this condition is not satisfied by human

*Source: Philosophy and Public Affairs* 2, no. 1 (1972), pp. 29–65. Reprinted by permission of publisher. The author is grateful to a number of people, particularly the editors of *Philosophy and Public Affairs*, Rodelia Hapke, and Walter Kaufmann, for their helpful comments. It should not, of course, be inferred that they share the views expressed in this essay.

fetuses and infants, and thus that they do not have a right to life. So unless there are other substantial objections to abortion and infanticide, one is forced to conclude that these practices are morally acceptable ones. In contrast, it may turn out that our treatment of adult members of other species—cats, dogs, polar bears—is morally indefensible. For it is quite possible that such animals do possess properties that endow them with a right to life.

## I. ABORTION AND INFANTICIDE

One reason the question of the morality of infanticide is worth examining is that it seems very difficult to formulate a completely satisfactory liberal position on abortion without coming to grips with the infanticide issue. The problem the liberal encounters is essentially that of specifying a cutoff point which is not arbitrary: at what stage in the development of a human being does it cease to be morally permissible to destroy it? It is important to be clear about the difficulty here. The conservative's objection is not that since there is a continuous line of development from a zygote to a newborn baby, one must conclude that if it is seriously wrong to destroy a newborn baby it is also seriously wrong to destroy a zygote or any intermediate stage in the development of a human being. His point is rather that if one says it is wrong to destroy a newborn baby but not a zygote or some intermediate stage in the development of a human being, one should be prepared to point to a *morally relevant* difference between a newborn baby and the earlier stage in the development of a human being.

Precisely the same difficulty can, of course, be raised for a person who holds that infanticide is morally permissible. The conservative will ask what morally relevant differences there are between an adult human being and a newborn baby. What makes it morally permissible to destroy a baby, but wrong to kill an adult? So the challenge remains. But I will argue that in this case there is an extremely plausible answer.

Reflecting on the morality of infanticide forces one to face up to this challenge. In the case of abortion a number of events—quickening or viability, for instance—might be taken as cutoff points, and it is easy to overlook the fact that one of these events involves any morally significant change in the developing human. In contrast, if one is going to defend infanticide, one has to get very clear about what makes something a person, what gives something a right to life.

One of the interesting ways in which the abortion issue differs from most other moral issues is that the plausible positions on abortion appear to be extreme positions. For if a human fetus is a person, one is inclined to say that, in general, one would be justified in killing it only to save the life of the mother.[1] Such is the extreme conservative position.[2] On the other hand, if the fetus is not a person, how can it be seriously wrong to destroy it? Why would one need to point to special circumstances to justify such action? The upshot is that there is no room for a moderate position on the issue of abortion such as one finds, for example, in the *Model Penal Code* recommendations.[3]

Aside from the light it may shed on the abortion question, the issue of infanticide is both interesting and important in its own right. The theoretical interest has been mentioned: it forces one to face up to the question of what makes something a person. The practical importance need not be labored. Most people would prefer to raise children who do not suffer from gross deformities or from severe physical, emotional, or intellectual handicaps. If it could be shown that there is no moral objection to infanticide the happiness of society could be significantly and justifiably increased.

Infanticide is also of interest because of the strong emotions it arouses. The typical reaction to infanticide is like the reaction to incest or cannibalism, or the reaction of previous generations to masturbation or oral sex. The response, rather than appealing to carefully formulated moral principles, is primarily visceral. When philosophers themselves respond in this way, offering no arguments, and dismissing infanticide out of hand, it is reasonable to suspect that one is dealing with a taboo rather than with a rational prohibition.[4] I shall attempt to show that this is in fact the case.

## II. TERMINOLOGY: "PERSON" VERSUS "HUMAN BEING"

How is the term "person" to be interpreted? I shall treat the concept of a person as a purely moral concept, free of all descriptive content (whereas "human" is a purely factual concept). Specifically, in my usage the sentence "X is a person" will be synonymous with the sentence "X has a (serious) moral right to life.". . .

The tendency to use expressions like "person" and "human being" interchangeably is an unfortunate one. For one thing, it tends to lend covert support to antiabortionist positions. Given such usage, one who holds a liberal view of abortion is put in the position of maintaining that fetuses, at least up to a certain point, are not human beings. Even philosophers are led astray by this usage. . . .

It should now be clear why the common practice of using expressions such as "person" and "human being" interchangeably in discussions of abortion is unfortunate. It would perhaps be best to avoid the term "human" altogether, employing instead some expression that is more naturally interpreted as referring to a certain type of biological organism characterized in physiological terms, such as "member of the species *Homo sapiens*." My own approach will be to use the term "human" only in contexts where it is not philosophically dangerous.

## III. THE BASIC ISSUE: WHEN IS A MEMBER OF THE SPECIES *HOMO SAPIENS* A PERSON?

Settling the issue of the morality of abortion and infanticide will involve answering the following questions: What properties must something have to be a person, i.e., to have a serious right to life? At what point in the development of a member of the species *Homo sapiens* does the organism possess the properties that make it a person? The first question raises a moral issue. To answer it is to decide what basic moral principles involving the ascription of a right to life one ought to accept.[5] The second question raises a purely factual issue, since the properties in question are properties of a purely descriptive sort.

Some writers seem quite pessimistic about the possibility of resolving the question of the morality of abortion. Indeed, some have gone so far as to suggest that the question of whether the fetus is a person is in principle unanswerable: "we seem to be stuck with the indeterminateness of the fetus' humanity.[6] An understanding of some of the sources of this pessimism will, I think, help us to tackle the problem. Let us begin by considering the similarity a number of people have noted between the issue of abortion and the issue of Negro slavery. The question here is why it should be more difficult to decide whether abortion and infanticide are acceptable than it was to decide whether slavery was acceptable. The answer seems to be that in the case of slavery there are moral principles of a quite uncontroversial sort that settle the issue. Thus most people would agree to some such principle as the following: No organism that has experiences, that is capable of thought and of using language, and that has harmed no one, should be made a slave. In the case of abortion, on the other hand, conditions that are generally agreed to be sufficient grounds for ascribing a right to life to something do not suffice to settle the issue. It is easy to specify other, purportedly sufficient conditions that will settle the issue, but no one has been successful in putting forward considerations that will convince others to accept those additional moral principles.

I do not share the general pessimism about the possibility of resolving the issue of abortion and infanticide because I believe it is possible to point to a very plausible moral principle dealing with the question of *necessary* conditions for something's having a right to life, where the conditions in question will provide an answer to the question of the permissibility of abortion and infanticide.

There is a second cause of pessimism that should be noted before proceeding. It is tied up with the fact that the development of an organism is one of gradual and continuous change. Given this continuity, how is one to draw a line at one point and declare it permissible to destroy a member of *Homo sapiens* up to, but not beyond, that point? Won't there be an arbitrariness about any point that is chosen? I will return to this worry shortly. It does not present a serious difficulty once the basic moral principles relevant to the ascription of a right to life to an individual are established.

Let us turn now to the first and most fundamental question: What properties must something have in order to be a person, i.e., to have a serious right to life? The claim I wish to defend is this: An organism possesses a serious right to life only if it possesses the concept of a self as a continuing subject of experiences and other mental states, and believes that it is itself such a continuing entity.

My basic argument in support of this claim, which I will call the self-consciousness requirement, will be clearest, I think, if I first offer a simplified version of the argument, and then consider a modification that seems desirable.

The simplified version of my argument is this. To ascribe a right to an individual is to assert something about the prima facie obligations of other individuals to act, or to refrain from acting, in certain ways. However, the obligations in question are conditional ones, being dependent upon the existence of certain desires of the individual to whom the right is ascribed. Thus if an individual asks one to destroy something to which he has a right, one does not violate his right to that thing if one proceeds to destroy it. This suggests the following analysis: "A has a right to X" is roughly synonymous with "If A desires X, then others are under a prima facie obligation to refrain from actions that would deprive him of it."[7]

Although this analysis is initially plausible, there are reasons for thinking it not entirely correct. I will consider these later. Even here, however, some expansion is necessary, since there are features of the concept of a right that are important in the present context, and that ought to be dealt with more explicitly. In particular, it seems to be a conceptual truth that things that lack consciousness, such as ordinary machines, cannot have rights. Does this conceptual truth follow from the above analysis of the concept of a right? The answer depends on how the term "desire" is interpreted. If one adopts a completely behavioristic interpretation of "desire," so that a machine that searches for an electrical outlet in order to get its batteries recharged is described as having a desire to be recharged, then it will not follow from this analysis that objects that lack consciousness cannot have rights. On the other hand, if "desire" is interpreted in such a way that desires are states necessarily standing in some sort of relationship to states of consciousness, it will follow from the analysis that a machine that is not capable of being conscious, and consequently of having desires, cannot have any rights. I think those who defend analyses of the concept of a right along the lines of this one do have in mind an interpretation of the term "desire" that involves reference to something more than behavioral dispositions. However, rather than relying on this, it seems preferable to make such an interpretation explicit. The following analysis is a natural way of doing that: "A has a right to X" is roughly synonymous with "A is the sort of thing that is a subject of experiences and other mental states, A is capable of desiring X, and if A does desire X, then others are under a prima facie obligation to refrain from actions that would deprive him of it."

The next step in the argument is basically a matter of applying this analysis to the concept of a right to life. Unfortunately the expression "right to life" is not entirely a happy one, since it suggests that the right in question concerns the continued existence of a biological organism. That this is incorrect can be brought out by considering possible ways of violating an individual's right to life. Suppose, for example, that by some technology of the future the brain of an adult human were to be completely reprogrammed, so that the organism wound up with memories (or rather, apparent memories), beliefs, attitudes, and personality traits completely different from those associated with it before it was subjected to reprogramming. In such a case one would surely say that an individual had been destroyed, that an adult human's right to life had been violated, even though no biological organism had been killed. This example shows that the expression "right to life" is misleading, since what one is really concerned about is not just the continued existence of a biological organism, but the right of a subject of experiences and other mental states to continue to exist.

Given this more precise description of the right with which we are here concerned, we are now in a position to apply the analysis of the concept of a right stated above. When we do so we find that the statement "A has a right to continue to exist as a subject of experiences and other mental states" is roughly synonymous with the statement "A is a subject of experiences and other mental states, A is capable of desiring to continue to exist as a subject of experiences and other mental states, and if A does desire to continue to exist as such an entity, then others are under a prima facie obligation not to prevent him from doing so."

The final stage in the argument is simply a matter of asking what must be the case if something is to be capable of having a desire to continue existing as a subject of experiences and other mental states. The basic point here is that the desires a thing can have are limited by the concepts it possesses. For the fundamental way of describing a given desire is as a desire that a certain proposition be true.[8] Then, since one cannot desire that a certain proposition be true unless one understands it, and since one cannot understand it without possessing the concepts involved in it, it follows that the desires one can have are limited by the concepts one possesses. Applying this to the present case results in the conclusion that an entity cannot be the sort of thing that can desire that a subject of experiences and other mental states exist unless it possesses the concept of such a subject. Moreover, an entity cannot desire that it itself *continue* existing as a subject of experiences and other mental states unless it believes that it is now such a subject. This completes the justification of the claim that it is a necessary condition of something's having a serious right to life that it possess the concept of a self as a continuing subject of experiences, and that it believe that it is itself such an entity. . . .

## IV.  SOME CRITICAL COMMENTS ON ALTERNATIVE PROPOSALS

I now want to compare the line of demarcation I am proposing with the cutoff points traditionally advanced in discussions of abortion. My fundamental claim will be that none of these cutoff points can be defended by appeal to plausible, basic moral principles. The main suggestions as to the point past which it is seriously wrong to destroy something that will develop into an adult member of the species *Homo sapiens* are these: (a) conception; (b) the attainment of human form; (c) the achievement of the ability to move about spontaneously; (d) viability; (e) birth.[9] The corresponding moral principles suggested by these cutoff points are as follows: (1) It is seriously wrong to kill an organism, from a zygote on, that belongs to the species *Homo sapiens*. (2) It is seriously wrong to kill an organism that belongs to *Homo sapiens* and that has achieved human form. (3) It is seriously wrong to kill an organism that is a member of *Homo sapiens* and that is capable of spontaneous movement. (4) It is seriously wrong to kill an organism that belongs to *Homo sapiens* and that is capable of existing outside the womb. (5) It is seriously wrong to kill an organism that is a member of *Homo sapiens* that is no longer in the womb.

My first comment is that it would not do *simply* to omit the reference to membership in the species *Homo sapiens* from the above principles, with the exception of principle (2). For then the principles would be applicable to animals in general, and one would be forced to conclude that it was seriously wrong to abort a cat fetus, or that it was seriously wrong to abort a motile cat fetus, and so on.

The second and crucial comment is that none of the five principles given above can plausibly be viewed as a *basic* moral principle. To accept any of them as such would be akin to accepting as a basic moral principle the proposition that it is morally permissible to enslave black members of the species *Homo sapiens* but not white members. Why should it be seriously wrong to kill an unborn member of the species *Homo sapiens* but not seriously wrong to kill an unborn kitten? Difference in species is not per se a morally relevant difference. If one holds that it is seriously wrong to kill an unborn member of the species *Homo sapiens* but not an unborn kitten, one should be prepared to point to some property that is morally significant and that is possessed by unborn members of *Homo sapiens* but not by unborn kittens. Similarly, such a property must be identified if one believes it seriously wrong to kill unborn members of *Homo sapiens* that have achieved viability but not seriously wrong to kill unborn kittens that have achieved that state.

What property might account for such a difference? That is to say, what *basic* moral principles might a person who accepts one of these five principles appeal to in support of his secondary moral judgment? Why should events such as the achievement of human form, or the achievement of the ability to move about, or the achievement of viability, or birth serve to endow something with a right to life? What the liberal must do is to show that these events involve changes, or are associated with changes, that are morally relevant.

Let us now consider reasons why the events involved in cutoff points (b) through (e) are not morally relevant, beginning with the last two: viability and birth. The fact that an organism is not physiologically dependent upon another organism, or is capable of such physiological independence, is surely irrelevant to whether the organism has a right to life. In defense of this contention, consider a speculative case where a fetus is able to learn a language while in the womb. One would surely not say that the fetus had no right to life until it emerged from the womb, or until it was capable of existing outside the womb. A less speculative example is the case of Siamese twins who have learned to speak. One doesn't want to say that since one of the twins would die were the two to be separated, it therefore has no right to life. Consequently it seems difficult to disagree with the conservative's claim that an organism which lacks a right to life before birth or before becoming viable cannot acquire this right immediately upon birth or upon becoming viable.

This does not, however, completely rule out viability as a line of demarcation. For instead of defending viability as a cutoff point on the ground that only then does a fetus acquire a right to life, it is possible to argue rather that when one organism is physiologically dependent upon another, the former's right to life may conflict with the latter's right to use its body as it will, and moreover, that the latter's right to do what it wants with its body may often take precedence over the other organism's right to life. Thomson has defended this view: "I am arguing only that having a right to life does not guarantee having either a right to the use of or a right to be allowed continued use of another person's body—even if one needs it for life itself. So the right to life will not serve the opponents of abortion in the very simple and clear way in which they seem to have thought it would."[10] I believe that Thomson is right in contending that philosophers have been altogether too casual in assuming that if one grants the fetus a serious right to life, one must accept a conservative position on abortion.[11] I also think the only defense of viability as a cutoff point which has any hope of success at all is one based on the considerations she advances. I doubt very much, however, that this defense of abortion is ultimately tenable. I think that one can grant even stronger assumptions than those made by Thomson and still argue persuasively for a semiconservative view. What I have in mind is this. Let it be granted, for the sake of argument, that a women's right to free her body of parasites which will inhibit her freedom of action and possibly impair her health is stronger than the parasite's right to life, and is so even if the parasite has as much right to life as an adult human. One can still argue that abortion ought not to be permitted. For if A's right is stronger than B's, and it is impossible to satisfy both, it does not follow that A's should be satisfied rather than B's. It may be possible to compensate A if his right isn't satisfied, but impossible to compensate B if his right isn't satisfied. In such a case the best thing to do may be to satisfy B's claim and to compensate A. Abortion may be a case in point. If the fetus has a right to life and the right is not satisfied, there is certainly no way the fetus can be compensated. On the other hand, if the woman's right to rid her body of harmful and annoying parasites is not satisfied, she can be compensated. Thus it would seem that the just thing to do would be to prohibit abortion, but to compensate women for the burden of carrying a parasite to term. Then, however, we are back at a (modified) conservative position.[12] Our conclusion must be that it appears unlikely there is any satisfactory defense either of viability or of birth as cutoff points.

Let us now consider the third suggested line of demarcation, the achievement of the power to move about spontaneously. It might be argued that acquiring this power is a morally relevant event on the grounds that there is a connection between the concept of an agent and the concept of a person, and being motile is an indication that a thing is an agent.[13]

It is difficult to respond to this suggestion unless it is made more specific. Given that one's interest here is in defending a certain cutoff point, it is natural to interpret the proposal as suggesting that motility is a necessary condition of an organism's having a right to life. But this won't do, because one certainly wants to ascribe a right to life to adult humans who are completely paralyzed. Maybe the suggestion is rather that motility is a sufficient condition of something's having a right to life. However, it is clear that motility alone is not sufficient, since this would imply that all animals, and also certain machines, have a right to life. Perhaps, then, the most reasonable interpretation of the claim is that motility together with some other property is a sufficient condition of something's having a right to life, where the other property will have to be a property possessed by unborn members of the species *Homo sapiens* but not by unborn members of other familiar species.

The central question, then, is what this other property is. Until one is told, it is very difficult to evaluate either the moral claim that motility together with that property is a sufficient basis for ascribing to an organism a right to life or the factual claim that a motile human fetus possesses that property while a motile fetus belonging to some other species does not. A conservative would presumably reject motility as a cutoff point by arguing that whether an organism has a right to life depends only upon its potentialities, which are of course not changed by its becoming motile. If, on the other hand, one favors a liberal view of abortion, I think that one can attack this third suggested cutoff point, in its unspecified form, only by determining what properties are necessary, or what properties sufficient, for an individual to have a right to life. Thus I would base my rejection of motility as a cutoff point on my claim, defended above, that a necessary condition of an organism's possessing a right to life is that it conceive of itself as a continuing subject of experiences and other mental states.

The second suggested cutoff point—the development of a recognizably human form—can be dismissed fairly quickly. I have already remarked that membership in a particular species is not itself a morally relevant property. For it is obvious that if we encountered other "rational animals," such as Martians, the fact that their physiological makeup was very different from our own would not be grounds for denying them a right to life.[14] Similarly, it is clear that the development of human form is not in itself a morally relevant event. Nor do there seem to be any grounds for holding that there is some other change, associated with this event, that is morally relevant. The appeal of this second cutoff point is, I think, purely emotional.

The overall conclusion seems to be that it is very difficult to defend the cutoff points traditionally advanced by those who advocate either a moderate or a liberal position on abortion. The reason is that there do not seem to be any basic moral principles one can appeal to in support of the cutoff points in question. We must now consider whether the conservative is any better off.

## V.  REFUTATION OF THE CONSERVATIVE POSITION

Many have felt that the conservative's position is more defensible than the liberal's because the conservative can point to the gradual and continuous development of an organism as it changes from a zygote to an adult human being.

He is then in a position to argue that it is morally arbitrary for the liberal to draw a line at some point in this continuous process and to say that abortion is permissible before, but not after, that particular point. The liberal's reply would presumably be that the emphasis upon the continuity of the process is misleading. What the conservative is really doing is simply challenging the liberal to specify the properties a thing must have in order to be a person, and to show that the developing organism does acquire the properties at the point selected by the liberal. The liberal may then reply that the difficulty he has meeting this challenge should not be taken as grounds for rejecting his position. For the conservative cannot meet this challenge either; the conservative is equally unable to say what properties something must have if it is to have a right to life.

Although this rejoinder does not dispose of the conservative's argument, it is not without bite. For defenders of the view that abortion is always wrong have failed to face up to the question of the basic moral principles on which their position rests. They have been content to assert the wrongness of killing any organism, from a zygote on, if that organism is a member of the species *Homo sapiens*. But they have overlooked the point that this cannot be an acceptable *basic* moral principle, since difference in species is not in itself a morally relevant difference. The conservative can reply, however, that it is possible to defend his position—but not the liberal's—*without* getting clear about the properties a thing must possess if it is to have a right to life. The conservative's defense will rest upon the following two claims: first, that there is a property, even if one is unable to specify what it is, that (i) is possessed by adult humans and (ii) endows any organism possessing it with a serious right to life. Second, that if there are properties which satisfy (i) and (ii) above, at least one of those properties will be such that any organism potentially possessing that property has a serious right to life even now, simply by virtue of that potentiality, where an organism possesses a property potentially if it will come to have that property in the normal course of its development. The second claim—which I shall refer to as the potentiality principle—is critical to the conservative's defense. Because of it he is able to defend his position without deciding what properties a thing must possess in order to have a right to life. It is enough to know that adult members of *Homo sapiens* do have such a right. For then one can conclude that any organism which belongs to the species *Homo sapiens*, from a zygote on, must also have a right to life by virtue of the potentiality principle.

The liberal, by contrast, cannot mount a comparable argument. He cannot defend his position without offering at least a partial answer to the question of what properties a thing must possess in order to have a right to life.

The importance of the potentiality principle, however, goes beyond the fact that it provides support for the conservative's position. If the principle is unacceptable, then so is his position. For if the conservative cannot defend the view that an organism's having certain potentialities is sufficient grounds for ascribing to it a right to life, his claim that a fetus which is a member of *Homo sapiens* has a right to life can be attacked as follows. The reason an adult member of *Homo sapiens* has a right to life, but an infant ape does not, is that there are certain psychological properties which the former possesses and the latter lacks. Now, even if one is unsure exactly what these psychological properties are, it is clear that an organism in the early stages of development from a zygote into an adult member of *Homo sapiens* does not possess these properties. One need merely compare a human fetus with an ape fetus. What mental states does the former enjoy that the latter does not? Surely it is reasonable to hold that there are no significant differences in their respective mental lives—assuming that one wishes to ascribe any mental states at all to such organisms. (Does a zygote have a mental life? Does it have experiences? Or beliefs? Or desires?) There are, of course, physiological differences, but these are not in themselves morally significant. *If* one held that potentialities were relevant to the ascription of a right to life, one could argue that the physiological differences, though not morally significant in themselves, are morally significant by virtue of their causal consequences: they will lead to later psychological differences that are morally relevant, and for this reason the physiological differences are themselves morally significant. But if the potentiality principle is not available, this line of argument cannot be used, and there will then be no differences between a human fetus and an ape fetus that the conservative can use as grounds for ascribing a serious right to life to the former but not to the latter.

It is therefore tempting to conclude that the conservative view of abortion is acceptable if and only if the potentiality principle is acceptable. But to say that the conservative position can be defended if the potentiality principle is acceptable is to assume that the argument is over once it is granted that the fetus has a right to life, and, as was noted above, Thomson has shown that there are serious grounds for questioning this assumption. In any case, the important point here is that the conservative position on abortion is acceptable *only if* the potentiality principle is sound.

One way to attack the potentiality principle is simply to argue in support of the self-consciousness requirement—the claim that only an organism that conceives of itself as a continuing subject of experiences has a right to life. For this requirement, when taken together with the claim that there is at least one property, possessed by adult humans, such that any organism possessing it has a serious right to life, entails the denial of the potentiality principle. Or at least this is so if we add the uncontroversial empirical claim that an organism that will in the normal course of events develop into an adult human does not from the very beginning of its existence possess a concept of a continuing subject of experiences together with a belief that it is itself such an entity.

I think it best, however, to scrutinize the potentiality principle itself, and not to base one's case against it simply on the self-consciousness requirement. Perhaps the first point to note is that the potentiality principle should not be confused with principles such as the following: the value of an object is related to the value of the things into which it can develop. This "valuation principle" is rather vague. There are ways of making it more precise, but we need not consider these here. Suppose now that one were to speak not of a right to life, but of the value of life. It would then be easy to make the mistake of thinking that the valuation principle was relevant to the potentiality principle—indeed, that it entailed it. But an individual's right to life is not based on the value of his life. To say that the world would be better off if it contained fewer people is not to say that it would be right to achieve such a better world by killing some of the present inhabitants. *If* having a right to life were a matter of a thing's value, then a thing's potentialities, being connected with its expected value, would clearly be relevant to the question of what rights it had. Conversely, once one realizes that a thing's rights are not a matter of its value, I think it becomes clear that an organism's potentialities are irrelevant to the question of whether it has a right to life. . . .

## VI.  SUMMARY AND CONCLUSIONS

Let us return now to my basic claim, the self-consciousness requirement: An organism possesses a serious right to life only if it possesses the concept of a self as a continuing subject of experiences and other mental states, and believes that it is itself such a continuing entity. My defense of this claim has been twofold. I have offered a direct argument in support of it, and I have tried to show that traditional conservative and liberal views on abortion and infanticide, which involve a rejection of it, are unsound. I now want to mention one final reason why my claim should be accepted. Consider the example of killing, as opposed to torturing, newborn kittens. . . . [W]hile in the case of adult humans most people would consider it worse to kill an individual than to torture him for an hour, we do not usually view the killing of a newborn kitten as morally outrageous, although we would regard someone who tortured a newborn kitten for an hour as heinously evil. . . . [A] possible conclusion that might be drawn from this is that newborn kittens have a right not to be tortured, but do not have a serious right to life. If this is the correct conclusion, how is one to explain it? One merit of the self-consciousness requirement is that it provides an explanation of this situation. The reason a newborn kitten does not have a right to life is explained by the fact that it does not possess the concept of a self. But how is one to explain the kitten's having a right not to be tortured? The answer is that a desire not to suffer pain can be ascribed to something without assuming that it has any concept of a continuing self. For while something that lacks the concept of a self cannot desire that a self not suffer, it can desire that a given sensation not exist. The state desired—the absence of a particular sensation, or of sensations of a certain sort—can be described in a purely phenomenalistic language, and hence without the concept of a continuing self. So long as the newborn kitten possesses the relevant phenomenal concepts, it can truly be said to desire that a certain sensation not exist. So we can ascribe to it a right not to be tortured even though, since it lacks the concept of a continuing self, we cannot ascribe to it a right to life.

This completes my discussion of the basic moral principles involved in the issue of abortion and infanticide. But I want to comment upon an important factual question, namely, at what point an organism comes to possess the concept of a self as a continuing subject of experiences and other mental states, together with the belief that it is itself such a continuing entity. This is obviously a matter for detailed psychological investigation, but everyday observation makes it perfectly clear, I believe, that a newborn baby does not possess the concept of a continuing self, any more than a newborn kitten possesses such a concept. If so, infanticide during a time interval shortly after birth must be morally acceptable.

But where is the line to be drawn? What is the cutoff point? If one maintained, as some philosophers have, that an individual possesses concepts only if he can express these concepts in language, it would be a matter of everyday observation whether or not a given organism possessed the concept of a continuing self. Infanticide would then be permissible up to the time an organism learned how to use certain expressions. However, I think the claim that acquisition of concepts is dependent on acquisition of language is mistaken. For example, one wants to ascribe mental states of a conceptual sort—such as beliefs and desires—to organisms that are incapable of learning a language. This issue of prelinguistic understanding is clearly outside the scope of this discussion. My point is simply that *if* an organism can acquire concepts without thereby acquiring a way of expressing those concepts linguistically, the question of whether a given organism possesses the concept of a self as a continuing subject of experiences and other mental states, together with the belief that it is itself such a continuing entity, may be a question that requires fairly subtle experimental techniques to answer.

If this view of the matter is roughly correct, there are two worries one is left with at the level of practical moral decisions, one of which may turn out to be deeply disturbing. The lesser worry is where the line is to be drawn in the case of infanticide. It is not troubling because there is no serious need to know the exact point at which a human infant acquires a right to life. For in the vast majority of cases in which infanticide is desirable, its desirability will be apparent within a short time after birth. Since it is virtually certain that an infant at such a stage of its development does not possess the concept of a continuing self, and thus does not possess a serious right to life, there is excellent reason to believe that infanticide is morally permissible in most cases where it is otherwise desirable. The practical moral problem can thus be satisfactorily handled by choosing some period of time, such as a week after birth, as the interval during which infanticide will be permitted. This interval could then be modified once psychologists have established the point at which a human organism comes to believe that it is a continuing subject of experiences and other mental states.

The troubling worry is whether adult animals belonging to species other than *Homo sapiens* may not also possess a serious right to life. For once one says that an organism can possess the concept of a continuing self, together with the belief that it is itself such an entity, without having any way of expressing that concept and that belief linguistically, one has to face up to the question of whether animals may not possess properties that bestow a serious right to life upon them. The suggestion itself is a familiar one, and one that most of us are accustomed to dismiss very casually. The line of thought advanced here suggests that this attitude may turn out to be tragically mistaken. Once one reflects upon the question of the *basic* moral principles involved in the ascription of a right to life to organisms, one may find himself driven to conclude that our everyday treatment of animals is morally indefensible, and that we are in fact murdering innocent persons.

## NOTES

1. Judith Jarvis Thomson, in "A Defense of Abortion," *Philosophy and Public Affairs* 1, no. 1 (Fall 1971), pp. 47–66, has argued with great force and ingenuity that this conclusion is mistaken. I will comment on her argument later in this paper.
2. While this is the position conservatives tend to hold, it is not clear that it is the position they ought to hold. For if the fetus is a person it is far from clear that it is permissible to destroy it to save the mother. Two moral principles lend support to the view that it is the fetus which should live. First, other things being equal, should not one give something to a person who has had less rather than to a person who has had more? The mother has had a chance to live, while the fetus has not. The choice is thus between giving the mother more of an opportunity to live while giving the fetus none at all and giving the fetus an opportunity to enjoy life while not giving the mother a further opportunity to do so. Surely fairness requires the latter. Secondly, since the fetus has a greater life expectancy than the mother, one is in effect distributing more goods by choosing the life of the fetus over the life of the mother.

   The position I am here recommending to the conservative should not be confused with the official Catholic position. The Catholic church holds that it is seriously wrong to kill a fetus directly even if failure to do so will result in the death of *both* the mother and the fetus. This perverse value judgment is not part of the conservative's position.
3. Section 230.3 of the American Law Institute's *Model Penal Code* (Philadelphia, 1962). There is some interesting, though at times confused, discussion of the proposed code in *Model Penal Code—Tentative Draft No. 9* (Philadelphia: American Law Institute, 1959), pp. 146–62.
4. A clear example of such an unwillingness to entertain seriously the possibility that moral judgments widely accepted in one's own society may nevertheless be incorrect is provided by Roger Wertheimer's superficial dismissal of infanticide in "Understanding the Abortion Argument," *Philosophy and Public Affairs* 1, no. 1 (Fall 1971), pp. 69–70.
5. A moral principle accepted by a person is *basic for him* if and only if his acceptance of it is not dependent upon any of his (nonmoral) factual beliefs. That is, no change in his factual beliefs would cause him to abandon the principle in question.

6. Wertheimer, "Understanding the Abortion Argument," p. 88.

7. Compare the analysis defended by Brandt, *Ethical Theory*, pp. 434–41.

8. In everyday life one often speaks of desiring things, such as an apple or a newspaper. Such talk is elliptical, the context together with one's ordinary beliefs serving to make it clear that one wants to eat the apple and read the newspaper. To say that what one desires is that a certain proposition be true should not be construed as involving any particular ontological commitment. The point is merely that it is sentences such as "John wants it to be the case that he is eating an apple in the next few minutes" that provide a completely explicit description of a person's desires. If one fails to use such sentences one can be badly misled about what concepts are presupposed by a particular desire.

9. Another frequent suggestion as to the cutoff point not listed here is quickening. I omit it because it seems clear that if abortion after quickening is wrong, its wrongness must be tied up with the motility of the fetus, not with the mother's awareness of the fetus' ability to move about.

10. Thomson, "A Defense of Abortion," p. 56.

11. A good example of a failure to probe this issue is Brody, "Abortion and the Law."

12. Admittedly the modification is a substantial one, since given a society that refused to compensate women, a woman who had an abortion would not be doing anything wrong.

13. Compare Wertheimer, "Understanding the Abortion Argument," p. 79.

14. This requires qualification. If their central nervous systems were radically different from ours, it might be thought that one would not be justified in ascribing to them mental states of an experiential sort. And then, since it seems to be a conceptual truth that only things having experiential states can have rights, one would be forced to conclude that one was not justified in ascribing any rights to them.

# Involuntary Euthanasia of Defective Newborns

## *John A. Robertson*

*In this selection, law professor John Robertson rejects the claim of Michael Tooley that seriously defective human infants are not persons. He also rejects utilitarian and quality-of-life arguments that imply that such infants are better off not existing.*

*The strategy of argument used here may be characterized as "onus of proof." The claim that an infant is better off dead, Robertson argues, is difficult to substantiate from the point of view of an infant who has known no other life.*

Nontreatment of defective newborns has occurred throughout history, but only recently has the medical profession openly acknowledged the scope and alleged desirability of the practice. In 1973, Doctors Raymond S. Duff and A. G. M. Campbell documented 43 cases of withholding care from defective infants at the Yale–New Haven Hospital, thereby breaking what they characterized as "public and professional silence on a major social taboo." Subsequently, similar cases across the country have received widespread public attention . . .

[This article] considers two arguments in favor of withholding necessary but ordinary medical care from defective infants, and concludes that neither is persuasive. It then considers whether, given the appropriateness of failing to treat some infants, parents and physicians should be given discretion to make such decisions, and suggests an alternative solution to the issue of who should decide.

*Source:* "Involuntary Euthanasia of Defective Newborns: A Legal Analysis," *Stanford Law Review* 27 (1975), pp. 246–61. Copyright 1975 by the board of trustees of the LeLand Stanford Junior University. Reprinted by permission. The notes in this essay have been omitted because of their great length. For biographical information about John A. Robertson, see the introduction to Selection 11.

# ARGUMENTS IN FAVOR OF WITHHOLDING ORDINARY MEDICAL CARE FROM DEFECTIVE INFANTS

## Defective Infants Are Not Persons

Children born with congenital malformations may lack human form and the possibility of ordinary, psychosocial development. In many cases mental retardation is or will be so profound, and physical incapacity so great, that the term "persons" or "humanly alive" has odd or questionable meaning when applied to them. In these cases the infant's physical and mental defects are so severe that they will never know anything but a vegetative existence, with no discernible personality, sense of self, or capacity to interact with others. Withholding ordinary medical care in such cases, one may argue, is justified on the ground that these infants are not persons or human beings in the ordinary or legal sense of the term, and therefore do not possess the right of care that persons possess.

Central to this argument is the idea that living products of the human uterus can be classified into offspring that are persons, and those that are not. Conception and birth by human parents does not automatically endow one with personhood and its accompanying rights. Some other characteristic or feature must be present in the organism for personhood to vest, and this the defective infant arguably lacks. Lacking that property, an organism is not a person or deserving to be treated as such.

Before considering what "morally significant features" might distinguish persons from nonpersons, and examining the relevance of such features to the case of the defective infant, we must face an initial objection to this line of inquiry. The objection questions the need for any distinction among human offspring because of

> the monumental misuse of the concept of "humanity" in so many practices of discrimination and atrocity throughout history. Slavery, witchhunts, and wars have all been justified by their perpetrators on the grounds that they held their victims to be less than fully human. The insane and the criminal have for long periods been deprived of the most basic necessities for similar reasons, and been excluded from society . . .
>
>    . . . Even when entered upon with the best of intentions, and in the most guarded manner, the enterprise of basing the protection of human life upon such criteria and definitions is dangerous. To question someone's humanity or personhood is a first step to mistreatment and killing.[1]

Hence, according to this view, human parentage is a necessary and sufficient condition for personhood, whatever the characteristics of the offspring, because qualifying criteria inevitably lead to abuse and untold suffering to beings who are unquestionably human. Moreover, the human species is sufficiently different from other sentient species that assigning its members greater rights on birth alone is not arbitrary.

This objection is indeed powerful. The treatment accorded slaves in the United States, the Nazi denial of personal status to non-Aryans, and countless other incidents testify that man's inhumanity to man is indeed greatest when a putative nonperson is involved. Arguably, however, a distinction based on gross physical form, profound mental incapacity, and the very existence of personality or selfhood, besides having an empirical basis in the monstrosities and mutations known to have been born to women, is a basic and fundamental one. Rather than distinguishing among the particular characteristics that persons might attain through the contingencies of race, culture, and class, it merely separates out those who lack the potential for assuming any personal characteristics beyond breathing and consciousness.

This reply narrows the issue: should such creatures be cared for, protected, or regarded as "ordinary" humans? If such treatment is not warranted, they may be treated as nonpersons. The arguments supporting care in all circumstances are based on the view that all living creatures are sacred, contain a spark of the divine, and should be so regarded. Moreover, identifying those human offspring unworthy of care is a difficult task and will inevitably take a toll on those whose humanity cannot seriously be questioned. At this point the argument becomes metaphysical or religious and immune to resolution by empirical evidence, not unlike the controversy over whether a fetus is a person. It should be noted, however, that recognizing all human offspring as persons, like recognizing the fetus to be a person, does not conclude the treatment issue.

Although this debate can be resolved only by reference to religious or moral beliefs, a procedural solution may reasonably be considered. Since reasonable people can agree that we ordinarily regard human offspring as persons, and further, that defining categories of exclusion is likely to pose special dangers of abuse, a reasonable solution is to presume that all living human offspring are persons. This rule would be subject to exception only if can be shown beyond a reasonable doubt that certain offspring will never possess the minimal properties that reasonable persons ordinarily associate with human personality. If this burden cannot be satisfied, then the presumption of personhood obtains.

For this purpose I will address only one of the many properties proposed as a necessary condition of personhood—the capacity for having a sense of self—and consider whether its advocates present a cogent account of the nonhuman. Since other accounts may be more convincingly articulated, this discussion will neither exhaust nor conclude the issue. But it will illuminate the strengths and weaknesses of the personhood argument and enable us to evaluate its application to defective infants.

Michael Tooley has recently argued that a human offspring lacking the capacity for a sense of self lacks the rights to life or equal treatment possessed by other persons. In considering the morality of abortion and infanticide, Tooley considers "what properties a thing must possess in order to have a serious right to life," and he concludes that "having a right to life presupposes that one is capable of desiring to continue existing as a subject of experiences and other mental states. This in turn presupposes both that one has the concept of such a continuing entity and that one believes that one is oneself such an entity. So an entity that lacks such a consciousness of itself as a continuing subject of mental states does not have a right to life."[2]

However, this account is at first glance too narrow, for it appears to exclude all those who do not presently have a desire "to continue existing as a subject of experiences and other mental states." The sleeping or unconscious individual, the deranged, the conditioned, and the suicidal do not have such desires, though they might have had them or could have them in the future. Accordingly, Tooley emphasizes the capability of entertaining such desires, rather than their actual existence. But it is difficult to distinguish the capability for such desires in an unconscious, conditioned, or emotionally disturbed person from the capability existing in a fetus or infant. In all cases the capability is a future one; it will arise only if certain events occur, such as normal growth and development in the case of the infant, and removal of the disability in the other cases. The infant, in fact, might realize its capability long before disabled adults recover emotional balance or consciousness.

To meet this objection, Tooley argues that the significance of the capability in question is not solely its future realization (for fetuses and infants will ordinarily realize it), but also its previous existence and exercise. He seems to say that once the conceptual capability has been realized, one's right to desire continued existence permanently vests, even though the present capability for desiring does not exist, and may be lost for substantial periods or permanently. Yet, what nonarbitrary reasons require that we protect the past realization of conceptual capability but not its potential realization in the future? As a reward for its past realization? To mark our reverence and honor for someone who has realized that state? Tooley is silent on this point.

Another difficulty is Tooley's ambiguity concerning the permanently deranged, comatose, or conditioned. Often he phrases his argument in terms of a temporary suspension of the capability of conceptual thought. One wonders what he would say of someone permanently deranged, or with massive brain damage, or in a prolonged coma. If he seriously means that the past existence of a desire for life vests these cases with the right to life, then it is indeed difficult to distinguish the comatose or deranged from the infant profoundly retarded at birth. Neither will ever possess the conceptual capability to desire to be a continuing subject of experiences. A distinction based on reward or desert seems arbitrary, and protection of life applies equally well in both cases. Would Tooley avoid this problem by holding that the permanently comatose and deranged lose their rights after a certain point because conceptual capacity will never be regained? This would permit killing (or at least withholding of care) from the insane and comatose—doubtless an unappealing prospect. Moreover, we do not ordinarily think of the insane, and possibly the comatose, as losing personhood before their death. Although their personality or identity may be said to change, presumably for the worse, or become fragmented or minimal, we still regard them as specific persons. If a "self" in some minimal sense exists here then the profoundly retarded, who at least is conscious, also may be considered a self, albeit a minimal one. Thus, one may argue that Tooley fails to provide a convincing account of criteria distinguishing persons and nonpersons. He both excludes beings we ordinarily think of as persons—infants, deranged, conditioned, possibly the comatose—and fails to articulate criteria that convincingly distinguish the nonhuman. But, even if we were to accept Tooley's distinction that beings lacking the potential for desire and a sense of self are not persons who are owed the duty to be treated by ordinary medical means, this would not appear to be very helpful in deciding whether to treat the newborn with physical or mental defects. Few infants, it would seem, would fall into this class. First, those suffering from malformations, however gross, that do not affect mental capabilities would not fit the class of nonpersons. Second, frequently even the most severe cases of mental retardation cannot be reliably determined until a much later period; care thus could not justifiably be withheld in the neonatal period, although this principle would permit nontreatment at the time when nonpersonality is clearly established. Finally, the only group of defective newborns who would clearly qualify as nonpersons is anencephalics, who altogether lack a brain, or those so severely brain-damaged that it is immediately clear that a sense of self or personality can never develop. Mongols, myelomeningoceles, and other defective infants from whom ordinary care is now routinely withheld would not qualify as nonpersons. Thus, even the most coherent and cogent criteria of humanity are only marginally helpful in the situation of the defective infant. We must therefore consider whether treatment can be withheld on grounds other than the claim that such infants are not persons.

## No Obligation to Treat Exists When the Costs of Maintaining Life Greatly Outweigh the Benefits

If we reject the argument that defective newborns are not persons, the question remains whether circumstances exist in which the consequences of treatment as compared with nontreatment are so undesirable that the omission of care is justified . . .

. . . Many parents and physicians deeply committed to the loving care of the newborn think that treating severely defective infants causes more harm than good, thereby justifying the withholding of ordinary care. In their view the suffering and diminished quality of the child's life do not justify the social and economic costs of treatment. This claim has a growing commonsense appeal, but it assumes that the utility or quality of one's life can be measured and compared with other lives, and that health resources may legitimately be allocated to produce the greatest personal utility. This argument will now be analyzed from the perspective of the defective patient and others affected by his care.

## ARGUMENTS IN FAVOR OF RENDERING ORDINARY MEDICAL CARE TO DEFECTIVE INFANTS

### The Quality of the Defective Infant's Life

Comparisons of relative worth among persons, or between persons and other interests, raise moral and methodological issues that make any argument that relies on such comparisons extremely vulnerable. Thus the strongest claim for not treating the defective newborn is that treatment seriously harms the infant's own interests, whatever may be the effects on others. When maintaining his life involves great physical and psychosocial suffering for the patient, a reasonable person might conclude that such a life is not worth living. Presumably the patient, if fully informed and able to communicate, would agree. One then would be morally justified in withholding lifesaving treatment if such action served to advance the best interests of the patient.

Congenital malformations impair development in several ways that lead to the judgment that deformed retarded infants are "a burden to themselves." One is the severe physical pain, much of it resulting from repeated surgery, that defective infants will suffer. Defective children also are likely to develop other pathological features, leading to repeated fractures, dislocations, surgery, malfunctions, and other sources of pain. The shunt, for example, inserted to relieve hydrocephalus, a common problem in defective children, often becomes clogged, necessitating frequent surgical interventions.

Pain, however, may be intermittent and manageable with analgesics. Since many infants and adults experience great pain, and many defective infants do not, pain alone, if not totally unmanageable, does not sufficiently show that a life is so worthless that death is preferable. More important are the psychosocial deficits resulting from the child's handicaps. Many defective children never can walk even with prosthesis, never interact with normal children, never appreciate growth, adolescence, or the fulfillment of education and employment, and seldom are even able to care for themselves. In cases of severe retardation, they may be left with a vegetative existence in a crib, incapable of choice or the most minimal response to stimuli. Parents or others may reject them, and much of their time will be spent in hospitals, in surgery, or fighting the many illnesses that beset them. Can it be said that such a life is worth living?

There are two possible responses to the quality-of-life argument. One is to accept its premises but to question the degree of suffering in particular cases, and thus restrict the justification for death to the most extreme cases. The absence of opportunities for schooling, career, and interaction may be the fault of social attitudes and the failings of healthy persons, rather than a necessary result of congenital malformations. Psychosocial suffering occurs because healthy, normal persons reject or refuse to relate to the defective, or hurry them to poorly funded institutions. Most nonambulatory, mentally retarded persons can be trained for satisfying roles. One cannot assume that a nonproductive existence is necessarily unhappy: even social rejection and nonacceptance can be mitigated. Moreover, the psychosocial ills of the handicapped often do not differ in kind from those experienced by many persons. With training and care, growth, development, and a full range of experiences are possible for most people with physical and mental handicaps. Thus, the claim that death is a far better fate than life cannot in most cases be sustained.

This response, however, avoids meeting the quality-of-life argument on its strongest grounds. Even if many defective infants can experience growth, interaction, and most human satisfactions if nurtured, treated, and trained, some infants are so severely retarded or grossly deformed that their response to love and care, in fact their capacity to be conscious, is always minimal. Although mongoloid and nonambulatory spina bifida children may experience an existence we would hesitate to adjudge worse than death, the profoundly retarded, nonambulatory, blind, deaf infant who will spend his few years in the back-ward cribs of a state institution is clearly a different matter.

To repudiate the quality-of-life argument, therefore, requires a defense of treatment in even these extreme cases. Such a defense would question the validity of any surrogate or proxy judgments of the worth or quality of life when the wishes of the person in question cannot be ascertained. The essence of the quality-of-life argument is a proxy's judgment that no reasonable person can prefer the pain, suffering, and loneliness of, for example, life in a crib at an IQ level of 20, to an immediate, painless death.

But in what sense can the proxy validly conclude that a person with different wants, needs, and interests, if able to speak, would agree that such a life were worse than death? At the start one must be skeptical of the proxy's claim to objective disinterestedness. If the proxy is also the parent or physician, as has been the case in pediatric euthanasia, the impact of treatment on the proxy's interests, rather than solely on those of the child, may influence his assessment. But even if the proxy were truly neutral and committed only to caring for the child, the problem of egocentricity and knowing another's mind remains. Compared with the situation and life prospects of a "reasonable man," the child's potential quality of life indeed appears dim. Yet a standard based on healthy, ordinary development may be entirely inappropriate to this situation. One who has never known the pleasures of mental operation, ambulation, and social interaction surely does not suffer from their loss as much as one who has. While one who has known these capacities may prefer death to a life without them, we have no assurance that the handicapped person, with no point of comparison, would agree. Life, and life alone, whatever its limitations, might be of sufficient worth to him.

One should also be hesitant to accept proxy assessments of quality of life because the margin of error in such predictions may be very great. For instance, while one expert argues that by a purely clinical assessment he can accurately forecast the minimum degree of future handicap an individual will experience, such forecasting is not infallible, and risks denying care to infants whose disability might otherwise permit a reasonably acceptable quality of life. Thus given the problems in ascertaining another's wishes, the proxy's bias to personal or culturally relative interests, and the unreliability of predictive criteria, the quality-of-life argument is open to serious question. Its strongest appeal arises in the case of a grossly deformed, retarded, institutionalized child, or one with incessant unmanageable pain, where continued life is itself torture. But these cases are few, and cast doubt on the utility of any such judgment. Even if the judgment occasionally may be defensible, the potential danger of quality-of-life assessments may be a compelling reason for rejecting this rationale for withholding treatment.

## The Suffering of Others

In addition to the infant's own suffering, one who argues that the harm of treatment justifies violation of the defective infant's right to life usually relies on the psychological, social, and economic costs of maintaining his existence to family and society. In their view the minimal benefit of treatment to persons incapable of full social and physical development does not justify the burdens that care of the defective infant imposes on parents, siblings, health professionals, and other patients. Matson, a noted pediatric neurosurgeon, states that "it is the doctor's and the community's responsibility to provide [custodial] care and to minimize suffering; but, at the same time, it is also their responsibility not to prolong such individual, familial, and community suffering unnecessarily, and not to carry out multiple procedures and prolonged, expensive, acute hospitalization in an infant whose chance for acceptable growth and development is negligible."[3]

Such a frankly utilitarian argument raises problems. It assumes that because of the greatly curtailed orbit of his existence, the costs or suffering of others is greater than the benefit of life to the child. This judgment, however, requires a coherent way of measuring and comparing interpersonal utilities, a logical-practical problem that utilitarianism has never surmounted. But even if such comparisons could reliably show a net loss from treatment, the fact remains that the child must sacrifice his life to benefit others. If the life of one individual, however useless, may be sacrificed for the benefit of any person, however useful, or for the benefit of any number of persons, then we have acknowledged the principle that rational utility may justify any outcome. As many philosophers have demonstrated, utilitarianism can always permit the sacrifice of one life for other interests, given the appropriate arrangement of utilities on the balance sheet. In the absence of principled grounds for such a decision, the social equation involved in mandating direct, involuntary euthanasia becomes a difference of degree, not of kind, and we reach the point where protection of life depends solely on social judgments of utility.

These objections may well be determinative. But if we temporarily bracket them and examine the extent to which care of the defective infant subjects others to suffering, the claim that inordinate suffering outweighs the infant's interest in life is rarely plausible. In this regard we must examine the impact of caring for defective infants on the family, health professions, and society at large.

**The Family**

The psychological impact and crisis created by birth of a defective infant is devastating. Not only is the mother denied the normal tension release from the stresses of pregnancy, but both parents feel a crushing blow to their dignity, self-esteem, and self-confidence. In a very short time, they feel grief for the loss of the normal expected child, anger at fate, numbness, disgust, waves of helplessness, and disbelief. Most feel personal blame for the defect, or blame their spouse. Adding to the shock is fear that social position and mobility are permanently endangered. The transformation of a "joyously awaited experience into one of catastrophe and profound psychological threat" often will reactivate unresolved maturational conflicts. The chances for social pathology—divorce, somatic complaints, nervous and mental disorders—increase, and hard-won adjustment patterns may be permanently damaged.

The initial reactions of guilt, grief, anger, and loss, however, cannot be the true measure of family suffering caused by care of a defective infant, because these costs are present whether or not the parents choose treatment. Rather, the question is to what degree treatment imposes psychic and other costs greater than would occur if the child were not treated. The claim that care is more costly rests largely on the view that parents and family suffer inordinately from nurturing such a child.

Indeed, if the child is treated and accepted at home, difficult and demanding adjustments must be made. Parents must learn how to care for a disabled child, confront financial and psychological uncertainty, meet the needs of other siblings, and work through their own conflicting feelings. Mothering demands are greater than with a normal child, particularly if medical care and hospitalization are frequently required. Counseling or professional support may be nonexistent or difficult to obtain. Younger siblings may react with hostility and guilt, older with shame and anger. Often the normal feedback of child growth that renders the turmoil of childrearing worthwhile develops more slowly or not at all. Family resources can be depleted (especially if medical care is needed), consumption patterns altered, or standards of living modified. Housing may have to be found closer to a hospital, and plans for further children changed. Finally, the anxieties, guilt, and grief present at birth may threaten to recur or become chronic.

Yet, although we must recognize the burdens and frustrations of raising a defective infant, it does not necessarily follow that these costs require nontreatment, or even institutionalization. Individual and group counseling can substantially alleviate anxiety, guilt, and frustration and enable parents to cope with underlying conflicts triggered by the birth and the adaptations required. Counseling also can reduce psychological pressures on siblings, who can be taught to recognize and accept their own possibly hostile feelings and the difficult position of their parents. They may even be taught to help their parents care for the child.

The impact of increased financial costs also may vary. In families with high income or adequate health insurance, the financial costs are manageable. In others, state assistance may be available. If severe financial problems arise or pathological adjustments are likely, institutionalization, though undesirable for the child, remains an option. Finally, in many cases, the experience of living through a crisis is a deepening and enriching one, accelerating personality maturation, and giving one a new sensitivity to the needs of spouse, siblings, and others. As one parent of a defective child states: "In the last months I have come closer to people and can understand them more. I have met them more deeply. I did not know there were so many people with troubles in the world."

Thus, while social attitudes regard the handicapped child as an unmitigated disaster, in reality the problem may not be insurmountable, and often may not differ from life's other vicissitudes. Suffering there is, but seldom is it so overwhelming or so imminent that the only alternative is death of the child.

## Health Professionals

Physicians and nurses also suffer when parents give birth to a defective child, though, of course, not to the degree of the parents. To the obstetrician or general practitioner the defective birth may be a blow to his professional identity. He has the difficult task of informing the parents of the defects, explaining their causes, and dealing with the parents' resulting emotional shock. Often he feels guilty for failing to produce a normal baby. In addition, the parents may project anger or hostility on the physician, questioning his professional competence or seeking the services of other doctors. The physician also may feel that his expertise and training are misused when employed to maintain the life of an infant whose chances for a productive existence are so diminished. By neglecting other patients, he may feel that he is prolonging rather than alleviating suffering.

Nurses, too, suffer role strain from care of the defective newborn. Intensive-care-unit nurses may work with only one or two babies at a time. They face the daily ordeals of care—the progress and relapses—and often must deal with anxious parents who are themselves grieving or ambivalent toward the child. The situation may trigger a nurse's own ambivalence about death and mothering, in a context in which she is actively working to keep alive a child whose life prospects seem minimal.

Thus, the effects of care on physicians and nurses are not trivial, and must be intelligently confronted in medical education or in management of a pediatric unit. Yet to state them is to make clear that they can but weigh lightly in the decision of whether to treat a defective newborn. Compared with the situation of the parents, these burdens seem insignificant, are short term, and most likely do not evoke such profound emotions. In any case, these difficulties are hazards of the profession—caring for the sick and dying will always produce strain. Hence, on these grounds alone it is difficult to argue that a defective person may be denied the right to life.

## Society

Care of the defective newborn also imposes societal costs, the utility of which is questioned when the infant's expected quality of life is so poor. Medical resources that can be used by infants with a better prognosis, or throughout the health-care system generally, are consumed in providing expensive surgical and intensive-care services to infants who may be severely retarded, never lead active lives, and die in a few months or years. Institutionalization imposes costs on taxpayers and reduces the resources available for those who might better benefit from it, while reducing further the quality of life experienced by the institutionalized defective.

One answer to these concerns is to question the impact of the costs of caring for defective newborns. Precise data showing the costs to taxpayers or the trade-offs with health and other expenditures do not exist. Nor would ceasing to care for the defective necessarily lead to a reallocation within the health budget that would produce net savings in suffering or life; in fact, the released resources might not be reallocated for health at all. In any case, the trade-offs within the health budget may well be small. With advances in prenatal diagnosis of genetic disorders many deformed infants who would formerly require care will be aborted beforehand. Then, too, it is not clear that the most technical and expensive procedures always constitute the best treatment for certain malformations. When compared with the almost 7 percent of the GNP now spent on health, the money in the defense budget, or tax revenues generally, the public resources required to keep defective newborns alive seem marginal, and arguably worth the commitment to life that such expenditures reinforce. Moreover, as the Supreme Court recently recognized, conservation of the taxpayer's purse does not justify serious infringement of fundamental rights. Given legal and ethical norms against sacrificing the lives of nonconsenting others, and the imprecisions in diagnosis and prediction concerning the eventual outcomes of medical care, the social cost argument does not compel nontreatment of defective newborns . . .

## NOTES

1. Sissela Bok, "Ethical Problems of Abortion," *Hastings Center Studies* 2 (January 1974), pp. 33, 41.
2. Michael Tooley, "Abortion and Infanticide," *Philosophy and Public Affairs* 2:1 (1972), pp. 37, 51.
3. Matson, "Surgical Treatment of Myelomeningocele," *Pediatrics* 42 (1968), pp. 225, 226.

## PART SEVEN

# Experimentation and Animals

# All Animals Are Equal

## Peter Singer

*Philosopher Peter Singer shook up the medical world in 1975 with* Animal Liberation, *which has become a classic. In the following selection, Singer presents his argument based on equal consideration of the interests of beings capable of feeling pain and
having interests that matter. Critics often focus on his conclusion while ignoring his
actual arguments. He specifically does not claim, as some critics imply, that nonhuman animals share all the same qualities as humans.*

In recent years a number of oppressed groups have campaigned vigorously
for equality. The classic instance is the Black Liberation movement, which
demands an end to the prejudice and discrimination that has made blacks
second-class citizens. The immediate appeal of the Black Liberation movement and its initial, if limited, success made it a model for other oppressed
groups to follow. We became familiar with liberation movements for Spanish-
Americans, gay people, and a variety of other minorities. When a majority
group—women—began their campaign, some thought we had come to the
end of the road. Discrimination on the basis of sex, it has been said, is the last
universally accepted form of discrimination, practiced without secrecy or pre-
tense even in those liberal circles that have long prided themselves on their
freedom from prejudice against racial minorities.

One should always be wary of talking of "the last remaining form of discrimination." If we have learnt anything from the liberation movements, we
should have learnt how difficult it is to be aware of latent prejudice in our attitudes to particular groups until this prejudice is forcefully pointed out.

A liberation movement demands an expansion of our moral horizons
and an extension or reinterpretation of the basic moral principle of equality.

*Source: Philosophic Exchange* 1, no. 5 (Summer 1974). Reprinted by permission of the author, who
holds copyright. For biographical information on Peter Singer, see the introduction to Selection 7.

Practices that were previously regarded as natural and inevitable come to be seen as the result of an unjustifiable prejudice. Who can say with confidence that all his or her attitudes and practices are beyond criticism? If we wish to avoid being numbered amongst the oppressors, we must be prepared to re-think even our most fundamental attitudes. We need to consider them from the point of view of those most disadvantaged by our attitudes, and the prac-tices that follow from these attitudes. If we can make this unaccustomed men-tal switch we may discover a pattern in our attitudes and practices that con-sistently operates so as to benefit one group—usually the one to which we ourselves belong—at the expense of another. In this way we may come to see that there is a case for a new liberation movement. My aim is to advocate that we make this mental switch in respect of our attitudes and practices towards a very large group of beings: members of species other than our own—or, as we popularly though misleadingly call them, animals. In other words, I am urging that we extend to other species the basic principle of equality that most of us recognize should be extended to all members of our own species.

All this may sound a little far-fetched, more like a parody of other libera-tion movements than a serious objective. In fact, in the past the idea of "The Rights of Animals" really has been used to parody the case for women's rights. When Mary Wollstonecraft, a forerunner of later feminists, published her *Vindication of the Rights of Women* in 1792, her ideas were widely regarded as absurd, and they were satirized in an anonymous publication entitled *A Vindication of the Rights of Brutes*. The author of this satire (actually Thomas Taylor, a distinguished Cambridge philosopher) tried to refute Woll-stonecraft's reasonings by showing that they could be carried one stage fur-ther. If sound when applied to women, why should the arguments not be ap-plied to dogs, cats, and horses? They seemed to hold equally well for these "brutes"; yet to hold that brutes had rights was manifestly absurd; therefore the reasoning by which this conclusion had been reached must be unsound, and if unsound when applied to brutes, it must also be unsound when applied to women, since the very same arguments had been used in each case.

One way in which we might reply to this argument is by saying that the case for equality between men and women cannot validly be extended to non-human animals. Women have a right to vote, for instance, because they are just as capable of making rational decisions as men are; dogs, on the other hand, are incapable of understanding the significance of voting, so they cannot have the right to vote. There are many other obvious ways in which men and women resemble each other closely, while humans and other animals differ greatly. So, it might be said, men and women are similar beings and should have equal rights, while humans and nonhumans are different and should not have equal rights.

The thought behind this reply to Taylor's analogy is correct up to a point, but it does not go far enough. There *are* important differences between humans and other animals, and these differences must give rise to *some* differences in the rights that each have. Recognizing this obvious fact, however, is no barrier to the case for extending the basic principle of equality to nonhuman animals.

The differences that exist between men and women are equally undeniable, and the supporters of Women's Liberation are aware that these differences may give rise to different rights. Many feminists hold that women have the right to an abortion on request. It does not follow that since these same people are campaigning for equality between men and women they must support the right of men to have abortions too. Since a man cannot have an abortion, it is meaningless to talk of his right to have one. Since a pig can't vote, it is meaningless to talk of its right to vote. There is no reason why either Women's Liberation or Animal Liberation should get involved in such nonsense. The extension of the basic principle of equality from one group to another does not imply that we must treat both groups in exactly the same way, or grant exactly the same rights to both groups. Whether we should do so will depend on the nature of the members of the two groups. The basic principle of equality, I shall argue, is equality of consideration; and equal consideration for different beings may lead to different treatment and different rights.

So there is a different way of replying to Taylor's attempt to parody Wollstonecraft's arguments, a way which does not deny the differences between humans and nonhumans, but goes more deeply into the question of equality and concludes by finding nothing absurd in the idea that the basic principle of equality applies to so-called "brutes." I believe that we reach this conclusion if we examine the basis on which our opposition to discrimination on grounds of race or sex ultimately rests. We will then see that we would be on shaky ground if we were to demand equality for blacks, women, and other groups of oppressed humans while denying equal consideration to nonhumans.

When we say that all human beings, whatever their race, creed, or sex, are equal, what is it that we are asserting? Those who wish to defend a hierarchical, inegalitarian society have often pointed out that by whatever test we choose, it simply is not true that all humans are equal. Like it or not, we must face the fact that humans come in different shapes and sizes; they come with differing moral capacities, differing intellectual abilities, differing amounts of benevolent feeling and sensitivity to the needs of others, differing abilities to communicate effectively, and differing capacities to experience pleasure and pain. In short, if the demand for equality were based on the actual equality of all human beings, we would have to stop demanding equality. It would be an unjustifiable demand.

Still, one might cling to the view that the demand for equality among human beings is based on the actual equality of the different races and sexes. Although humans differ as individuals in various ways, there are no differences between the races and sexes *as such*. From the mere fact that a person is black, or a woman, we cannot infer anything else about that person. This, it may be said, is what is wrong with racism and sexism. The white racist claims that whites are superior to blacks, but this is false—although there are differences between individuals, some blacks are superior to some whites in all of the capacities and abilities that could conceivably be relevant. The opponent of sexism would say the same: a person's sex is no guide to his or her abilities, and this is why it is unjustifiable to discriminate on the basis of sex.

This is a possible line of objection to racial and sexual discrimination. It is not, however, the way that someone really concerned about equality would choose, because taking this line could, in some circumstances, force one to accept a most inegalitarian society. The fact that humans differ as individuals, rather than as races or sexes, is a valid reply to someone who defends a hierarchical society like, say, South Africa, in which all whites are superior in status to all blacks. The existence of individual variations that cut across the lines of race or sex, however, provides us with no defence at all against a more sophisticated opponent of equality, one who proposes that, say, the interests of those with I.Q. ratings above 100 be preferred to the interests of those with I.Q.s below 100. Would a hierarchical society of this sort really be so much better than one based on race or sex? I think not. But if we tie the moral principle of equality to the factual equality of the different races or sexes, taken as a whole, our opposition to racism and sexism does not provide us with any basis for objecting to this kind of inegalitarianism.

There is a second important reason why we ought not to base our opposition to racism and sexism on any kind of factual equality, even the limited kind which asserts that variations in capacities and abilities are spread evenly between the different races and sexes: we can have no absolute guarantee that these abilities and capacities really are distributed evenly, without regard to race or sex, among human beings. So far as actual abilities are concerned, there do seem to be certain measurable differences between both races and sexes. These differences do not, of course, appear in each case, but only when averages are taken. More important still, we do not yet know how much of these differences is really due to the different genetic endowments of the various races and sexes, and how much is due to environmental differences that are the result of past and continuing discrimination. Perhaps all of the important differences will eventually prove to be environmental rather than genetic. Anyone opposed to racism and sexism will certainly hope that this will be so, for it will make the task of ending discrimination a lot easier; nevertheless it would be dangerous to rest the case against racism and sexism on the belief that all significant differences are environmental in origin. The opponent of, say, racism who takes this line will be unable to avoid conceding that if differences in ability did after all prove to have some genetic connection with race, racism would in some way be defensible.

It would be folly for the opponent of racism to stake his whole case on a dogmatic commitment to one particular outcome of a difficult scientific issue which is still a long way from being settled. While attempts to prove that differences in certain selected abilities between races and sexes are primarily genetic in origin have certainly not been conclusive, the same must be said of attempts to prove that these differences are largely the result of environment. At this stage of the investigation we cannot be certain which view is correct, however much we may hope it is the latter.

Fortunately, there is no need to pin the case for equality to one particular outcome of this scientific investigation. The appropriate response to those who claim to have found evidence of genetically based differences in ability between the races or sexes is not to stick to the belief that the genetic explanation must be wrong, whatever evidence to the contrary may turn up: instead we should make it quite clear that the claim to equality does not depend on intelligence, moral capacity, physical strength, or similar matters of fact. Equality is a moral ideal, not a simple assertion of fact. There is no logically compelling reason for assuming that a factual difference in ability between two people justifies any difference in the amount of consideration we give to satisfying their needs and interests. The principle of the equality of human beings is not a description of an alleged actual equality among humans: it is a prescription of how we should treat animals.

Jeremy Bentham incorporated the essential basis of moral equality into his utilitarian system of ethics in the formula "Each to count for one and none for more than one." In other words, the interests of every being affected by an action are to be taken into account and given the same weight as the like interests of any other being. A later utilitarian, Henry Sidgwick, put the point in this way: "The good of any one individual is of no more importance, from the point of view (if I may say so) of the Universe, than the good of any other."[1] More recently, the leading figures in contemporary moral philosophy have shown a great deal of agreement in specifying as a fundamental presupposition of their moral theories some similar requirement which operates so as to give everyone's interests equal consideration—although they cannot agree on how this requirement is best formulated.[2]

It is an implication of this principle of equality that our concern for others ought not to depend on what they are like, or what abilities they possess— although precisely what this concern requires us to do may vary according to the characteristics of those affected by what we do. It is on this basis that the case against racism and the case against sexism must both ultimately rest; and it is in accordance with this principle that speciesism is also to be condemned.[3] If possessing a higher degree of intelligence does not entitle one human to use another for his own ends, how can it entitle humans to exploit nonhumans?

Many philosophers have proposed the principle of equal consideration of interests, in some form or other, as a basic moral principle; but, as we shall see in more detail shortly, not many of them have recognised that this principle applies to members of other species as well as to our own. Bentham was one of the few who did realize this. In a forward-looking passage, written at a time when black slaves in the British dominions were still being treated much as we now treat nonhuman animals, Bentham wrote:

> The day *may* come when the rest of the animal creation may acquire those rights which never could have been witholden from them but by the hand of tyranny. The French have already discovered that the blackness of the skin is no reason why a human being should be abandoned without redress to the caprice of a tormentor. It may one day come to be recognized that the number of the legs, the villosity of the skin, or the termination of the *os sacrum*, are reasons equally insufficient for abandoning a sensitive being to the same fate. What else is it that should trace the insuperable line? Is it the faculty of reason, or perhaps the faculty of discourse? But a full-grown horse or dog is beyond

comparison a more rational, as well as a more conversable animal, than an infant of a day, or a week, or even a month, old. But suppose they were otherwise, what would it avail? The question is not, Can they reason? nor Can they *talk?* but, *Can they suffer?*[4]

In this passage Bentham points to the capacity for suffering as the vital characteristic that gives a being the right to equal consideration. The capacity for suffering—or more strictly, for suffering and/or enjoyment or happiness— is not just another characteristic like the capacity for language, or for higher mathematics. Bentham is not saying that those who try to mark "the insuperable line" that determines whether the interests of a being should be considered happen to have selected the wrong characteristic. The capacity for suffering and enjoying things is a prerequisite for having interests at all, a condition that must be satisfied before we can speak of interests in any meaningful way. It would be nonsense to say that it was not in the interests of a stone to be kicked along the road by a schoolboy. A stone does not have interests because it cannot suffer. Nothing that we can do to it could possibly make any difference to its welfare. A mouse, on the other hand, does have an interest in not being tormented, because it will suffer if it is.

If a being suffers, there can be no moral justification for refusing to take that suffering into consideration. No matter what the nature of the being, the principle of equality requires that its suffering be counted equally with the like suffering—in so far as rough comparisons can be made—of any other being. If a being is not capable of suffering, or of experiencing enjoyment or happiness, there is nothing to be taken into account. This is why the limit of sentience (using the term as a convenient, if not strictly accurate, shorthand for the capacity to suffer or experience enjoyment or happiness) is the only defensible boundary of concern for the interests of others. To mark this boundary by some characteristic like intelligence or rationality would be to mark it in an arbitrary way. Why not choose some other characteristic, like skin color?

The racist violates the principle of equality by giving greater weight to the interests of members of his own race, when there is a clash between their interests and the interests of those of another race. Similarly the speciesist allows the interests of his own species to override the greater interests of members of other species. The pattern is the same in each case. Most human beings are speciesists. I shall now very briefly describe some of the practices that show this.

For the great majority of human beings, especially in urban, industrialized societies, the most direct form of contact with members of other species is at mealtimes: we eat them. In doing so we treat them purely as means to our ends. We regard their life and well-being as subordinate to our taste for a particular kind of dish. I say "taste" deliberately—this is purely a matter of pleasing our palate. There can be no defence of eating flesh in terms of satisfying nutritional needs, since it has been established beyond doubt that we could satisfy our need for protein and other essential nutrients far more efficiently with a diet that replaced animal flesh by soy beans, or products derived from soy beans, and other high-protein vegetable products.[5]

It is not merely the act of killing that indicates what we are ready to do to other species in order to gratify our tastes. The suffering we inflict on the animals while they are alive is perhaps an even clearer indication of our speciesism than the fact that we are prepared to kill them.[6] In order to have meat on the table at a price that people can afford, our society tolerates methods of meat production that confine sentient animals in cramped, unsuitable conditions for the entire durations of their lives. Animals are treated like machines that convert fodder into flesh, and any innovation that results in a higher "conversion ratio" is liable to be adopted. As one authority on the subject has said, "cruelty is acknowledged only when profitability ceases"[7] . . .

Since, as I have said, none of these practices cater for anything more than our pleasures of taste, our practice of rearing and killing other animals in order to eat them is a clear instance of the sacrifice of the most important interests of other beings in order to satisfy trivial interests of our own. To avoid speciesism we must stop this practice, and each of us has a moral obligation to cease supporting the practice. Our custom is all the support that the meat industry needs. The decision to cease giving it that support may be difficult, but it is no more difficult than it would have been for a white Southerner to go against the traditions of his society and free his slaves: if we do not change our dietary habits, how can we censure those slaveholders who would not change their own way of living?

The same form of discrimination may be observed in the widespread practice of experimenting on other species in order to see if certain substances are safe for human beings, or to test some psychological theory about the effect of severe punishment on learning, or to try out various new compounds just in case something turns up . . .

In the past, argument about vivisection has often missed the point, because it has been put in absolutist terms: Would the abolitionist be prepared to let thousands die if they could be saved by experimenting on a single animal? The way to reply to this purely hypothetical question is to pose another: Would the experimenter be prepared to perform his experiment on an orphaned human infant, if that were the only way to save many lives? (I say "orphan" to avoid the complication of parental feelings, although in doing so I am being overfair to the experimenter, since the nonhuman subjects of experiments are not orphans.) If the experimenter is not prepared to use an orphaned human infant, then his readiness to use nonhumans is simple discrimination, since adult apes, cats, mice, and other mammals are more aware of what is happening to them, more self-directing, and, so far as we can tell, at least as sensitive to pain, as any human infant. There seems to be no relevant characteristic that human infants possess that adult mammals do not have to the same or a higher degree. (Someone might try to argue that what makes it wrong to experiment on a human infant is that the infant will, in time and if left alone, develop into more than the nonhuman, but one would then, to be consistent, have to oppose abortion, since the fetus has the same potential as the infant—indeed, even contraception and abstinence might be wrong on this ground—since the egg and sperm, considered jointly, also have

the same potential. In any case, this argument still gives us no reason for selecting a nonhuman, rather than a human with severe and irreversible brain
damage, as the subject for our experiments.)

The experimenter, then, shows a bias in favor of his own species whenever he carries out an experiment on a nonhuman for a purpose that he would
not think justified him in using a human being at an equal or lower level of
sentience, awareness, ability to be self-directing, etc. No one familiar with the
kind of results yielded by most experiments on animals can have the slightest
doubt that if this bias were eliminated the number of experiments performed
would be a minute fraction of the number performed today.

Experimenting on animals and eating their flesh are perhaps the two
major forms of speciesism in our society. By comparison, the third and last
form of speciesism is so minor as to be insignificant, but it is perhaps of some
special interest to those for whom this article was written. I am referring to
speciesism in contemporary philosophy.

Philosophy ought to question the basic assumptions of the age. Thinking
through, critically and carefully, what most people take for granted is, I believe, the chief task of philosophy, and it is this task that makes philosophy a
worthwhile activity. Regrettably, philosophy does not always live up to its
historic role. Philosophers are human beings, and they are subject to all the
preconceptions of the society to which they belong. Sometimes they succeed in
breaking free of the prevailing ideology: more often they become its most sophisticated defenders. So, in this case, philosophy as practiced in the universi-
ties today does not challenge anyone's preconceptions about our relations
with other species. By their writings, those philosophers who tackle problems
that touch upon the issue reveal that they make the same unquestioned assumptions as most other humans, and what they say tends to confirm the
reader in his or her comfortable speciesist habits.

I could illustrate this claim by referring to the writings of philosophers in
various fields—for instance, the attempts that have been made by those interested in rights to draw the boundary of the sphere of rights so that it runs parallel to the biological boundaries of the species *Homo sapiens,* including infants
and even mental defectives, but excluding those other beings of equal or
greater capacity who are so useful to us at mealtimes and in our laboratories. I
think it would be a more appropriate conclusion to this article, however, if I
concentrated on the problem with which we have been centrally concerned,
the problem of equality.

It is significant that the problem of equality, in moral and political philosophy, is invariably formulated in terms of human equality. The effect of this is
that the question of the equality of other animals does not confront the
philosopher, or student, as an issue itself—and this is already an indication of
the failure of philosophy to challenge accepted beliefs. Still, philosophers have
found it difficult to discuss the issue of human equality without raising, in a
paragraph or two, the question of the status of other animals. The reason for
this, which should be apparent from what I have said already, is that if humans are to be regarded as equal to one another, we need some sense of

"equal" that does not require any actual, descriptive equality of capacities, talents, or other qualities. If equality is to be related to any actual characteristics of humans, these characteristics must be some lowest common denominator, pitched so low that no human lacks them—but then the philosopher comes up against the catch that any such set of characteristics which covers *all* humans will not be possessed *only by humans.* In other words, it turns out that in the only sense in which we can truly say, as an assertion of fact, that all humans are equal, at least some members of other species are also equal—equal, that is, to each other and to humans. If, on the other hand, we regard the statement "All humans are equal" in some nonfactual way, perhaps as a prescription, then, as I have already argued, it is even more difficult to exclude nonhumans from the sphere of equality.

This result is not what the egalitarian philosopher originally intended to assert. Instead of accepting the radical outcome to which their own reasonings naturally point, however, most philosophers try to reconcile their beliefs in human equality and animal inequality by arguments that can only be described as devious.

As a first example, I take William Frankena's well-known article "The Concept of Social Justice." Frankena opposes the idea of basing justice on merit, because he sees that this could lead to highly inegalitarian results. Instead he proposes the principle that "all men are to be treated as equals, not because they are equal, in any respect, but simply because they are human. They are human because they have emotions and desires, and are able to think, and hence are capable of enjoying a good life in a sense in which other animals are not."[8]

But what is this capacity to enjoy the good life which all humans have, but no other animals? Other animals have emotions and desires and appear to be capable of enjoying a good life. We may doubt that they can think—although the behavior of some apes, dolphins, and even dogs suggests that some of them can—but what is the relevance of thinking? Frankena goes on to admit that by "the good life" he means "not so much the morally good life as the happy or satisfactory life," so thought would appear to be unnecessary for enjoying the good life; in fact to emphasize the need for thought would make difficulties for the egalitarian, since only some people are capable of leading intellectually satisfying lives, or morally good lives. This makes it difficult to see what Frankena's principle of equality has to do with simply being *human.* Surely every sentient being is capable of leading a life that is happier or less miserable than some alternative life, and hence has a claim to be taken into account. In this respect the distinction between humans and nonhumans is not a sharp division, but rather a continuum along which we move gradually, and with overlaps between the species, from simple capacities for enjoyment and satisfaction, or pain and suffering, to more complex ones.

Faced with a situation in which they see a need for some basis for the moral gulf that is commonly thought to separate humans and animals, but can find no concrete difference that will do the job without undermining the equality of humans, philosophers tend to waffle. They resort to high-sounding phrases like "the intrinsic dignity of the human individual";[9] they talk of the "intrinsic worth of all men" as if men (humans?) had some worth that other beings did not;[10] or they say that humans, and only humans, are "ends in themselves," while "everything other than a person can only have value for a person."[11]

This idea of a distinctive human dignity and worth has a long history; it can be traced back directly to the Renaissance humanists, for instance to Pico della Mirandola's *Oration on the Dignity of Man*. Pico and other humanists based their estimate of human dignity on the idea that man possessed the central, pivotal position in the "Great Chain of Being" that led from the lowliest forms of matter to God himself; this view of the universe, in turn, goes back to both classical and Judeo-Christian doctrines. Contemporary philosophers have cast off these metaphysical and religious shackles and freely invoke the dignity of mankind without needing to justify the idea at all. Why should we not attribute "intrinsic dignity" or "intrinsic worth" to ourselves? Fellow humans are unlikely to reject the accolades we so generously bestow on them, and those to whom we deny the honor are unable to object. Indeed, when one thinks only of humans, it can be very liberal, very progressive, to talk of the dignity of all human beings. In so doing, we implicitly condemn slavery, racism, and other violations of human rights. We admit that we ourselves are in some fundamental sense on a par with the poorest, most ignorant members of our own species. It is only when we think of humans as no more than a small sub-group of all the beings that inhabit our planet that we may realize that in elevating our own species we are at the same time lowering the relative status of all other species.

The truth is that the appeal to the intrinsic dignity of human beings appears to solve the egalitarian's problems only as long as it goes unchallenged. Once we ask *why* it should be that all humans—including infants, mental defectives, psychopaths, Hitler, Stalin, and the rest—have some kind of dignity or worth that no elephant, pig, or chimpanzee can ever achieve, we see that this question is as difficult to answer as our original request for some relevant fact that justifies the inequality of humans and other animals. In fact, these two questions are really one: talk of intrinsic dignity or moral worth only takes the problem back one step, because any satisfactory defence of the claim that all and only humans have intrinsic dignity would need to refer to some relevant capacities or characteristics that all and only humans possess. Philosophers frequently introduce ideas of dignity, respect, and worth at the point at which other reasons appear to be lacking, but this is hardly good enough. Fine phrases are the last resource of those who have run out of arguments.

In case there are those who still think it may be possible to find some relevant characteristic that distinguishes all humans from all members of other species, I shall refer again, before I conclude, to the existence of some humans who quite clearly are below the level of awareness, self-consciousness, intelligence, and sentience, of many nonhumans. I am thinking of humans with severe and irreparable brain damage, and also of infant humans. To avoid the

complication of the relevance of a being's potential, however, I shall hence-
forth concentrate on permanently retarded humans.

Philosophers who set out to find a characteristic that will distinguish humans from other animals rarely take the course of abandoning these groups of
humans by lumping them in with the other animals. It is easy to see why they
do not. To take this line without re-thinking our attitudes to other animals
would entail that we have the right to perform painful experiments on retarded humans for trivial reasons; similarly it would follow that we had the
right to rear and kill these humans for food. To most philosophers these consequences are as unacceptable as the view that we should stop treating nonhumans in this way.

Of course, when discussing the problem of equality it is possible to ignore
the problem of mental defectives, or brush it aside as if somehow insignificant.[12] This is the easiest way out. What else remains? My final example of
speciesism in contemporary philosophy has been selected to show what happens when a writer is prepared to face the question of human equality and
animal inequality without ignoring the existence of mental defectives, and
without resorting to obscurantist mumbo-jumbo. Stanley Benn's clear and
honest article "Egalitarianism and Equal Consideration of Interests"[13] fits this
description.

Benn, after noting the usual "evident human inequalities," argues, correctly I think, for equality of consideration as the only possible basis for egalitarianism. Yet Benn, like other writers, is thinking only of "equal consideration
of human interests." Benn is quite open in his defence of this restriction of
equal consideration:

> not to possess human shape *is* a disqualifying condition. However faithful or
> intelligent a dog may be, it would be a monstrous sentimentality to attribute
> to him interests that could be weighed in an equal balance with those of
> human beings . . . if, for instance, one had to decide between feeding a hun-
> gry baby or a hungry dog, anyone who chose the dog would generally be
> reckoned morally defective, unable to recognize a fundamental inequality of
> claims.
>
> This is what distinguishes our attitude to animals from our attitude to im-
> beciles. It would be odd to say that we ought to respect equally the dignity or
> personality of the imbecile and of the rational man . . . but there is nothing
> odd about saying that we should respect their interests equally, that is, that
> we should give to the interests of each the same serious consideration as
> claims to considerations necessary for some standard of well-being that we
> can recognize and endorse.

Benn's statement of the basis of the consideration we should have for imbeciles seems to me correct, but why should there be any fundamental inequality of claims between a dog and a human imbecile? Benn sees that if
equal consideration depended on rationality, no reason could be given against
using imbeciles for research purposes, as we now use dogs and guinea pigs.
This will not do: "But of course we do distinguish imbeciles from animals in
this regard," he says. That the common distinction is justifiable is something

Benn does not question; his problem is how it is to be justified. The answer he gives is this:

> we respect the interests of men and give them priority over dogs not *insofar* as they are rational, but because rationality is the human norm. We say it is *unfair* to exploit the deficiencies of the imbecile who falls short of the norm, just as it would be unfair, and not just ordinarily dishonest, to steal from a blind man. If we do not think in this way about dogs, it is because we do not see the irrationality of the dog as a deficiency or a handicap, but as normal for the species. The characteristics, therefore, that distinguish the normal man from the normal dog make it intelligible for us to talk of other men having interests and capacities, and therefore claims, of precisely the same kind as we make on our own behalf. But although these characteristics may provide the point of the distinction between men and other species, they are not in fact the qualifying conditions for membership, or the distinguishing criteria of the class of morally considerable persons; and this is precisely because a man does not become a member of a different species, with its own standards of normality, by reason of not possessing these characteristics.

The final sentence of this passage gives the argument away. An imbecile, Benn concedes, may have no characteristics superior to those of a dog; nevertheless this does not make the imbecile a member of "a different species," as the dog is. *Therefore* it would be "unfair" to use the imbecile for medical research as we use the dog. But why? That the imbecile is not rational is just the way things have worked out, and the same is true of the dog—neither is any more responsible for their mental level. If it is unfair to take advantage of an isolated defect, why is it fair to take advantage of a more general limitation? I find it hard to see anything in this argument except a defence of preferring the interests of members of our own species because they are members of our own species. To those who think there might be more to it, I suggest the following mental exercise. Assume that it has been proven that there is a difference in the average, or normal, intelligence quotient for two different races, say whites and blacks. Then substitute the term "white" for every occurrence of "men" and "black" for every occurrence of "dog" in the passage quoted; and substitute "high I.Q." for "rationality" and, when Benn talks of "imbeciles," replace this term by "dumb whites"—that is, whites who fall well below the normal white I.Q. score. Finally, change "species" to "race." Now re-read the passage. It has become a defence of a rigid, no-exceptions division between whites and blacks, based on I.Q. scores, *notwithstanding an admitted overlap* between whites and blacks in this respect. The revised passage is, of course, outrageous, and this is not only because we have made fictitious assumptions in our substitutions. The point is that in the original passage Benn was defending a rigid division in the amount of consideration due to members of different species, despite admitted cases of overlap. If the original did not, at first reading, strike us as being as outrageous as the revised version does, this is largely because although we are not racists ourselves, most of us are speciesists. Like the other articles, Benn's stands as a warning of the ease with which the best minds can fall victim to a prevailing ideology.

**NOTES**

1. Henry Sidgwick, *The Methods of Ethics,* 7th ed. (London, MacMillan, 1874), p. 382.
2. For example, R. M. Hare, *Freedom and Reason* (Oxford: Oxford University Press, 1963); and John Rawls, *A Theory of Justice* (Cambridge, MA: Harvard University Press, 1972). For a brief account of the essential agreement on this issue between these and other positions, see R. M. Hare, "Rules of War and Moral Reasoning," *Philosophy and Public Affairs* I, no. 2 (1972).
3. I owe the term "speciesism" to Richard Ryder.
4. Jeremy Bentham, *Introduction to the Principles of Morals and Legislation,* chap. 17.
5. In order to produce one pound of protein in the form of beef or veal, we must feed twenty-one pounds of protein to the animal. Other forms of livestock are slightly less inefficient, but the average ratio in the United States is still 1:8. It has been estimated that the amount of protein lost to humans in this way is equivalent to 90 percent of the annual world protein deficit. For a brief account, see Frances Moore Lappe, *Diet for a Small Planet* (New York: Friends of the Earth/Ballantine, 1971), pp. 4–11.
6. Although one might think that killing a being is obviously the ultimate wrong one can do to it, I think that the infliction of suffering is a clearer indication of speciesism because it might be argued that at least part of what is wrong with killing a human is that most humans are conscious of their existence over time and have desires and purposes that extend into the future—see, for instance, M. Tooley, "Abortion and Infanticide," *Philosophy and Public Affairs,* vol. 2, no. 1 (1972). Of course, if one took this view one would have to hold—as Tooley does—that killing a human infant or mental defective is not in itself wrong and is less serious than killing certain higher mammals that probably do have a sense of their own existence over time.
7. Ruth Harrison, *Animal Machines* (London: Stuart, 1964). For an account of farming conditions, see Peter Singer, "Down on the Factory Farm," *Animal Liberation* (New York: New York Review, 1975).
8. William Frankena, "The Concept of Social Justice," in *Social Justice,* ed. R. Brandt (Prentice-Hall, Englewood Cliffs, 1962), p. 19.
9. Ibid., p. 23.
10. H. A. Bedau, "Egalitarianism and the Idea of Equality," in *Nomos IX: Equality,* ed. J. R. Pennock and J. W. Chapman (New York, 1967).
11. G. Vlastos, "Justice and Equality," in Brandt, *Social Justice,* p. 48.
12. For example, Bernard Williams, "The Idea of Equality," in *Philosophy, Politics, and Society,* 2d ser., ed. P. Laslett and W. Runciman (Oxford: Blackwell, 1962), p. 118; Rawls, *A Theory of Justice,* pp. 509–10.
13. Stanley Benn, "Egalitarianism and Equal Consideration of Interests," in Pennock and Chapman, *Nomos IX: Equality,* p. 62 ff.

## PART EIGHT

# Just Allocation of Scarce Medical Resources

# The Allocation of Exotic Medical Lifesaving Therapy

## Nicholas Rescher

*In 1962 a committee in Seattle had to decide who got a scarce artificial kidney (he-modialysis machine) and lived, and who did not and died. As such, it was called "The God Committee." Its criterion for selection was "social worth." In 1963 Washington state's Boeing Corporation began subsidizing access for many of the state's citizens. In 1972 the U.S. Congress decided to pay for the machines for all Americans through the Medicare program. Some would say that this move set a precedent for not making hard choices and not establishing some standard for allocation.*

*The issue remains unresolved, as the following selections illustrate. An early classic by Nicholas Rescher lays out a defensible and plausible decision procedure involving several stages: medical screening to eliminate incompatible candidates (criteria of exclusion), then criteria of inclusion, and finally, among all the remaining candidates, a lottery. Thus Rescher incorporates medical, utilitarian, and Kantian elements into his procedures for selection.*

*Nicholas Rescher has been one of the most prolific writers of his generation on a wide, rich variety of philosophical topics. For many years he was the editor of the distinguished* American Philosophical Quarterly. *He is professor of philosophy at the University of Pittsburgh.*

## I. THE PROBLEM

Technological progress has in recent years transformed the limits of the possible in medical therapy. However, the elevated state of sophistication of modern medical technology has brought the economists' classic problem of scarcity in its wake as an unfortunate side product. The enormously sophisticated and

Source: Ethics 79 (April 1969). Reprinted by permission of the author and the University of Chicago Press. Footnotes in this selection have been edited.

complex equipment and the highly trained teams of experts requisite for its utilization are scarce resources in relation to potential demand. The administrators of the great medical institutions that preside over these scarce resources thus come to be faced increasingly with the awesome choice: *Whose life to save?*

A (somewhat hypothetical) paradigm example of this problem may be sketched within the following set of definitive assumptions: We suppose that persons in some particular medically morbid condition are "mortally afflicted": it is virtually certain that they will die within a short time period (say ninety days). We assume that some very complex course of treatment (e.g., a heart transplant) represents a substantial probability of life prolongation for persons in this mortally afflicted condition. We assume that the facilities available in terms of human resources, mechanical instrumentalities, and requisite materials (e.g., hearts in the case of a heart transplant) make it possible to give a certain treatment—this "exotic (medical) lifesaving therapy," or ELT for short—to a certain, relatively small number of people. And finally we assume that a substantially greater pool of people in the mortally afflicted condition is at hand. The problem then may be formulated as follows: How is one to select within the pool of afflicted patients the ones to be given the ELT treatment in question; how to select those "whose lives are to be saved"? Faced with many candidates for an ELT process that can be made available to only a few, doctors and medical administrators confront the decision of who is to be given a chance at survival and who is, in effect, to be condemned to die.

As has already been implied, the "heroic" variety of spare-part surgery can pretty well be assimilated to this paradigm. One can foresee the time when heart transplantation, for example, will have become pretty much a routine medical procedure, albeit on a very limited basis, since a cardiac surgeon with the technical competence to transplant hearts can operate at best a rather small number of times each week and the elaborate facilities for such operations will most probably exist on a modest scale. Moreover, in "spare-part" surgery there is always the problem of availability of the "spare parts" themselves. A report in one British newspaper gives the following picture: "Of the 150,000 who die of heart disease each year [in the U.K.], Mr. Donald Longmore, research surgeon at the National Heart Hospital [in London] estimates that 22,000 might be eligible for heart surgery. Another 30,000 would need heart and lung transplants. But there are probably only between 7,000 and 14,000 potential donors a year."[1] Envisaging this situation in which at the very most something like one in four heart-malfunction victims can be saved, we clearly confront a problem in ELT allocation.

A perhaps even more drastic case in point is afforded by long-term hemodialysis, an ongoing process by which a complex device—an "artificial kidney machine"—is used periodically in cases of chronic renal failure to substitute for a non-functional kidney in "cleaning" potential poisons from the blood. Only a few major institutions have chronic hemodialysis units, whose complex operation is an extremely expensive proposition. For the present and the foreseeable future the situation is that "the number of places available for chronic hemodialysis is hopelessly inadequate."[2]

The traditional medical ethos has insulated the physician against facing the very existence of this problem. When swearing the Hippocratic Oath, he commits himself to work for the benefit of the sick in "whatsoever house I enter."[3] In taking this stance, the physician substantially renounces the explicit choice of saving certain lives rather than others. Of course, doctors have always in fact had to face such choices on the battlefield or in times of disaster, but there the issue had to be resolved hurriedly, under pressure, and in circumstances in which the very nature of the case effectively precluded calm deliberation by the decision maker as well as criticism by others. In sharp contrast, however, cases of the type we have postulated in the present discussion arise predictably, and represent choices to be made deliberately and "in cold blood."

It is, to begin with, appropriate to remark that this problem is not fundamentally a medical problem. For when there are sufficiently many afflicted candidates for ELT then—so we may assume—there will also be more than enough for whom the purely medical grounds for ELT allocation are decisively strong in any individual case, and just about equally strong throughout the group. But in this circumstance a selection of some afflicted patients over and against others cannot *ex hypothesi* be made on the basis of purely medical considerations.

The selection problem, as we have said, is in substantial measure not a medical one. It is a problem *for* medical men, which must somehow be solved by them, but that does not make it a medical issue—any more than the problem of hospital building is a medical issue. As a problem it belongs to the category of philosophical problems—specifically a problem of moral philosophy or ethics. Structurally, it bears a substantial kinship with those issues in this field that revolve about the notorious whom-to-save-on-the-lifeboat and whom-to-throw-to-the-wolves-pursuing-the-sled questions. But whereas questions of this just-indicated sort are artificial, hypothetical, and far-fetched, the ELT issue poses a *genuine* policy question for the responsible administrators in medical institutions, indeed a question that threatens to become commonplace in the foreseeable future.

Now what the medical administrator needs to have, and what the philosopher is presumably *ex officio* in a position to help in providing, is a body of *rational guidelines* for making choices in these literally life-or-death situations. This is an issue in which many interested parties have a substantial stake, including the responsible decision maker who wants to satisfy his conscience that he is acting in a reasonable way. Moreover, the family and associates of the man who is turned away—to say nothing of the man himself—have the right to an acceptable explanation. And indeed even the general public wants to know that what is being done is fitting and proper. All of these interested parties are entitled to insist that a reasonable code of operating principles provides a defensible rationale for making the life-and-death choices involved in ELT.

## II. THE TWO TYPES OF CRITERIA

Two distinguishable types of criteria are bound up in the issue of making ELT choices. We shall call these *Criteria of Inclusion* and *Criteria of Comparison*, respectively. The distinction at issue here requires some explanation. We can think of the selection as being made by a two-stage process: (1) the selection from among all possible candidates (by a suitable screening process) of a group to be taken under serious consideration as candidates for therapy, and then (2) the actual singling out, within this group, of the particular individuals to whom therapy is to be given. Thus the first process narrows down the range of comparative choices by eliminating *en bloc* whole categories of potential candidates. The second process calls for a more refined case-by-case comparison of those candidates that remain. By means of the first set of criteria one forms a selection group; by means of the second set, an actual selection is made within this group.

Thus what we shall call a "selection system" for the choice of patients to receive therapy of the ELT type will consist of criteria of these two kinds. Such a system will be acceptable only when the reasonableness of its component criteria can be established.

## III. ESSENTIAL FEATURES OF AN ACCEPTABLE ELT SELECTION SYSTEM

To qualify as reasonable, an ELT selection must meet two important "regulative" requirements: it must be *simple* enough to be readily intelligible, and it must be *plausible,* that is, patently reasonable in a way that can be apprehended easily and without involving ramified subtleties. Those medical administrators responsible for ELT choices must follow a modus operandi that virtually all the people involved can readily understand to be acceptable (at a reasonable level of generality, at any rate). Appearances are critically important here. It is not enough that the choice be made in a *justifiable* way; it must be possible for people—*plain* people—to "see" (i.e., understand without elaborate teaching or indoctrination) that *it is justified,* insofar as any mode of procedure can be justified in cases of this sort.

One "constitutive" requirement is obviously an essential feature of a reasonable selection system: all of its component criteria—those of inclusion and those of comparison alike—must be reasonable in the sense of being *rationally defensible.* The ramifications of this requirement call for detailed consideration. But one of its aspects should be noted without further ado: it must be *fair*—it must treat relevantly like cases alike, leaving no room for "influence" or favoritism, etc.

## IV. THE BASIC SCREENING STAGE: CRITERIA OF INCLUSION (AND EXCLUSION)

Three sorts of considerations are prominent among the plausible criteria of inclusion/exclusion at the basic screening stage: the constituency factor, the progress-of-science factor, and the prospect-of-success factor.

## A. The Constituency Factor

It is a "fact of life" that ELT can be available only in the institutional setting of a hospital or medical institute or the like. Such institutions generally have normal clientele boundaries. A veterans' hospital will not concern itself primarily with treating nonveterans, a children's hospital cannot be expected to accommodate the "senior citizen," an army hospital can regard college professors as outside its sphere. Sometimes the boundaries are geographic—a state hospital may admit only residents of a certain state. (There are, of course, indefensible constituency principles—say, race or religion, party membership, or ability to pay; and there are cases of borderline legitimacy, e.g., sex.) A medical institution is justified in considering for ELT only persons within its own constituency, provided this constituency is constituted upon a defensible basis. Thus the hemodialysis selection committee in Seattle "agreed to consider only those applications who were residents of the state of Washington. They justified this stand on the grounds that since the basic research . . . had been done at . . . a state-supported institution—the people whose taxes had paid for the research should be its first beneficiaries."[4]

While thus insisting that constituency considerations represent a valid and legitimate factor in ELT selection, I do feel there is much to be said for minimizing their role in life-or-death cases. Indeed a refusal to recognize them at all is a significant part of medical tradition, going back to the very oath of Hippocrates. They represent a departure from the ideal arising with the institutionalization of medicine, moving it away from its original status as an art practiced by an individual practitioner.

## B. The Progress-of-Science Factor

The needs of medical research can provide a second valid principle of inclusion. The research interests of the medical staff in relation to the specific nature of the cases at issue is a significant consideration. It may be important for the progress of medical science—and thus of potential benefit to many persons in the future—to determine how effective the ELT at issue is with diabetics or persons over sixty or with a negative RH factor. Considerations of this sort represent another type of legitimate factor in ELT selection. A very definitely *borderline* case under this head would revolve around the question of a patient's willingness to pay, not in monetary terms, but in offering himself as an experimental subject, say by contracting to return at designated times for a series of tests substantially unrelated to his own health, but yielding data of importance to medical knowledge in general.

## C. The Prospect-of-Success Factor

It may be that while the ELT at issue is not without *some* effectiveness in general, it has been established to be highly effective only with patients in certain specific categories (e.g., females under forty of a specific blood type). This difference in effectiveness—in the absolute or in the probability of success—is (we assume) so marked as to constitute virtually a difference in kind rather than in degree. In this case, it would be perfectly legitimate to adopt the general rule of making the ELT at issue available only or primarily to persons in this substantial-promise-of-success category. (It is on grounds of this sort that young children and persons over fifty are generally ruled out as candidates for hemodialysis.)

We have maintained that the three factors of constituency, progress of science, and prospect of success represent legitimate criteria of inclusion for ELT selection. But it remains to examine the considerations which legitimate them. The legitimating factors are in the final analysis practical or pragmatic in nature. From the practical angle it is advantageous—indeed to some extent necessary—that the arrangements governing medical institutions should embody certain constituency principles. It makes good pragmatic and utilitarian sense that progress-of-science considerations should be operative here. And, finally, the practical aspect is reinforced by a whole host of other considerations—including moral ones—in supporting the prospect-of-success criterion. The workings of each of these factors are of course conditioned by the ever-present element of limited availability. They are operative only in this context; that is, prospect of success is a legitimate consideration at all only because we are dealing with a situation of scarcity.

## V. THE FINAL SELECTION STAGE:
## CRITERIA OF SELECTION

Five sorts of elements must, as we see it, figure primarily among the plausible criteria of selection that are to be brought to bear in further screening the group constituted after application of the criteria of inclusion: the relative- likelihood-of-success factor, the life-expectancy factor, the family-role factor, the potential-contributions factor, and the services-rendered factor. The first two represent the *biomedical* aspect, the second three the *social* aspect.

### A.  The Relative-Likelihood-of-Success Factor

It is clear that the relative likelihood of success is a legitimate and appropriate factor in making a selection within the group of qualified patients that are to receive ELT. This is obviously one of the considerations that must count very significantly in a reasonable selection procedure.

The present criterion is of course closely related to item C of the preceding section. There we were concerned with prospect-of-success considerations categorically and *en bloc*. Here at present they come into play in a particularized case-by-case comparison among individuals. If the therapy at issue is not a once-and-for-all proposition and requires ongoing treatment, cognate consid-erations must be brought in. Thus, for example, in the case of a chronic ELT procedure such as hemodialysis it would clearly make sense to give priority to patients with a potentially reversible condition (who would thus need treat-ment for only a fraction of their remaining lives).

## B.  The Life-Expectancy Factor

Even if the ELT is "successful" in the patient's case he may, considering his age and/or other aspects of his general medical condition, look forward to only a very short probable future life. This is obviously another factor that must be taken into account.

## C.  The Family-Role Factor

A person's life is a thing of importance not only to himself but to others—friends, associates, neighbors, colleagues, etc. But his (or her) relationship to his immediate family is a thing of unique intimacy and significance. The na-ture of his relationship to his wife, children, and parents, and the issue of their financial and psychological dependence upon him, are obviously matters that deserve to be given weight in the ELT selection process. Other things being anything like equal, the mother of minor children must take priority over the middle-aged bachelor.

## D.  The Potential-Future-Contributions Factor (Prospective Service)

In "choosing to save" one life rather than another, "the society," through the mediation of the particular medical institution in question—which should certainly look upon itself as a trustee for the social interest—is clearly war-ranted in considering the likely pattern of future *services to be rendered* by the patient (adequate recovery assumed), considering his age, talent, training, and past record of performance. In its allocations of ELT, society "invests" a scarce resource in one person as against another and is thus entitled to look to the probable prospective "return" on its investment.

It may well be that a thoroughly egalitarian society is reluctant to put someone's social contribution into the scale in situations of the sort at issue. One popular article states that "the most difficult standard would be the can-didate's value to society," and goes on to quote someone who said: "You can't just pick a brilliant painter over a laborer. The average citizen would be quickly eliminated."[5] But what if it were not a brilliant painter but a brilliant surgeon or medical researcher that was at issue? One wonders if the author of the *obiter dictum* that one "can't just pick" would still feel equally sure of his ground. In any case, the fact that the standard is difficult to apply is certainly no reason for not attempting to apply it. The problem of ELT selection is inevitably burdened with difficult standards.

Some might feel that in assessing a patient's value to society one should ask not only who if permitted to continue living can make the greatest contribution to society in some creative or constructive way, but also who by dying would leave behind the greatest burden on society in assuming the discharge of their residual responsibilities. Certainly the philosophical utilitarian would give equal weight to both these considerations. Just here is where I would part ways with orthodox utilitarianism. For—though this is not the place to do so—I should be prepared to argue that a civilized society has an obligation to promote the furtherance of positive achievements in cultural and related areas even if this means the assumption of certain added burdens.

## E. The Past-Services-Rendered Factor
## (Retrospective Service)

A person's services to another person or group have always been taken to constitute a valid basis for a claim upon this person or group—of course a moral and not necessarily a legal claim. Society's obligation for the recognition and reward of services rendered—an obligation whose discharge is also very possibly conducive to self-interest in the long run—is thus another factor to be taken into account. This should be viewed as a morally necessary correlative of the previously considered factor of *prospective* service. It would be morally indefensible of society in effect to say: "Never mind about services you rendered yesterday—it is only the services to be rendered tomorrow that will count with us today." We live in very future-oriented times, constantly preoccupied in a distinctly utilitarian way with future satisfactions. And this disinclines us to give much recognition to past services. But parity considerations of the sort just adduced indicate that such recognition should be given *on grounds of equity*. No doubt a justification for giving weight to services rendered can also be attempted along utilitarian lines. ("The reward of past services rendered spurs people on to greater future efforts and is thus socially advantageous in the long-run future.") In saying that past services should be counted "on grounds of equity"—rather than "on grounds of utility"—I take the view that even if this utilitarian defense could somehow be shown to be fallacious, I should still be prepared to maintain the propriety of taking services rendered into account. The position does not rest on a utilitarian basis and so would not collapse with the removal of such a basis.

As we have said, these five factors fall into three groups: the biomedical factors A and B, the familial factor C, and the social factors D and E. With items A and B the need for a detailed analysis of the medical considerations comes to the fore. The age of the patient, his medical history, his physical and psychological condition, his specific disease, etc., will all need to be taken into exact account. These biomedical factors represent technical issues: they call for the physicians' expert judgment and the medical statisticians' hard data. And they are ethically uncontroversial factors—their legitimacy and appropriateness are evident from the very nature of the case.

Greater problems arise with the familial and social factors. They involve intangibles that are difficult to judge. How is one to develop subcriteria for weighing the relative social contributions of (say) an architect or a librarian or a mother of young children? And they involve highly problematic issues. (For example, should good moral character be rated a plus and bad a minus in judging services rendered?) And there is something strikingly unpleasant in grappling with issues of this sort for people brought up in times greatly inclined towards maxims of the type "Judge not!" and "Live and let live!" All the same, in the situation that concerns us here such distasteful problems must be faced, since a failure to choose to save some is tantamount to sentencing all. Unpleasant choices are intrinsic to the problem of ELT selection; they are of the very essence of the matter.[6]

But is reference to all these factors indeed inevitable? The justification for taking account of the medical factors is pretty obvious. But why should the social aspect of services rendered and to be rendered be taken into account at all? The answer is that they must be taken into account not from the *medical* but from the *ethical* point of view. Despite disagreement on many fundamental issues, moral philosophers of the present day are pretty well in consensus that the justification of human actions is to be sought largely and primarily—if not exclusively—in the principles of utility and of justice. But utility requires reference to services to be rendered, and justice calls for a recognition of services that have been rendered. Moral considerations would thus demand recognition of these two factors. (This, of course, still leaves open the question of whether the point of view provides a valid basis of action: Why base one's actions upon moral principles?—or, to put it bluntly—Why be moral? The present paper is, however, hardly the place to grapple with so fundamental an issue, which has been canvassed in the literature of philosophical ethics since Plato.)

## VI. MORE THAN MEDICAL ISSUES ARE INVOLVED

An active controversy has of late sprung up in medical circles over the question of whether nonphysician laymen should be given a role in ELT selection (in the specific context of chronic hemodialysis). One physician writes: "I think that the assessment of the candidates should be made by a senior doctor on the [dialysis] unit, but I am sure that it would be helpful to him—both in sharing responsibility and in avoiding personal pressure—if a small unnamed group of people [presumably including laymen] officially made the final decision. I visualize the doctor bringing the data to the group, explaining the points in relation to each case, and obtaining their approval of his order of priority."[7]

Essentially this procedure of a selection committee of laymen has for some years been in use in one of the most publicized chronic dialysis units, that of the Swedish Hospital of Seattle, Washington.[8] Many physicians are apparently reluctant to see the choice of allocation of medical therapy pass out of strictly medical hands. Thus in a recent symposium on the "Selection of Patients for Haemodialysis,"[9] Dr. Ralph Shakman writes: "Who is to implement the selection? In my opinion it must ultimately be the responsibility of the consultants in charge of the renal units . . . I can see no reason for delegating this responsibility to lay persons. Surely the latter would be better employed if they could be persuaded to devote their time and energy to raise more and more money for us to spend on our patients."[10] Other contributors to this symposium strike much the same note. Dr. F. M. Parsons writes: "In an attempt to overcome . . . difficulties in selection some have advocated introducing certain specified lay people into the discussions. Is it wise? I doubt whether a committee of this type can adjudicate as satisfactorily as two medical colleagues, particularly as successful therapy involves close cooperation between doctor and patient."[11] And Dr. M. A. Wilson writes in the same symposium: "The suggestion has been made that lay panels should select individuals for dialysis from among a group who are medically suitable. Though this would relieve the doctor-in-charge of a heavy load of responsibility, it would place the burden on those who have no personal knowledge and have to base their judgments on medical or social reports. I do not believe this would result in better decisions for the group or improve the doctor-patient relationship in individual cases."

But no amount of flag waving about the doctor's facing up to his responsibility—or prostrations before the idol of the doctor-patient relationship and reluctance to admit laymen into the sacred precincts of the conference chambers of medical consultations—can obscure the essential fact that ELT selection is not a wholly medical problem. When there are more than enough places in an ELT program to accommodate all who need it, then it will clearly be a medical question to decide who does have the need and which among these would successfully respond. But when an admitted gross insufficiency of places exists, when there are ten or fifty or one hundred highly eligible candidates for each place in the program, then it is unrealistic to take the view that purely medical criteria can furnish a sufficient basis for selection. The question of ELT selection becomes serious as a phenomenon of scale—because, as more candidates present themselves, strictly medical factors are increasingly less adequate as a selection criterion precisely because by numerical category-crowding there will be more and more cases whose "status is much the same" so far as purely medical considerations go.

The ELT selection problem clearly poses issues that transcend the medical sphere because—in the nature of the case—many residual issues remain to be dealt with once *all* of the medical questions have been faced. Because of this there is good reason why laymen as well as physicians should be involved in the selection process. Once the medical considerations have been brought to bear, fundamental social issues remain to be resolved. The instrumentalities of ELT have been created through the social investment of scarce resources, and the interests of the society deserve to play a role in their utilization. As representatives of their social interests, lay opinions should function to complement and supplement medical views once the proper arena of medical considerations is left behind. Those physicians who have urged the presence of lay members on selection panels can, from this point of view, be recognized as having seen the issue in proper perspective.

One physician has argued against lay representation on selection panels for hemodialysis as follows: "If the doctor advises dialysis and the lay panel refuses, the patient will regard this as a death sentence passed by an anonymous court from which he has no right of appeal."[12] But this drawback is not specific to the use of a lay panel. Rather, it is a feature inherent in every *selection* procedure, regardless of whether the selection is done by the head doctor of the unit, by a panel of physicians, etc. No matter who does the selecting among patients recommended for dialysis, the feelings of the patient who has been rejected (and knows it) can be expected to be much the same, provided that he recognizes the actual nature of the choice (and is not deceived by the possibly convenient but ultimately poisonous fiction that because the selection was made by physicians it was made entirely on medical grounds).

In summary, then, the question of ELT selection would appear to be one that is in its very nature heavily laden with issues of medical research, practice, and administration. But it will not be a question that can be resolved on solely medical grounds. Strictly social issues of justice and utility will invariably arise in this area—questions going outside the medical area in whose resolution medical laymen can and should play a substantial role.

## VII. THE INHERENT IMPERFECTION (NON-OPTIMALITY) OF ANY SELECTION SYSTEM

Our discussion to this point of the design of a selection system for ELT has left a gap that is a very fundamental and serious omission. We have argued that five factors must be taken into substantial and explicit account:

A. *Relative likelihood of success.* Is the chance of the treatment's being "successful" to be rated as high, good, average, etc.?

B. *Expectancy of future life.* Assuming the "success" of the treatment, how much longer does the patient stand a good chance (75 percent or better) of living—considering his age and general condition?

C. *Family role.* To what extent does the patient have responsibilities to others in his immediate family?

D. *Social contributions to be rendered.* Are the patient's past services to his society outstanding, substantial, average, etc.?

E. *Social contributions to be rendered.* Considering his age, talents, training, and past record of performance, is there a substantial probability that the patient will—*adequate recovery being assured*—render in the future services to his society that can be characterized as outstanding, substantial, average, etc.?

This list is clearly insufficient for the construction of a reasonable selection system, since that would require not only *that these factors be taken into account* (somehow or other), but—going beyond this—would specify a *specific set of procedures for taking account of them.* The specific procedures that would constitute such a system would have to take account of the interrelationship of these factors (e.g., B and E), and to set out exact guidelines as to the relevant weight that is to be given to each of them. This is something our discussion has not as yet considered.

In fact, I should want to maintain that there is no such thing here as a single rationally superior selection system. The position of affairs seems to me to be something like this: (1) It is necessary (for reasons already canvassed) to have a system, and to have a system that is rationally defensible, and (2) to be rationally defensible, this system must take the factors A–E into substantial and explicit account. But (3) the exact manner in which a rationally defensible system takes account of these factors cannot be fixed in any one specific way on the basis of general considerations. Any of the variety of ways that give A–E "their due" will be acceptable and viable. One cannot hope to find within this range of workable systems some one that is optimal in relation to the alternatives. There is no one system that does "the (uniquely) best"—only a variety of systems that do "as well as one can expect to do" in cases of this sort.

The situation is structurally very much akin to that of rules of partition of an estate among the relations of a decedent. It is important *that there be* such rules. And it is reasonable that spouse, children, parents, siblings, etc., be taken account of in these rules. But the question of the exact method of division—say that when the decedent has neither living spouse nor living children then his estate is to be divided, dividing 60 percent between parents, 40 percent between siblings versus dividing 90 percent between parents, 10 percent between siblings—cannot be settled on the basis of any general abstract considerations of reasonableness. Within broad limits, a *variety* of resolutions are all perfectly acceptable—so that no one procedure can justifiably be regarded as "the (uniquely) best" because it is superior to all others.

## VIII. A POSSIBLE BASIS FOR A REASONABLE SELECTION SYSTEM

Having said that there is no such thing as *the optimal* selection system for ELT, I want now to sketch out the broad features of what I would regard as *one acceptable* system.

The basis for the system would be a point rating. The scoring here at issue would give roughly equal weight to the medical considerations (A and B) in comparison with the extramedical considerations (C = family role, D = services rendered, and E = services to be rendered), also giving roughly equal weight to the three items involved here (C, D, and E). The result of such a scoring procedure would provide the essential starting point of our ELT selection mechanism. I deliberately say "starting point" because it seems to me that one should not follow the results of this scoring in an *automatic* way. I would propose that the actual selection should only be guided but not actually be dictated by this scoring procedure, along lines now to be explained.

## IX. THE DESIRABILITY OF INTRODUCING AN ELEMENT OF CHANCE

The detailed procedure I would propose—not of course as optimal (for reasons we have seen), but as eminently acceptable—would combine the scoring procedure just discussed with an element of chance. The resulting selection system would function as follows:

1. First the criteria of inclusion of Section IV above would be applied to constitute a *first phase selection group*—which (we shall suppose) is substantially larger than the number *n* of persons who can actually be accommodated with ELT.
2. Next the criteria of selection of Section V are brought to bear via a scoring procedure of the type described in Section VIII. On this basis a *second phase selection group* is constituted which is only *somewhat* larger—say by a third or a half—than the critical number *n* at issue.
3. If this second-phase selection group is relatively homogeneous as regards rating by the scoring procedure—that is, if there are no really major disparities within this group (as would be likely if the initial group was significantly larger than *n*)—then the final selection is made by *random* selection of *n* persons from within this group.

This introduction of the element of chance—in what could be dramatized as a "lottery of life and death"—must be justified. The fact is that such a procedure would bring with it three substantial advantages.

First, as we have argued above (in Section VII), any acceptable selection system is inherently nonoptimal. The introduction of the element of chance prevents the results that life-and-death choices are made by the automatic application of an admittedly imperfect selection method.

Second, a recourse to chance would doubtless make matters easier for the rejected patient and those who have a specific interest in him. It would surely be quite hard for them to accept his exclusion by relatively mechanical application of objective criteria in whose implementation subjective judgment is involved. But the circumstances of life have conditioned us to accept the workings of chance and to tolerate the element of luck (good or bad): human life is an inherently contingent process. Nobody, after all, has an absolute right to ELT—but most of us would feel that we have "every bit as much right" to it as anyone else in significantly similar circumstances. The introduction of the element of chance assures a like handling of like cases over the widest possible area that seems reasonable in the circumstances.

Third (and perhaps least), such a recourse to random selection does much to relieve the administrators of the selection system of the awesome burden of ultimate and absolute responsibility.

These three considerations would seem to build up a substantial case for introducing the element of chance into the mechanism of the system for ELT selection in a way limited and circumscribed by other weightier considerations, along some such lines as those set forth above.[13]

It should be recognized that this injection of *man-made* chance supplements the element of *natural* chance that is present inevitably and in any case (apart from the role of chance in singling out certain persons as victims for the affliction at issue). As F. M. Parsons has observed: "any vacancies [in an ELT program—specifically hemodialysis] will be filled immediately by the first suitable patients, even though their claims for therapy may subsequently prove less than those of other patients refused later."[14] Life is a chancy business, and even the most rational of human arrangements can cover this over to a very limited extent at best.

## NOTES

1. Christine Doyle, "Spare-Part Heart Surgeons Worried by Their Success," *Observer,* May 12, 1968.
2. J. D. N. Nabarro, "Selection of Patients for Haemodialysis," *British Medical Journal,* March 11, 1967, p. 623. See data from a forthcoming paper, "Home Dialysis," by C. M. Conty and H. V. Murdaugh. See also R. A. Baillod et al., "Overnight Haemodialysis in the Home," *Proceedings of the European Dialysis and Transplant Association* (1965), pp. 99 ff.
3. For the Hippocratic oath see *Hippocrates: Works,* vol. 1 (Loeb Library; London: Macmillan, 1959), p. 298.
4. Shana Alexander, "They Decide Who Lives, Who Dies," *Life,* November 9, 1962, p. 107.
5. Lawrence Lader, "Who Has the Right to Live?" *Good Housekeeping,* January 1968, p. 144.
6. This is the symposium on "Selection of Patients for Haemodialysis," *British Medical Journal* (March 11, 1967), pp. 622–24. F. M.
7. J. D. N. Nabarro, *op. cit.,* p. 622.
8. See Shana Alexander, *op cit.*

  9. *British Medical Journal* (March 11, 1967), pp. 622–24.
10. *Ibid.*, p. 624.
11. "Selection of Patients for Haemodialysis," *op. cit.* (n. 6 above), p. 623.
12. M. A. Wilson, "Selection of Patients for Haemodialysis," *op cit.*, p. 624.
13. See S. Gorovitz, "Ethics and the Allocation of Medical Resources," *Medical Research Engineering,* V [1966], p. 7).
14. "Selection of Patients for Haemodialysis," *op. cit.*, p. 623.

# Alcoholics and Liver Transplantation

## Carl Cohen, Martin Benjamin, and the Ethics and Social Impact Committee of the Transplant and Health Policy Center, Ann Arbor, Michigan

*The "God Committee's" social-worth standard gave way to Medicare's free dialysis machine for all Americans in renal failure. In other areas, however, the idea of using social worth as a basis for allocating scarce medical resources persists, especially in cases involving people whom society considers responsible for their own illness. Should public policy reward, punish, or be neutral about damage to people's lungs as a result of heavy smoking, or damage to people's livers as a result of heavy drinking? Liver transplants can cost $250,000. Alcoholics Anonymous considers alcoholism a disease for which victims are no more responsible than are victims of diabetes; others, such as philosopher Herbert Fingarette, believe that alcoholic behavior is mostly voluntary and controllable.*

*In 1991 physicians Mark Siegler and Alvin Moss argued (in the same journal and issue as the following selection) that alcoholics with end-stage liver disease should receive lower priority for liver transplants than nonalcoholics. Their position seems to endorse the position that alcoholics are less deserving than nonalcoholics and to deny that alcoholism is a real disease.*

*In the following selection philosophers Carl Cohen and Martin Benjamin challenge the moral basis of the physicians' argument. First, they dispute the claim that alcoholics deserve less than others. Second, they argue that there is no evidence that transplanting a liver to an alcoholic will result in fewer years per life per liver. If this second claim is true, denial of livers to alcoholics rests only on the moral claim.*

*Source: Journal of the American Medical Association,* 265, no. 10 (March 13, 1991), pp. 1299–1301. Reprinted by permission of the publisher.

*With experimental lung transplants for smokers now underway, the degree to which people are responsible for their health and sickness, and the degree to which public policy will reward or punish "sinful" behaviors, remain core issues in medical ethics.*

*Carl Cohen is professor of philosophy at the University of Michigan School of Medicine; Martin Benjamin is professor of philosophy at Michigan State University.*

Alcoholic cirrhosis of the liver—severe scarring due to the heavy use of alcohol—is by far the major cause of end-stage liver disease.[1] For persons so afflicted, life may depend on receiving a new, transplanted liver. The number of alcoholics in the United States needing new livers is great, but the supply of available livers for transplantation is small. *Should those whose end-stage liver disease was caused by alcohol abuse be categorically excluded from candidacy for liver transplantation?* This question, partly medical and partly moral, must now be confronted forthrightly. Many lives are at stake.

Reasons of two kinds underlie a widespread unwillingness to transplant livers into alcoholics: First, there is a common conviction—explicit or tacit—that alcoholics are morally blameworthy, their condition the result of their own misconduct, and that such blameworthiness disqualifies alcoholics in unavoidable competition for organs with others equally sick but blameless. Second, there is a common belief that because of their habits, alcoholics will not exhibit satisfactory survival rates after transplantation, and that, therefore, good stewardship of a scarce lifesaving resource requires that alcoholics not be considered for liver transplantation. We examine both of these arguments.

## THE MORAL ARGUMENT

A widespread condemnation of drunkenness and a revulsion for drunks lie at the heart of this public policy issue. Alcoholic cirrhosis—unlike other causes of end-stage liver disease—is brought on by a person's conduct, by heavy drinking. Yet if the dispute here were only about whether to treat someone who is seriously ill because of personal conduct, we would not say—as we do not in cases of other serious diseases resulting from personal conduct—that such conduct disqualifies a person from receiving desperately needed medical attention. Accident victims injured because they were not wearing seat belts are treated without hesitation; reformed smokers who become coronary bypass candidates partly because they disregarded their physicians' advice about tobacco, diet, and exercise are not turned away because of their bad habits. But new livers are a scarce resource, and transplanting a liver into an alcoholic may, therefore, result in death for a competing candidate whose liver disease was wholly beyond his or her control. Thus we seem driven, in this case unlike in others, to reflect on the weight given to the patient's personal conduct. And heavy drinking—unlike smoking, or overeating, or failing to wear a seat belt—is widely regarded as morally wrong.

Many contend that alcoholism is not a moral failing but a disease. Some authorities have recently reaffirmed this position, asserting that alcoholism is "best regarded as a chronic disease."[2] But this claim cannot be firmly established and is far from universally believed. Whether alcoholism is indeed a disease, or a moral failing, or both, remains a disputed matter surrounded by intense controversy.[3]

Even if it is true that alcoholics suffer from a somatic disorder, many people will argue that this disorder results in deadly liver disease only when coupled with a weakness of will—a weakness for which part of the blame must fall on the alcoholic. This consideration underlies the conviction that the alcoholic needing a transplanted liver, unlike a nonalcoholic competing for the same liver, is at least partly responsible for his or her need. Therefore, some conclude, the alcoholic's personal failing is rightly considered in deciding upon his or her entitlement to this very scarce resource.

Is this argument sound? We think it is not. Whether alcoholism is a moral failing, in whole or in part, remains uncertain. But even if we suppose that it is, it does not follow that we are justified in categorically denying liver transplants to those alcoholics suffering from end-stage cirrhosis. We could rightly preclude alcoholics from transplantation only if we assume that qualification for a new organ requires some level of moral virtue or is canceled by some level of moral vice. But there is absolutely no agreement—and there is likely to be none—about what constitutes moral virtue and vice and what rewards and penalties they deserve. The assumption that undergirds the moral argument for precluding alcoholics is thus unacceptable. Moreover, even if we could agree (which, in fact, we cannot) upon the kind of misconduct we would be looking for, the fair weighting of such a consideration would entail highly intrusive investigations into patients' moral habits—investigations universally thought repugnant. Moral evaluation is wisely and rightly excluded from all deliberations of who should be treated and how.

Indeed, we do exclude it. We do not seek to determine whether a particular transplant candidate is an abusive parent or a dutiful daughter, whether candidates cheat on their income taxes or their spouses, or whether potential recipients pay their parking tickets or routinely lie when they think it is in their best interests. We refrain from considering such judgments for several good reasons: (1) We have genuine and well-grounded doubts about comparative degrees of voluntariness and, therefore, *cannot pass judgment fairly.* (2) Even if we could assess degrees of voluntariness reliably, we *cannot know what penalties different degrees of misconduct deserve.* (3) *Judgments of this kind could not be made consistently in our medical system*—and a fundamental requirement of a fair system in allocating scarce resources is that it treat all in need of certain goods on the same standard, without unfair discrimination by group.

If alcoholics should be penalized because of their moral fault, then all others who are equally at fault in causing their own medical needs should be similarly penalized. To accomplish this, we would have to make vigorous and sustained efforts to find out whose conduct has been morally weak or sinful and to what degree. That inquiry, as a condition for medical care or for the receipt of goods in short supply, we certainly will not and should not undertake.

The unfairness of such moral judgments is compounded by other accidental factors that render moral assessment especially difficult in connection with alcoholism and liver disease. Some drinkers have a greater predisposition for alcohol abuse than others. And for some who drink to excess, the predisposition to cirrhosis is also greater; many grossly intemperate drinkers do not suffer grievously from liver disease. On the other hand, alcohol consumption that might be considered moderate for some may cause serious liver disease in others. It turns out, in fact, that the disastrous consequences of even low levels of alcohol consumption may be much more common in women than in men.[4] Therefore, penalizing cirrhotics by denying them transplant candidacy would have the effect of holding some groups arbitrarily to a higher standard than others and would probably hold women to a higher standard of conduct than men.

Moral judgments that eliminate alcoholics from candidacy thus prove unfair and unacceptable. The alleged (but disputed) moral misconduct of alcoholics with end-stage liver disease does not justify categorically excluding them as candidates for liver transplantation.

## MEDICAL ARGUMENT

Reluctance to use available livers in treating alcoholics is due in some part to the conviction that, because alcoholics would do poorly after transplant as a result of their bad habits, good stewardship of organs in short supply requires that alcoholics be excluded from consideration.

This argument also fails, for two reasons: First, it fails because the premise—that the outcome for alcoholics will invariably be poor relative to other groups—is at least doubtful and probably false. Second, it fails because, even if the premise were true, it could serve as a good reason to exclude alcoholics only if it were an equally good reason to exclude other groups having a prognosis equally bad or worse. But equally low survival rates have not excluded other groups; fairness therefore requires that this group not be categorically excluded either.

In fact, the data regarding the post-transplant histories of alcoholics are not yet reliable. Evidence gathered in 1984 indicated that the 1-year survival rate for patients with alcoholic cirrhosis was well below the survival rate for other recipients of liver transplants, excluding those with cancer.[5] But a 1988 report, with a larger (but still small) sample number, shows remarkably good results in alcoholics receiving transplants: 1-year survival is 73.2 percent—and of 35 carefully selected (and possibly nonrepresentative) alcoholics who received transplants and lived 6 months or longer, only two relapsed into alcohol abuse.[6] Liver transplantation, it would appear, can be a very sobering experience. Whether this group continues to do as well as a comparable group of nonalcoholic liver recipients remains uncertain. But the data, though not supporting the broad inclusion of alcoholics, do suggest that medical considerations do not now justify categorically excluding alcoholics from liver transplantation.

A history of alcoholism is of great concern when considering liver transplantation, not only because of the impact of alcohol abuse upon the entire system of the recipient, but also because the life of an alcoholic tends to be beset by general disorder. Returning to heavy drinking could ruin a new liver, though probably not for years. But relapse into heavy drinking would quite likely entail the inability to maintain the routine of multiple medication, daily or twice-daily, essential for immunosuppression and survival. As a class, alcoholic cirrhotics may therefore prove to have substantially lower survival rates after receiving transplants. All such matters should be weighed, of course. But none of them gives any solid reason to exclude alcoholics from consideration categorically.

Moreover, even if survival rates for alcoholics selected were much lower than normal—a supposition now in substantial doubt—what could fairly be concluded from such data? Do we exclude from transplant candidacy members of other groups known to have low survival rates? In fact we do not. Other things being equal, we may prefer not to transplant organs in short supply into patients afflicted, say, with liver cell cancer, knowing that such cancer recurs not long after a new liver is implanted.[7] Yet in some individual cases we do it. Similarly, some transplant recipients have other malignant neoplasms or other conditions that suggest low survival probability. Such matters are weighed in selecting recipients, but they are insufficient grounds to categorically exclude an entire group. This shows that the argument for excluding alcoholics on the basis of survival probability rates alone is simply not just.

## THE ARGUMENTS DISTINGUISHED

In fact, the exclusion of alcoholics from transplant candidacy probably results from an intermingling, perhaps at times a confusion, of the moral and medical arguments. But if the moral argument indeed does not apply, no combination of it with probable survival rates can make it applicable. Survival data, carefully collected and analyzed, deserve to be weighed in selecting candidates. These data do not come close to precluding alcoholics from consideration. Judgments of blameworthiness, which ought to be excluded generally, certainly should be excluded when weighing the impact of those survival rates. Some people with a strong antipathy to alcohol abuse and abusers may, without realizing it, be relying on assumed unfavorable data to support a fixed moral judgment. The arguments must be untangled. Actual results with transplanted alcoholics must be considered without regard to moral antipathies.

The upshot is inescapable: there are no good grounds at present—moral or medical—to disqualify a patient with end-stage liver disease from consideration for liver transplantation simply because of a history of heavy drinking.

## SCREENING AND SELECTING OF LIVER
## TRANSPLANT CANDIDATES

In the initial evaluation of candidates for any form of transplantation, the central questions are whether patients (1) are sick enough to need a new organ and (2) enjoy a high enough probability of benefiting from this limited resource. At this stage the criteria should be noncomparative.[8] Even the initial screening of patients must, however, be done individually and with great care.

The screening process for those suffering from alcoholic cirrhosis must be especially rigorous—not for moral reasons, but because of factors affecting survival, which are themselves influenced by a history of heavy drinking— and even more by its resumption. Responsible stewardship of scarce organs requires that the screening for candidacy take into consideration the manifold impact of heavy drinking on long-term transplant success. Cardiovascular problems brought on by alcoholism and other systematic contraindications must be looked for. Psychiatric and social evaluation is also in order, to determine whether patients understand and have come to terms with their condition and whether they have the social support essential for continuing immunosuppression and follow-up care.

Precisely which factors should be weighed in this screening process have not been firmly established. Some physicians have proposed a specified period of alcohol abstinence as an "objective"criterion for selection—but the data supporting such a criterion are far from conclusive, and the use of this criterion to exclude a prospective recipient is at present medically and morally arbitrary.[9]

Indeed, one important consequence of overcoming the strong presumption against considering alcoholics for liver transplantation is the research opportunity it presents and the encouragement it gives to the quest for more reliable predictors of medical success. As that search continues, some defensible guidelines for case-by-case determination have been devised, based on factors associated with sustained recovery from alcoholism and other considerations related to liver transplantation success in general. Such guidelines appropriately include (1) refined diagnosis by those trained in the treatment of alcoholism, (2) acknowledgment by the patient of a serious drinking problem, (3) social and familial stability, and (4) other factors experimentally associated with long-term sobriety.[10]

The experimental use of guidelines like these, and their gradual refinement over time, may lead to more reliable and more generally applicable predictors. But those more refined predictors will never be developed until prejudices against considering alcoholics for liver transplantation are overcome.

Patients who are sick because of alleged self-abuse ought not be grouped for discriminatory treatment—unless we are prepared to develop a detailed calculus of just deserts for health care based on good conduct. Lack of sympathy for those who bring serious disease upon themselves is understandable, but the temptation to institutionalize that emotional response must be tempered by our inability to apply such considerations justly and by our duty *not* to apply them unjustly. In the end, some patients with alcoholic cirrhosis may be judged, after careful evaluation, as good risks for a liver transplant.

## OBJECTION AND REPLY

Providing alcoholics with transplants may present a special "political" problem for transplant centers. The public perception of alcoholics is generally negative. The already low rate of organ donation, it may be argued, will fall even lower when it becomes known that donated organs are going to alcoholics. Financial support from legislatures may also suffer. One can imagine the effect on transplantation if the public were to learn that the liver of a teenager killed by a drunken driver had been transplanted into an alcoholic patient. If selecting even a few alcoholics as transplant candidates reduces the number of lives saved overall, might that not be good reason to preclude alcoholics categorically?

No. The fear is understandable, but excluding alcoholics cannot be rationally defended on that basis. Irresponsible conduct attributable to alcohol abuse should not be defended. No excuses should be made for the deplorable consequences of drunken behavior, from highway slaughter to familial neglect and abuse. But alcoholism must be distinguished from those consequences; not all alcoholics are morally irresponsible, vicious, or neglectful drunks. If there is a general failure to make this distinction, we must strive to overcome that failure, not pander to it.

Public confidence in medical practice in general, and in organ transplantation in particular, depends on the scientific validity and moral integrity of the policies adopted. Sound policies will prove publicly defensible. Shaping present health care policy on the basis of distorted public perceptions or prejudices will, in the long run, do more harm than good to the process and to the reputation of all concerned.

Approximately one in every ten Americans is a heavy drinker, and approximately one family in every three has at least one member at risk for alcoholic cirrhosis.[11] The care of alcoholics and the just treatment of them when their lives are at stake are matters a democratic polity may therefore be expected to act on with concern and reasonable judgment over the long run. The allocation of organs in short supply does present vexing moral problems; if thoughtless or shallow moralizing would cause some to respond very negatively to transplanting livers into alcoholic cirrhotics, that cannot serve as good reason to make such moralizing the measure of public policy.

We have argued that there is now no good reason, either moral or medical, to preclude alcoholics categorically from consideration for liver transplantation. We further conclude that it would therefore be unjust to implement that categorical preclusion simply because others might respond negatively if we do not.

# NOTES

1. "NIH Consensus Conference on Liver Transplantation," *JAMA* 250 (1983), pp. 2961–64.
2. F. L. Klerman, "Treatment of Alcoholism," *New England Journal of Medicine* 320 (1989), pp. 394–96.
3. G. E. Vaillant, *The National History of Alcoholism* (Cambridge, MA: Harvard University Press, 1983); E. M. Jellinek, *The Disease Concept of Alcoholism* (New Haven: Yale University Press, 1960).
4. M. Berglund, "Mortality in Alcoholics Related to Clinical State at First Admission: A Study of 537 Deaths," *Psychiatrica Scandinavica* 70 (1984), pp. 407–16.
5. B. F. Scharschmidt, "Human Liver Transplantation: Analysis of Data on 540 Patients from Four Centers," *Hepatology* 4 (1984), pp. 95–111.
6. T. E. Starzl, D. Van Thiel, A. G. Tazkis, et al., "Orthotopic Liver Transplantation for Alcoholic Cirrhosis," *JAMA* 260 (1988), pp. 2542–44.
7. R. D. Gordon, S. Iwatsuki, A. G. Tazkis, et al., "The Denver-Pittsburgh Liver Transplant Series," *Clinical Transplants,* ed. P. I. Terasaki (Los Angeles: UCLA Tissue-Typing Laboratory, 1987), pp. 43–49; R. D. Gordon, S. Iwatsuki, and C. O. Esquivel, "Liver Transplantation," in *Organ Transplantation and Replacement,* ed. C. J. Cerilli (Philadelphia: J. B. Lippincott, 1988), pp. 511–34.
8. J. F. Childress, "Who Shall Live When Not All Can Live? *Soundings* 53 (1970), pp. 339–62; T. E. Starzl, R. D. Gordon, S. Tazkis, et al., "Equitable Allocation of Extrarenal Organs: With Special Reference to the Liver," *Transplant Proceedings* 20 (1988), pp. 131–38.
9. S. Schenker, H. S. Perkins, and M. F. Sorrell, "Should Patients with End-Stage Alcoholic Liver Disease Have a New Liver?" *Hepatology* 11 (1990), pp. 314–19; *Allen v. A. Mansour,* U.S. District Court for the Eastern District of Michigan, Southern Division, 86-73429 (1986).
10. T. P. Beresford, J. G. Turcotte, R. Merion, et al., "A Rational Approach to Liver Transplantation for the Alcoholic Patient," *Psychosomatics* 31 (1990), pp. 241–54.
11. R. M. Rose and J. E. Barret, eds., *Alcoholism: Origins and Outcome* (New York: Raven Press, 1988).

# Rationing Failure: Ethical Lessons of Retransplantation

## Peter A. Ubel, Robert M. Arnold,
## and Arthur L. Caplan

*At a convention of medical ethicists in Memphis in 1992, Peter Ubel's presentation from the following paper was the talk of the meeting. A new allocation problem and a new, philosophically interesting variation of the "rule of rescue" had been discovered.*

*The rule of rescue is a departure from rationality in allocating scarce medical resources. First identified in the 1970s by pioneering medical ethicist Albert Jonsen, it states that the patient who manages to get "rescued" by media attention (such as a photogenic child in liver failure whose parents get him on television) is the patient who will get the scarce organ.*

*In this variation, the rule of rescue involves giving one or more successive organ transplants to an identified, "rescued" patient, while the anonymous, statistical patients who are not in the system are ignored. Ethically, the transplant team feels it would be "patient abandonment" not to perform a successive transplant on someone whom the team has already saved, although the person who does not get the next organ has needs that are just as real. A crucial medical fact remains that patients who receive a second or third heart or liver do worse than first-time recipients, so that maximization of life-per-organ comes from transplanting only first-timers.*

*Robert M. Arnold, MD, is an associate professor of medicine and also teaches in the Center for Medical Ethics at the University of Pittsburgh. Peter Ubel, MD, also teaches at the University of Pittsburgh Medical Center. Philosopher Arthur Caplan is one of the best-known bioethicists in America. A frequent commentator*

*Source: Journal of the American Medical Association, 270, no. 20 (November 24, 1993), pp. 2469–74. Reprinted with permission of the author and publisher. The authors thank Mark Wieclair, PhD, and Paula Greeno, MBA, for comments on earlier drafts of this essay; and Frances Kamm, PhD, for helpful discussions of her work in this area. Peter Ubel's work was supported by the DeCamp Foundation at the University of Chicago and by a National Institutes of Health grant at the University of Pittsburgh.*

*on television and radio, he has written a nationally syndicated column on bioethical issues. He is trustee professor and director of the Center for Bioethics at the University of Pennsylvania.*

Vital organ transplantation has captured the attention of the medical community and the public in part because of the tragic choices the transplant community must make every day. The demand for vital cadaver organs far exceeds the supply, forcing the transplant community to decide who should get available lifesaving organs. At the end of 1991, over 1,500 people were on waiting lists seeking cadaver livers, and over 2,000 were seeking hearts; of those patients, 9.9 percent awaiting livers and 16.7 percent awaiting hearts were removed from the waiting lists because they died before transplant organs became available.[1] Because of this unavoidable shortage, the transplant community has had to literally decide—by choosing who gets an organ—who lives or dies.

Despite the great amount of attention focused on transplant allocation, few have remarked at length about the special issues raised by the allocation of organs to retransplant candidates. This made some sense initially, both because retransplantation was a rapidly progressing field, with uncertain efficacy in many patient groups, and because many were hopeful that enough organs could be procured to reduce the scarcity of available organs.[2] But this inattention is no longer justifiable. The shortage of cadaveric transplant organs has grown with time rather than decreased.[3] Meanwhile, retransplantation has become a large part of transplant practice, accounting for 20 percent of all liver transplants and 10 percent of heart transplants, excluding heart-lung transplants.[4] And experience with retransplantation has accumulated to the point where its relative efficacy is clear: retransplant candidates do not do as well as primary transplant recipients.[5]

In cases of unavoidable scarcity, many believe that there is a moral obligation to distribute the scarce resources to those most likely to benefit from them. Yet present transplant policy seems to violate this maxim. The allocation system distributes 10 to 20 percent of available hearts and livers to retransplant patients, a group of individuals who have not only received the resource already, but who are also less likely to benefit from a new organ. At first glance, it appears that the allocation system, by offering retransplantation to so many patients, risks being both unfair and ineffective.

In this article, we explore how a just allocation system ought to distribute scarce hearts and livers among primary transplant and retransplant candidates. First, we describe how the present system allocates organs to primary transplant and retransplant candidates. Then, we examine three differences between primary transplantation and retransplantation that may affect the priority that retransplant candidates should receive in vying for available organs: (1) the special obligations that transplant teams have not to abandon patients on whom they have already performed a transplant, (2) the fairness of allowing a few individuals to get multiple transplants while some die awaiting their first, and (3) the magnitude of difference in efficacy between primary trans-plantation and retransplantation. We conclude that because of this last differ-ence, we ought to reassess the way we distribute organs among primary trans-plant and retransplant candidates. We argue that the present allocation system should be changed so that retransplant candidates no longer get the same ac-cess to transplant organs as those awaiting their first transplant.

## THE SYSTEM TO ALLOCATE HEARTS AND LIVERS

The system that allocates cadaver hearts and livers to primary transplant and retransplant candidates is coordinated by the United Network for Organ Shar-ing (UNOS), which supervises the procurement of organs and the formulation of patient waiting lists, monitors the conduct of surgeons and transplant cen-ters in utilizing cadaver organs, and distributes cadaver organs among trans-plant centers.

To enter the system, patients must first be diagnosed as having end-stage heart or liver failure. Patients who may need a transplant are then referred to a transplant center. At the center, patients are evaluated by a transplant team. These transplant teams, made up of physicians, nurses, social workers, and others, decide whether potential candidates meet medical standards of organ failure while remaining healthy enough to survive and adapt to a transplant. Thus, for example, transplant teams may reject a patient with end-stage heart disease who also has a serious, chronic infection. Transplant teams must also decide whether the patient has enough family support, money, competency, and personal stability to manage the complicated posttransplant regimen. These considerations are given significant weight in evaluating patients, as 5.6 percent of patients undergoing evaluation for a cardiac transplant are turned down for psychosocial reasons.[6]

Once deemed to be suitable transplant candidates, patients are placed on a waiting list, where they compete with other patients for available organs. Based on the UNOS Articles of Incorporation of June 27, 1991, cadaver livers are allocated according to a point system, which ranks candidates according to degree of ABO blood-group compatibility (an immunologic measurement), ex-tent of medical urgency (with critically ill candidates denoted as status 4), and amount of time on the waiting list (Table 1). In addition, priority is given to potential recipients in the same locality or region as the harvesting site. Distri-bution follows the order shown in Table 1.

Unlike cadaver livers, cadaver hearts are not allocated according to a point system. However, in other ways the systems are quite similar. Like liver candidates, heart transplant candidates are ranked according to ABO compati-bility, medical urgency (with critically ill candidates listed as status 1), time on the waiting list, and local and regional priority. In addition, because hearts cannot be preserved over long distances as effectively as livers, hearts are also allocated according to the distance between the recipient hospital and the donor. Thus, distribution follows the order listed in Table 2.

**TABLE 1** Rules for Distributing Cadaver Livers

Order of Liver Allocation[a]
  Local, status 4
  Local, all other
  Regional, status 4
  Regional, all other
  National, status 4
  National, all other

Point System for Liver Allocation

| | | |
|---|---|---|
| ABO blood-group compatibility | | |
|   Identical match | 10 points | |
|   Compatible | 5 points | |
|   Incompatible | 0 points | |
| Time waiting | | |
|   Longest waiting time | 10 points | |
|   Others | Percentile of line position $\times 10$[b] | |
| Degree of medical urgency | | |
|   Status 7 (inactive) | 0 points | |
|   Status 1 (normal) | 6 points | |
|   Status 2 (ill outpatients) | 12 points | |
|   Status 3 (hospitalized) | 18 points | |
|   Status 4 (intensive care unit) | 24 points | |

a. Distributed within each group according to number of points, in descending order.
b. Example: 50th percentile = 5 points.

**TABLE 2** Order of Heart Allocation[a]

Local, status 1
Local, status 2
Regional, status 1
Regional, status 2
Zone A, status 1, heart recipients
Zone A, heart-lung recipients
Zone B, status 1, heart recipients
Zones B and C, heart-lung recipients
Zone A, status 2, heart recipients
Zone B, status 2, heart recipients
Zone C, status 1, heart recipients
Zone C, status 2, heart recipients

a. In order of descending amount of waiting time, with preference in each category for blood-group-compatible (A, AB, B, O) candidates. Zones indicate the following distances between the recipient hospital and the donor: zone A, less than 800 km: zone B, 800 to 1,600 km: and zone C, more than 1,600 km.
*Source:* UNOS Articles of Incorporation, June 27, 1991.

By ranking the candidates according to these criteria, the transplant community is attempting to balance fairness, efficacy, and urgency. By factoring waiting time into allocation decisions, the lists resemble an egalitarian, "First come, first served" allocation approach.[7] All else equal, it seems fair to give organs to those who have been waiting the longest. However, this egalitarianism is balanced by attention to important measures of transplant effectiveness. Thus, the waiting lists distribute organs according to ABO matching and, for hearts, cadaver organ ischemic time, because these criteria are important predictors of transplant success. Finally, the waiting list gives great weight to the preoperative medical condition of the candidate. The emphasis on giving organs to those most urgently ill arises from a sense that, all else equal, we ought to give the organs to those who will die soonest without them.

One other fact is important to know for our purposes. Once on the list, primary transplant and retransplant candidates are treated identically. No points are awarded to or deducted from liver candidates because they have already received a transplant, nor are heart retransplant candidates given any special position on their waiting list.

## SPECIAL OBLIGATIONS TO RETRANSPLANT CANDIDATES

There are reasons to question whether retransplant candidates should be accorded the same treatment as primary transplant candidates. While most theories of justice would hold that equals should be treated equally, retransplant candidates differ from primary transplant candidates in several important ways. Do these differences merit changing the relative priorities of those needing primary transplants or retransplants?

There are several reasons some might argue that retransplant candidates should be given higher priority in receiving available organs. First, one might claim that the transplant system owes these patients another chance at receiving a transplant to make up for the suffering caused by the failure of their previous transplant. But this claim fails. Decisions to transplant or retransplant would be very hard to base on a scale of comparative misery. To begin with, it would be impossible to calculate how much different candidates had suffered. Even if this could be measured, allocation based on the amount of suffering would raise important moral problems. Should stoic transplant candidates receive lower priority because they have suffered less than other candidates?

Second, some argue that transplant teams have a special duty not to abandon their patients.[8] In general, health care workers are expected to protect the best interests of their patients.[9] This duty persists even when the chances of success seem remote.[10] Surgeons feel an even stronger duty to help patients on whom they have operated. This is likely to affect how transplant teams feel about transplant candidates on whom they have previously performed a transplant.

While these factors understandably create a sense of obligation among some who work on transplant teams, such feelings should not alter allocation priorities. It is not immoral for transplant teams to want their patients to do well. Nor can or should transplant teams avoid emotional attachments to their patients. But if such commitments determined how organs were allocated, we would end up favoring patients who are better at forming relationships with transplant teams. Those who are less likely to become close to team members, whether because of personality, appearance, race, language skills, or socioeconomic background, would be less likely to receive organs. In matters of unavoidable scarcity, health care workers' advocacy duties must be balanced by attention to justice.[11]

This conclusion stands even if members of the transplant team feel responsible for the failure of the previous transplant. While most failed transplants do not result from transplant team error, transplant team members may nonetheless blame themselves. This is a very human reaction to an unfortunate event. But although transplant failures are unfortunate, it would be unfair to respond by penalizing others who await transplant organs. Those whose organs fail as a result of natural causes are no less deserving of a transplant than those few whose illness is iatrogenic.

## IS RETRANSPLANTATION FAIR?

Those who would argue that we should give higher priority to retransplant candidates are unconvincing. Allocating priorities should not be affected by how much one has suffered or how well one has bonded to a transplant team. On the other hand, others might argue that retransplant candidates should get lower priority in receiving organs, because they have already had their chance at getting a transplant. Is it fair for some to receive more than one transplant while others die waiting for their first organ?

### "It's My Turn!": A Hypothetical Case

Imagine two individuals who have equally dire need of a new liver to survive. Both reach the point of needing the liver at the same time, and are coincidentally placed on the transplant waiting list. They are judged, as best as can be determined, to have an equal chance of surviving and benefiting from a new liver. An organ becomes available equally suitable for either candidate. Should their names be placed in a hat and one selected? What if one were to learn of the lottery and complain: "She has already received a liver transplant. I should get a crack at one liver before she gets a second!"

### Theories of Just Allocation

In order to evaluate this claim, we need to examine some common views of justice. Theories of justice are developed, at least in part, to find criteria to determine fair ways to distribute scarce goods. Some of the more common allocation criteria include utility, need, merit, age, social worth, ability to pay, personal responsibility, and quality of life. None of these criteria would favor the primary transplant candidate. For example, utilitarian theories hold that goods should be allocated in ways that maximize total happiness or utility.[12] Because our hypothetical case assumes that the two patients would have similar benefits from a transplant (in length and quality of life), utilitarianism would direct us to toss a coin. Similarly, a needs-based theory of just allocation would find each patient in equally desperate need. Those who think we should allocate goods according to age, social worth, personal responsibility, or ability to pay also would not look on the number of previous transplants as a relevant allocation criterion.

Theories of justice based on what a rational planner would choose behind a veil of ignorance could be used either to support or to penalize retransplant candidates.[13] It would be rational to choose a system that gives preference to those who have already received a transplant, assuring that once a patient has received a transplant he or she would have a better chance of staying alive. But it would also be rational to choose a system that allows more people to get a chance at transplantation at the expense of decreasing the opportunity for retransplant candidates to get organs. These theories are therefore not much help in deciding how to treat retransplant candidates.

Some might respond that these theories of justice do not capture the real issue. A more commonsense view of justice dictates that we all deserve an equal slice of the health care pie. That is, all else equal, we should not be giving out scarce pieces of pie to those who have already had some, while others await their first piece. This argument has an intuitive appeal. We do not have enough hearts and livers to go around, so we should not let anyone hog those that are available. However, this analogy breaks down. It asks us to base allocation of organs on a very narrow view of the health care pie—the pie of transplant organs—while ignoring other medical services and social goods that can affect health, such as income, education, and access to primary care. The primary transplant candidate in the hypothetical case may have grown up with all of life's advantages while the retransplant candidate has had to struggle to overcome poverty, absent parents, and inadequate access to health care. Fairness may just as well dictate that we should allocate organs according to how many health care goods one has had access to. If so, then primary transplant candidates would no longer have moral priority over retransplant candidates. Fairness based on an idea of a "fair slice of the pie" does not favor either candidate.

In summary, if retransplantation were as likely to succeed as primary transplantation, then theories of justice or ideas about what is a fair slice of the health care pie could not be used to favor primary transplant candidates over those needing retransplantation.

## EFFICACY DATA: POSTTRANSPLANT SURVIVAL

There is one other important difference between primary transplant and retransplant patients that might support an argument to give retransplant candidates lower priority. Retransplant patients are less likely to live 1 year after

**TABLE 3** Liver Transplant Patient Survival Rates,
October 1, 1987–December 31, 1991

| Transplant No. | No. Receiving Transplants | 1-year Survival (%) |
|---|---|---|
| | All Transplants | |
| 1 | 8539 | 76.5 |
| 2 | 1226 | 54.0 |
| 3 | 155 | 43.3 |
| | On Life Support | |
| 1 | 1158 | 60.1 |
| 2 | 710 | 46.7 |
| 3 | 93 | 35.3 |

*Source:* Steve Belle, PhD, United Network for Organ Sharing Scientific Registry.

their transplant. Should this decreased efficacy have a bearing on the priority that ought be given to retransplant candidates?

Before we discuss this question further, we must look at the data on retransplant survival. We have chosen to look at 1-year survival because it is an important, though minimal, measure of transplant success. In addition, there are good data on 1-year survival of retransplant patients, and there is not much information on other measures of retransplant success, such as quality of life.

## Liver Retransplantation

Data on the survival of patients receiving primary, secondary, and tertiary liver transplants have been compiled by UNOS.[14] The data show a significant 1-year survival advantage for primary transplant recipients (Table 3). The data continue to show a 10 to 30 percent 1-year survival advantage for primary transplant recipients when primary transplant and retransplant recipients are stratified according to the severity of their medical condition preoperatively, as shown in Table 3 for status 6 recipients (on life support prior to transplant). This survival advantage increases another 10 percent when primary transplant recipients are compared with tertiary transplant recipients (76.5 percent 1-year survival for primary transplant recipients versus 43.3 percent for tertiary recipients).

The survival advantage for primary transplant recipients holds at even the most experienced transplant centers.[15] For example, the largest reported experience with liver retransplantation in the cyclosporine era comes from the University of Pittsburgh, which has published data on 69 retransplant operations.[16] They compared 1-year survival in primary transplant and retransplant patients. For adults, primary transplant recipients had a statistically significant survival advantage, with 63.5 percent surviving versus 42.3 percent of retransplant recipients ($P = .026$). In children, primary transplant recipients had a similar advantage, with 76.8 percent surviving versus 56.5 percent of retransplant recipients ($P = .042$).

**TABLE 4** Heart Transplant Patient Survival Rates, October 1, 1987–December 31, 1991

| Group | No. Receiving Transplants | 1-year Survival (%) |
|---|---|---|
| Primary Transplant vs. Retransplant | | |
| First transplant | 4830 | 81.6 |
| Retransplant | 86 | 56.7 |
| All Patients | | |
| Work or school, full-time | 53 | 95.0 |
| Work or school, part-time | 142 | 84.4 |
| Homebound | 2176 | 84.1 |
| Hospitalized | 486 | 81.9 |
| Intensive care unit | 1174 | 83.0 |
| Life support | 793 | 73.8 |
| Unknown | 93 | 75.1 |
| Overall | 4917 | 81.6 |

Source: Steve Belle, PhD, United Network for Organ Sharing Scientific Registry.

## Cardiac Retransplantation

The United Network for Organ Sharing has also collected data comparing heart transplantation and retransplantation.[17] As with liver transplants, the data show a significant survival advantage for primary transplant recipients (Table 4). Retransplant candidates have a 25 percent lower 1-year survival rate than primary transplant recipients; UNOS has not stratified these data according to the preoperative condition of primary transplant and retransplant recipients. However, even if all retransplant candidates were in intensive care units (ICUs) preoperatively, their survival rate would still be significantly less than that of equally ill primary transplant candidates. This is so because the 1-year survival rate for all ICU patients receiving transplants is 73 percent, compared with a 56.7 percent 1-year survival rate for retransplant patients. Thus, even adjusting for preoperative condition, retransplant candidates do not do as well as primary transplant candidates.

The survival advantage for primary transplant recipients holds at even the most experienced transplant center. At Stanford University, one recent study compared the success of 288 patients receiving primary heart transplantation and 23 requiring retransplantation.[18] Of these 23 patients, 14 required transplantation because of accelerated graft atherosclerosis and the other 9 because of acute allograft rejection. The latter group had a significantly higher perioperative mortality than did primary transplant recipients. The acute allograft rejection group had 44 percent 1-year survival versus 81 percent for primary transplant. Patients undergoing retransplantation for accelerated graft atherosclerosis had a similar survival rate as primary transplant recipients (85 percent versus 81 percent), but 5-year survival was worse in the retransplant group than in the primary transplant group, with only 1 of the 14 patients surviving at that time. In a different study, the same group calculated 1-, 2-, and 5-year graft survival rates of 55 percent, 25 percent, and 10 percent in those undergoing retransplantation for accelerated graft atherosclerosis.[19] This compares with patient survival rates for primary transplantation of 67 percent, 46 percent, and 13 percent, respectively.[20]

## JUSTICE AND EFFICACY

The available data show that heart and liver retransplant patients do not do as well as primary transplant recipients. Retransplant patients are 20 percent less likely to survive 1 year after transplantation. This raises an ethical dilemma: should a moderate difference in survival rates make a difference in how we allocate scarce organs?

Perhaps one way to answer this question is to look at how the present allocation system already uses efficacy data to allocate organs. Both hearts and livers are preferentially distributed to those whose ABO types match the available organs. This preference was built into the liver point system after studies showed improved graft survival in patients who received ABO-identical organs.[21] The Pittsburgh transplant group compared all their liver recipients between 1981 and 1986.[22] They found a 15 percent to 20 percent survival advantage for ABO-identical recipients compared with those who were mismatched or incompatible. This difference was slightly smaller after adjusting for severity of illness and removing those patients whose transplants failed due to technical problems. These findings are consistent with more recent data collected by UNOS, which show a 16 percent decrease in 1-year graft survival for ABO-incompatible recipients compared with those with ABO-identical organs.[23]

In cardiac transplantation, ABO matching has an even greater impact on outcome. Despite occasional successes,[24] transplantation of hearts into ABO-incompatible recipients is generally associated with a poor prognosis. A survey of cardiac transplant programs revealed that the majority of such patients experience hyperacute graft rejection, with only a 45 percent chance of gaining long-term survival.[25] The prognosis is better for ABO-mismatched but compatible recipients. In a large study in Houston, Texas, 1-year survival for ABO-identical and ABO-nonidentical recipients was 79.5 percent and 62.2 percent, respectively.[26]

Thus, ABO mismatching of heart and liver transplants is associated with moderate to large decreases in 1-year survival. The current UNOS system for allocating livers and hearts takes these survival differences into account by favoring ABO-identical recipients. As the Pittsburgh transplant group concluded: "liver transplantation across ABO blood groups is usually successful, but not without risk. We therefore continue to give preference to ABO compatibility in the selection of liver transplant recipients."[27] The transplant community thus acts as if justice is best served by distributing available organs to those more likely to benefit from them.

However, the survival advantage for ABO-identical heart and liver recipients over most mismatched recipients is no larger than that seen for primary transplant recipients over retransplant recipients. The transplant community has already factored moderate efficacy differences into the allocation system. It seems inconsistent to ignore similar efficacy differences between primary transplant and retransplant recipients.

## Should We Factor Efficacy into Allocation?

While we have shown that it is inconsistent to treat retransplantation status differently from ABO status (since both have a similar effect on transplant efficacy), we have not established that efficacy is a morally relevant allocation criterion. One might argue that we should not factor efficacy into the allocation scheme. However, a number of theories of justice argue that efficacy should be factored into an allocation system. For example, utilitarianism would urge us to distribute organs to accrue the greatest benefit, which would clearly require us to pay attention to efficacy. In addition, a rational planner, choosing an allocation system behind a veil of ignorance, would plausibly opt for a system that favored those most likely to benefit from a transplant. Rational planners, ignorant as to whether or not they will ever need a transplant or a retransplant, would increase their own chances of benefiting from a transplant by setting up a system that, all else equal, distributed scarce organs to those most likely to gain long-term survival from a transplant. It is hard to imagine any theory of justice credibly asserting that we should transplant scarce organs into people regardless of their chance of surviving. As others have argued at greater length, efficacy is a morally relevant criterion for distributing scarce transplant organs.[28]

## Balancing Urgency and Efficacy

A critical question for an allocation system is to find an appropriate balance between urgency and efficacy. Some will argue that the urgency of patients' needs for organs should always take precedence over their likelihood of having good outcomes. To turn a dying patient away because of a lower chance of survival, it is argued, violates our duty to help the most urgently ill patients. This is especially relevant to our discussion of retransplantation because retransplant recipients are sicker, on average, than primary transplant recipients.[29]

This objection to the use of efficacy in allocating organs assumes that efficacy and urgency are always at odds, forcing us to choose one or the other. However, this is not always the case. While it is true that urgently ill patients are less likely to gain long-term survival from a transplant,[30] they are also less likely to live without a transplant. For example, some candidates on the heart waiting list are healthy enough that their chance of living an additional year will not be significantly improved by a transplant.[31] In contrast, some urgently ill candidates have such high mortality without a transplant that transplantation greatly improves their chance of surviving 1 year. In these cases, allocating organs to those most urgently ill (who have the most to gain from an early transplant) may potentially increase the number of years of life added by a transplant. Only when the likelihood of surviving a transplant gets very low does priority to urgency decrease the amount of benefit brought by transplant. For example, one study estimates that this would occur when a heart transplant candidate's chance of 1-year survival fell below 50 percent.[32]

Balancing our duty to urgently ill patients and our duty to use scarce organs in ways that maximize their benefit depends on the complex interaction between patients' predicted prognoses with and without a transplant and the relative weight one places on performing transplants on urgently ill patients. Luckily, the argument for giving primary transplant patients higher priority for organs does not require making these complex calculations. At any level of urgency, retransplant recipients do not do as well as similarly ill primary transplant recipients.[33] As we show in Table 3, retransplant recipients do worse than primary transplant recipients even after controlling for their preoperative status. And this difference increases with each successive transplant. Equally ill patients receiving their third liver transplants do even worse than those receiving their second. Retransplantation is an independent risk factor for poor transplant outcome.

Because these primary transplant and retransplant candidates are of similar levels of illness, there is no greater duty to help one group over the other. Thus, efficacy should determine which group has priority in receiving organs. By giving retransplant candidates equal access to transplantable organs, our present policy does not do all it can to distribute organs efficaciously. We give organs to a group of people who have less chance of gaining long-term survival from a transplant. We ignore our duty to distribute scarce resources in ways that increase the chance that the resources will bring benefit.

## CONCLUSIONS

We have looked at several ways in which retransplant candidates differ from those awaiting their first transplant to see if any of these differences ought to affect how we allocate organs. Two of these differences do not hold up to close scrutiny. Allocation priorities should not be altered on the basis of any special obligations that transplant teams feel to support patients on whom they have already performed transplants. Nor does any sense of justice support a claim that it is unfair to give patients second or third organs while others await their first.

Only one difference holds up to scrutiny: retransplant candidates do not do as well as primary transplant recipients. The current allocation system factors ABO matching into the allocation scheme on the basis of its moderate effect on transplant outcomes. Consistency demands that other factors that are as, if not more, important in predicting 1-year survival should also be included in the allocation system. The system should be revised to separate specific groups of candidates with a significantly lower chance of gaining long-term survival from a transplant.

Retransplantation provides one example of the cutoffs the transplant community should make. Retransplant recipients at similar levels of urgency do significantly worse than primary transplant recipients, a difference that increases with each successive transplant. We need to revise the allocation system in a way that directs more organs to primary transplant candidates instead of retransplant candidates. Reasonable people can disagree about the best way to do this. But some type of change should be made so that we can bring more benefit with the few organs available for transplant.

We think that the waiting lists should be altered so that primary transplant candidates have a better chance of receiving organs than retransplant candidates. In addition, we think those needing a third or fourth transplant should be removed from the waiting lists altogether. Instead, we should only allow them a limited number of experimental transplants, in hopes of improving their future chances of survival, or let them receive organs that are, for various reasons, not appropriate for others. But we should no longer allow them to vie for scarce organs on an equal basis with those who have never received a transplant and whose chances of benefiting from a transplant are much greater.

Health care workers cannot always be expected to recognize when it is time to forgo heroic lifesaving measures. Indeed, their traditional role as patient advocates would seem to compel them to ignore the odds and do whatever they can to help their patients, especially when they have already performed a transplant on the patient. However, when such heroic measures require scarce resources that could be better used to help others, their good intentions can be unjust. A change in the allocation system will reduce the tension physicians feel to balance their duties to patients and society. It is time to change the system to limit the number of times we will offer transplants to patients whose previous transplants have failed.

## NOTES

1. R. W. Evans, C. E. Orians, and N. L. Ascher, "The Potential Supply of Organ Donors: An Assessment of the Efficiency of Organ Procurement Efforts in the United States," *JAMA* 267 (1992), pp. 239–46.
2. B. Cohen, "Organ Donor Shortage: European Situation and Possible Solutions," *Scand J Urol Nephrol* 92 (1985), pp. 77–80; M. A. Cwiek, "Presumed Consent as a Solution to the Organ Shortfall Problem," *Public Law Forum* 4 (1984), pp. 81–89; M. Miller, "A Proposed Solution to the Present Organ Donation Crisis Based on a Hard Look at the Past," *Circulation* 75 (1987), pp. 20–23; A. Spital, "The Shortage of Organs for Transplantation: Where Do We Go from Here?" *New England Journal of Medicine* 325 (1991), pp. 1243–46.
3. Evans, Orians, and Ascher, "Potential Supply."
4. Written communications, Steven Belle, PhD, United Network for Organ Sharing (UNOS)/University of Pittsburgh Liver Transplant Registry, December 14, 1992; Tim Breen, PhD, UNOS Heart Transplant Registry, September 25, 1992.

5. B. W. Shaw, R. D. Gordon, S. Iwatsuki, and T. E. Starzl, "Hepatic Retransplantation," *Transplant Proceedings* 17 (1985), pp. 264–71; W. J. Wall, D. R. Grant, C. N. Ghent, et al., "Liver Transplantation: The University Hospital–Children's Hospital of Western Ontario Experience," in *Clinical Transplants,* ed. P. Terasaki (Los Angeles: UCLA Tissue Typing Laboratory, 1988); J. R. Dein, P. E. Oyer, E. B. Stinson, V. A. Starnes, and N. E. Shumway, "Cardiac Retransplantation in the Cyclosporine Era," *Annals of Thoracic Surgery* 48 (1989), pp. 350–55; S. Z. Gao, J. S. Schroeder, S. Hunt, and E. B. Stinson, "Retransplantation for Severe Accelerated Coronary Artery Disease in Heart Transplant Recipients," *American Journal of Cardiology* 62 (1988), pp. 876–81; written communications, Steven Belle, December 14, 1992, and Tim Breen, September 25, 1992.
6. M. E. Olbrisch and J. L. Levenson, "Psychosocial Evaluation of Heart Transplant Candidates: An International Survey of Process, Criteria, and Outcomes," *Journal of Heart and Lung Transplant* 10 (1991), pp. 948–55.
7. G. Calabresi and P. Bobbit, *Tragic Choices: The Conflicts Society Confronts in the Allocation of Tragically Scarce Resources* (New York: W. W. Norton, 1978).
8. Written communication, Thomas E. Starzl, MD, PhD, University of Pittsburgh, January 28, 1993.
9. F. R. Abrams, "Patient Advocate or Secret Agent?" *JAMA* 256 (1986), pp. 1784–85; M. Angell, "Cost Containment and the Physician," *JAMA* 254 (1985), pp. 1203–7; E. J. Cassell, "Do Justice, Love Mercy: The Inappropriateness of the Concept of Justice Applied to Bedside Decisions," in *Justice and Health Care,* ed. E. E. Shelp (New York: D. Reidel, 1981); H. H. Hiatt, "Protecting the Medical Commons," *New England Journal of Medicine* 293 (1975), pp. 235–41.
10. J. LaPuma, C. K. Cassel, and H. Humphrey, "Ethics, Economics, and Endocarditis: The Physician's Role in Resource Allocation," *Archives of Internal Medicine* 148 (1988), pp. 1809–11.
11. C. Cassel, "Doctors and Allocation Decisions: A New Role in the New Medicare," *Journal of Health Political Policy Law* (1985), pp. 549–64; N. Daniels, "The Ideal Advocate and Limited Resources," *Theor Med* 8 (1987), pp. 69–80; N. S. Jecker, "Integrating Medical Ethics with Normative Theory: Patient Advocacy and Social Responsibility," *Theoretical Medicine* 11 (1990), pp. 125–39.
12. J. S. Mill, *Utilitarianism* (London: Collins, 1863).
13. N. Daniels, *Just Health Care* (New York: Cambridge University Press, 1985); J. Rawls, *A Theory of Justice* (Cambridge, MA: Harvard University Press, 1971).
14. Written communication, Steven Belle, December 14, 1992.
15. Shaw et al., "Hepatic Retransplantation"; Wall et al., "Liver Transplantation."
16. Shaw et al., "Hepatic Retransplantation."
17. Written communication, Tim Breen, September 25, 1992.
18. Dein et al., "Cardiac Retransplantation."

19. Gao et al., "Retransplantation for Severe Accelerated Coronary Artery Disease."
20. Dein et al., "Cardiac Retransplantation."
21. R. D. Gordon, S. Iwatsuki, C. O. Esquivel, et al., "Experience with Primary Liver Transplantation across ABO Blood Groups," *Transplant Proceedings* 19 (1987), pp. 179–83; R. L. Jenkins, B. A. Georgi, C. A. Gallik-Karlson, R. J. Rohrer, U. Khettry, and W. S. Dzik, "ABO Mismatch and Liver Transplantation," *Transplant Proceedings* 19 (1987), pp. 184–89.
22. Gordon et al., "Experience with Primary Liver Transplantation."
23. S. H. Belle, K. C. Beringer, J. B. Murphy, et al., "Liver Transplantation in the United States: 1988 to 1990," in Terasaki, *Clinical Transplants.*
24. R. J. Caruana, G. L. Zumbro, R. G. Hoff, R. N. Rao, and S. A. Daspit, "Successful Cardiac Transplantation across an ABO Blood Group Barrier," *Transplantation* 46 (1988), pp. 472–74.
25. D. K. C. Cooper, "A Clinical Survey of Cardiac Transplantation between ABO Blood-Group-Incompatible Recipients and Donors," *Transplant Proceedings* 22 (1990), p. 1457.
26. T. Nakatani, H. Aida, O. H. Frazier, and M. P. Macris, "Effect of ABO Blood Type on Survival of Heart Transplant Patients Treated with Cyclosporine," *Journal of Heart Transplantation* 8 (1989), pp. 827–33.
27. Gordon et al., "Experience with Primary Liver Transplantation."
28. J. F. Kilner, *Who Lives? Who Dies? Ethical Criteria in Patient Selection* (New Haven: Yale University Press, 1990).
29. Written communication, Tim Breen, September 25, 1992.
30. Written communication, Steven Belle, December 14, 1992.
31. L. W. Stevenson, M. A. Hamilton, I. H. Tillisch, et al., "Decreasing Survival Benefit from Cardiac Transplantation for Outpatients as the Waiting List Lengthens," *Journal of the American College of Cardiologists* 18 (1991), pp. 919–25.
32. L. W. Stevenson, S. L. Warner, M. A. Hamilton, et al., "Distribution of Donor Hearts to Maximize Transplant Candidate Survival," *Circulation* 84 suppl. II-352 (1991).
33. Written communication, Steven Belle, December 14, 1992.

## PART NINE

# Involuntary Psychiatric Treatment

# The Case for Involuntary Hospitalization of the Mentally Ill

## Paul Chodoff

*This essay and the next argue the two classic positions for and against involuntary hospitalization of the mentally ill. Here, psychiatrist Paul Chodoff argues against the strict standards for involuntary commitment set out in the U.S. Supreme Court's 1975 decision in* O'Connor v. Donaldson, *which said that a state may pass a law allowing involuntary commitment only if the mentally ill person is a danger to others or to himself. Chodoff argues that this "dangerousness" standard is too narrow and that benefit to the person himself from involuntary hospitalization should also be a justification for commitment.*

*Paul Chodoff, MD, is a psychiatrist in private practice and Clinical Professor of Psychiatry and Behavioral Sciences at George Washington University School of Medicine.*

I will begin this paper with a series of vignettes designed to illustrate graphically the question that is my focus: under what conditions, if any, does society have the right to apply coercion to an individual to hospitalize him against his will, by reason of mental illness?

> *Case 1.* A woman in her mid-50s, with no previous overt behavioral difficulties, comes to believe that she is worthless and insignificant. She is completely preoccupied with her guilt and is increasingly unavailable for the ordinary demands of life. She eats very little because of her conviction that the food should go to others whose need is greater than hers, and her physical condition progressively deteriorates. Although she will talk to others about herself, she insists that she is not sick, only bad. She refuses medication, and when hospitalization is suggested she also refuses that on the grounds that she

*Source:* From *American Journal of Psychiatry* 133, no. 5 (May 1976), pp. 496–501. Reprinted by permission of the author and publisher.

would be taking up space that otherwise could be occupied by those who merit treatment more than she.

*Case 2.* For the past 6 years the behavior of a 42-year-old woman has been disturbed for periods of 3 months or longer. After recovery from her most recent episode she has been at home, functioning at a borderline level. A month ago she again started to withdraw from her environment. She pays increasingly less attention to her bodily needs, talks very little, and does not respond to questions or attention from those about her. She lapses into a mute state and lies in her bed in a totally passive fashion. She does not respond to other people, does not eat, and does not void. When her arm is raised from the bed it remains for several minutes in the position in which it is left. Her medical history and a physical examination reveal no evidence of primary physical illness.

*Case 3.* A man with a history of alcoholism has been on a binge for several weeks. He remains at home doing little else than drinking. He eats very little. He becomes tremulous and misinterprets spots on the wall as animals about to attack him, and he complains of "creeping" sensations in his body, which he attributes to infestation by insects. He does not seek help voluntarily, insists there is nothing wrong with him, and despite his wife's entreaties he continues to drink.

*Case 4.* Passersby and station personnel observe that a young woman has been spending several days at Union Station in Washington, D.C. Her behavior appears strange to others. She is finally befriended by a newspaper reporter who becomes aware that her perception of her situation is profoundly unrealistic and that she is, in fact, delusional. He persuades her to accompany him to St. Elizabeth's Hospital, where she is examined by a psychiatrist who recommends admission. She refuses hospitalization and the psychiatrist allows her to leave. She returns to Union Station. A few days later she is found dead, murdered, on one of the surrounding streets.

*Case 5.* A government attorney in his late 30s begins to display pressured speech and hyperactivity. He is too busy to sleep and eats very little. He talks rapidly, becomes irritable when interrupted, and makes phone calls all over the country in furtherance of his political ambitions, which are to begin a campaign for the presidency of the United States. He makes many purchases, some very expensive, thus running through a great deal of money. He is rude and tactless to his friends, who are offended by his behavior, and his job is in jeopardy. In spite of his wife's pleas he insists that he does not have the time to seek or accept treatment, and he refuses hospitalization. This is not the first such disturbance for this individual; in fact, very similar episodes have been occurring at roughly 2-year intervals since he was 18 years old.

*Case 6.* Passersby in a campus area observe two young women standing together, staring at each other, for over an hour. Their behavior attracts attention, and eventually the police take the pair to a nearby precinct station for questioning. They refuse to answer questions and sit mutely, staring into space. The police request some type of psychiatric examination but are informed by the city attorney's office that state law (Michigan) allows persons to be held for observation only if they appear obviously dangerous to themselves or others. In

this case, since the women do not seem homicidal or suicidal, they do not qualify for observation and are released.

Less than 30 hours later the two women are found on the floor of their
campus apartment, screaming and writhing in pain with their clothes ablaze
from a self-made pyre. One woman recovers; the other dies. There is no conclusive evidence that drugs were involved.[1]

Most, if not all, people would agree that the behavior described in these
vignettes deviates significantly from even elastic definitions of normality.
However, it is clear that there would not be a similar consensus on how to
react to this kind of behavior and that there is a considerable and increasing
ferment about what attitude the organized elements of our society should take
toward such individuals. Everyone has a stake in this important issue, but the
debate about it takes place principally among psychiatrists, lawyers, the
courts, and law enforcement agencies.

Points of view about the question of involuntary hospitalization fall into
the following three principal groups: the "abolitionists," medical model psychiatrists, and civil liberties lawyers.

## THE ABOLITIONISTS

Those holding this position would assert that in none of the cases I have described should involuntary hospitalization be a viable option because, quite
simply, it should never be resorted to under any circumstances. As Szasz has
put it, "we should value liberty more highly than mental health no matter
how defined" and "no one should be deprived of his freedom for the sake of
his mental health."[2] Ennis has said that the goal "is nothing less than the abolition of involuntary hospitalization."[3]

Prominent among the abolitionists are the "anti-psychiatrists," who, somewhat surprisingly, count in their ranks a number of well-known psychiatrists.
For them mental illness simply does not exist in the field of psychiatry.[4] They
reject entirely the medical model of mental illness and insist that acceptance of
it relies on a fiction accepted jointly by the state and by psychiatrists as a device
for exerting social control over annoying or unconventional people. The anti-
psychiatrists hold that these people ought to be afforded the dignity of being
held responsible for their behavior and required to accept its consequences. In
addition, some members of this group believe that the phenomena of "mental
illness" often represent essentially a tortured protest against the insanities of an
irrational society.[5] They maintain that society should not be encouraged in its
oppressive course by affixing a pejorative label to its victims.

Among the abolitionists are some civil liberties lawyers who both assert
their passionate support of the magisterial importance of individual liberty
and react with repugnance and impatience to what they see as the abuses of
psychiatric practice in this field—the commitment of some individuals for
flimsy and possibly self-serving reasons and their inhumane warehousing in
penal institutions wrongly called "hospitals."

The abolitionists do not oppose psychiatric treatment when it is conducted with the agreement of those being treated. I have no doubt that they would try to gain the consent of the individuals described earlier to undergo treatment, including hospitalization. The psychiatrists in this group would be very likely to confine their treatment methods to psychotherapeutic efforts to influence the aberrant behavior. They would be unlikely to use drugs and would certainly eschew such somatic therapies as ECT. If efforts to enlist voluntary compliance with treatment failed, the abolitionists would not employ any means of coercion. Instead, they would step aside and allow social, legal, and community sanctions to take their course. If a human being should be jailed or a human life lost as a result of this attitude, they would accept it as a necessary evil to be tolerated in order to avoid the greater evil of unjustified loss of liberty for others.[6]

## THE MEDICAL MODEL PSYCHIATRISTS

I use this admittedly awkward and not entirely accurate label to designate the position of a substantial number of psychiatrists. They believe that mental illness is a meaningful concept and that under certain conditions its existence justifies the state's exercise, under the doctrine of *parens patriae,* of its right and obligation to arrange for the hospitalization of the sick individual even though coercion is involved and he is deprived of his liberty. I believe that these psychiatrists would recommend involuntary hospitalization for all six of the patients described earlier.

### The Medical Model

There was a time, before they were considered to be ill, when individuals who displayed the kind of behavior I described earlier were put in "ships of fools" to wander the seas or were left to the mercies, sometimes tender but often savage, of uncomprehending communities that regarded them as either possessed or bad. During the Enlightenment and the early nineteenth century, however, these individuals gradually came to be regarded as sick people to be included under the humane and caring umbrella of the Judeo-Christian attitude toward illness. This attitude, which may have reached its height during the era of moral treatment in the early nineteenth century, has had unexpected and ambiguous consequences. It became overextended and partially perverted, and these excesses led to the reaction that is so strong a current in today's attitude toward mental illness.

However, reaction itself can go too far, and I believe that this is already happening. Witness the disastrous consequences of the precipitate dehospitalization that is occurring all over the country. To remove the protective mantle of illness from these disturbed people is to expose them, their families, and their communities to consequences that are certainly maladaptive and possibly irreparable. Are we really acting in accordance with their best interests when we allow them to "die with their rights on" or when we condemn them to a "preservation of liberty which is actually so destructive as to constitute another form of imprisonment"?[7] Will they not suffer "if [a] liberty they cannot enjoy is made superior to a health that must sometimes be forced on them"?[8]

Many of those who reject the medical model out of hand as inapplicable to so-called mental illness have tended to oversimplify its meaning and have, in fact, equated it almost entirely with organic disease. It is necessary to recognize that it is a complex concept and that there is a lack of agreement about its meaning. Sophisticated definitions of the medical model do not require only the demonstration of unequivocal organic pathology. A broader formulation, put forward by sociologists and deriving largely from Talcott Parsons' description of the sick role, extends the domain of illness to encompass certain forms of social deviance as well as biological disorders.[9] According to this definition, the medical model is characterized not only by organicity but also by being negatively valued by society, by "nonvoluntariness," thus exempting its exemplars from blame, and by the understanding that physicians are the technically competent experts to deal with its effects.[10]

Except for the question of organic disease, the patients I described earlier conform well to this broader conception of the medical model. They are all suffering both emotionally and physically, they are incapable by an effort of will of stopping or changing their destructive behavior, and those around them consider them to be in an undesirable sick state and to require medical attention.

Categorizing the behavior of these patients as involuntary may be criticized as evidence of an intolerably paternalistic and antitherapeutic attitude that fosters the very failure to take responsibility for their lives and behavior that the therapist should uncover rather than encourage. However, it must also be acknowledged that these severely ill people are not capable at a conscious level of deciding what is best for themselves and that in order to help them examine their behavior and motivation, it is necessary that they be alive and available for treatment. Their verbal message that they will not accept treatment may at the same time be conveying other more covert messages— that they are desperate and want help even though they cannot ask for it.[11]

Although organic pathology may not be the only determinant of the medical model, it is of course an important one and it should not be avoided in any discussion of mental illness. There would be no question that the previously described patient with delirium tremens is suffering from a toxic form of brain disease. There are a significant number of other patients who require involuntary hospitalization because of organic brain syndrome due to various causes. Among those who are not overtly organically ill, most of the candidates for involuntary hospitalization suffer from schizophrenia or one of the major affective disorders. A growing and increasingly impressive body of evidence points to the presence of an important genetic-biological factor in these conditions; thus, many of them qualify on these grounds as illnesses.

Despite the revisionist efforts of the anti-psychiatrists, mental illness *does* exist. It does not by any means include all of the people being treated by psychiatrists (or by nonpsychiatrist physicians), but it does encompass those few desperately sick people for whom involuntary commitment must be considered. In the words of a recent article, "The problem is that mental illness is not a myth. It is not some palpable falsehood propagated among the populace by power-mad psychiatrists, but a cruel and bitter reality that has been with the human race since antiquity."[12]

## Criteria for Involuntary Hospitalization

Procedures for involuntary hospitalization should be instituted for individuals who require care and treatment because of diagnosable mental illness that produces symptoms, including marked impairment in judgment, that disrupt their intrapsychic and interpersonal functioning. All three of these criteria must be met before involuntary hospitalization can be instituted.

**1. Mental illness.**   This concept has already been discussed, but it should be repeated that only a belief in the existence of illness justifies involuntary commitment. It is a fundamental assumption that makes aberrant behavior a medical matter and its care the concern of physicians.

**2. Disruption of functioning.**   This involves combinations of serious and often obvious disturbances that are both intrapsychic (for example, the suffering of severe depression) and interpersonal (for example, withdrawal from others because of depression). It does not include minor peccadilloes or eccentricities. Furthermore, the behavior in question must represent symptoms of the mental illness from which the patient is suffering. Among these symptoms are actions that are imminently or potentially dangerous in a physical sense to self or others, as well as other manifestations of mental illness such as those in the cases I have described. This is not to ignore dangerousness as a criterion for commitment but rather to put it in its proper place as one of a number of symptoms of the illness. A further manifestation of the illness, and indeed, the one that makes involuntary rather than voluntary hospitalization necessary, is impairment of the patient's judgment to such a degree that he is unable to consider his condition and make decisions about it in his own interests.

**3. Need for care and treatment.**   The goal of physicians is to treat and cure their patients; however, sometimes they can only ameliorate the suffering of their patients and sometimes all they can offer is care. It is not possible to predict whether someone will respond to treatment; nevertheless, the need for treatment and the availability of facilities to carry it out constitute essential preconditions that must be met to justify requiring anyone to give up his freedom. If mental hospital patients have a right to treatment, then psychiatrists have a right to ask for treatability as a front-door as well as a back-door criterion for commitment.[13] All of the six individuals I described earlier could have been treated with a reasonable expectation of returning to a more normal state of functioning.

I believe that the objections to this formulation can be summarized as follows.

1. The whole structure founders for those who maintain that mental illness is a fiction.

2. These criteria are also untenable to those who hold liberty to be such a supreme value that the presence of mental illness per se does not constitute justification for depriving an individual of his freedom; only when such illness is manifested by clearly dangerous behavior may commitment be considered. For reasons to be discussed later, I agree with those psychiatrists who do not believe that dangerousness should be elevated to primacy above other manifestations of mental illness as a sine qua non for involuntary hospitalization.[14]

3. The medical model criteria are "soft" and subjective and depend on the fallible judgment of psychiatrists. This is a valid objection. There is no reliable blood test for schizophrenia and no method for injecting grey cells into psychiatrists. A relatively small number of cases will always fall within a grey area that will be difficult to judge. In those extreme cases in which the question of commitment arises, competent and ethical psychiatrists should be able to use these criteria without doing violence to individual liberties and with the expectation of good results. Furthermore, the possible "fuzziness" of some aspects of the medical model approach is certainly no greater than that of the supposedly "objective" criteria for dangerousness, and there is little reason to believe that lawyers and judges are any less fallible than psychiatrists.

4. Commitment procedures in the hands of psychiatrists are subject to intolerable abuses. Here, as Peszke said, "It is imperative that we differentiate between the principle of the process of civil commitment and the practice itself."[15] Abuses can contaminate both the medical and the dangerousness approaches, and I believe that the abuses stemming from the abolitionist view of no commitment at all are even greater. Measures to abate abuses of the medical approach include judicial review and the abandonment of indeterminate commitment. In the course of commitment proceedings and thereafter, patients should have access to competent and compassionate legal counsel. However, this latter safeguard may itself be subject to abuse if the legal counsel acts solely in the adversary tradition and undertakes to carry out the patient's wishes even when they may be destructive.

## Comment

The criteria and procedures outlined will apply most appropriately to initial episodes and recurrent attacks of mental illness. To put it simply, it is necessary to find a way to satisfy legal and humanitarian considerations and yet allow psychiatrists access to initially or acutely ill patients in order to do the best they can for them. However, there are some involuntary patients who have received adequate and active treatment but have not responded satisfactorily. An irreducible minimum of such cases, principally among those with brain disorders and process schizophrenia, will not improve sufficiently to be able to adapt to even a tolerant society.

The decision of what to do at this point is not an easy one, and it should certainly not be in the hands of psychiatrists alone. With some justification they can state that they have been given the thankless job of caring, often with inadequate facilities, for badly damaged people and that they are now being subjected to criticism for keeping these patients locked up. No one really knows what to do with these patients. It may be that when treatment has failed they exchange their sick role for what has been called the impaired role,[16] which implies a permanent negative evaluation of them coupled with a somewhat less benign societal attitude. At this point, perhaps a case can be made for giving greater importance to the criteria for dangerousness and releasing such patients if they do not pose a threat to others. However, I do not believe that the release into the community of these severely malfunctioning individuals will serve their interests even though it may satisfy formal notions of right and wrong.

It should be emphasized that the number of individuals for whom involuntary commitment must be considered is small (although, under the influence of current pressure, it may be smaller than it should be). Even severe mental illness can often be handled by securing the cooperation of the patient, and certainly one of the favorable effects of the current ferment has been to encourage such efforts. However, the distinction between voluntary and involuntary hospitalization is sometimes more formal than meaningful. How "voluntary" are the actions of an individual who is being buffeted by the threats, entreaties, and tears of his family?

I believe, however, that we are at a point (at least in some jurisdictions) where, having rebounded from an era in which involuntary commitment was too easy and employed too often, we are now entering one in which it is becoming very difficult to commit anyone, even in urgent cases. Faced with the moral obloquy that has come to pervade the atmosphere in which the decision to involuntarily hospitalize is considered, some psychiatrists, especially younger ones, have become, as Stone put it, "soft as grapes" when faced with the prospect of committing anyone under any circumstances.[17]

## THE CIVIL LIBERTIES LAWYERS

I use this admittedly inexact label to designate those members of the legal profession who do not in principle reject the necessity for involuntary hospitalization but who do reject or wish to diminish the importance of medical model criteria in the hands of psychiatrists. Accordingly, the civil liberties lawyers, in dealing with the problem of involuntary hospitalization, have enlisted themselves under the standard of dangerousness, which they hold to be more objective and capable of being dealt with in a sounder evidentiary manner than the medical model criteria. For them the question is not whether mental illness, even of disabling degree, is present, but only whether it has resulted in the probability of behavior dangerous to others or to self. Thus they would scrutinize the cases previously described for evidence of such dangerousness and would make the decision about involuntary hospitalization accordingly. They would probably feel that commitment is not indicated in most of these cases, since they were selected as illustrative of severe mental illness in which outstanding evidence of physical dangerousness was not present.

The dangerousness standard is being used increasingly not only to supplement criteria for mental illness but, in fact, to replace them entirely. The recent Supreme Court decision in *O'Connor v. Donaldson* is certainly a long step in this direction.[18] In addition, "dangerousness" is increasingly being understood to refer to the probability that the individual will inflict harm on himself or others in a specific physical manner rather than in other ways. This tendency has perhaps been carried to its ultimate in the *Lessard v. Schmidt* case in Wisconsin, which restricted suitability for commitment to the "extreme likelihood that if the person is not confined, he will do immediate harm to himself or others."[19] (This decision was set aside by the U.S. Supreme Court in 1974.) In a recent Washington, D.C., Superior Court case the instructions to the jury stated that the government must prove that the defendant was likely to cause "substantial physical harm to himself or others in the reasonably foreseeable future."[20]

For the following reasons, the dangerousness standard is an inappropriate and dangerous indicator to use in judging the conditions under which someone should be involuntarily hospitalized. Dangerousness is being taken out of its proper context as one among other symptoms of the presence of severe mental illness that should be the determining factor.

1. To concentrate on dangerousness (especially to others) as the sole criterion for involuntary hospitalization deprives many mentally ill persons of the protection and treatment that they urgently require. A psychiatrist under the constraints of the dangerousness rule, faced with an out-of-control manic individual whose frantic behavior the psychiatrist truly believes to be a disguised call for help, would have to say, "Sorry, I would like to help you but I can't because you haven't threatened anybody and you are not suicidal." Since psychiatrists are admittedly not very good at accurately predicting dangerousness to others, the evidentiary standards for commitment will be very stringent. This will result in mental hospitals' becoming prisons for a small population of volatile, highly assaultive, and untreatable patients.[21]

2. The attempt to differentiate rigidly (especially in regard to danger to self) between physical and other kinds of self-destructive behavior is artificial, unrealistic, and unworkable. It will tend to confront psychiatrists who want to help their patients with the same kind of dilemma they were faced with when justification for therapeutic abortion on psychiatric grounds depended on evidence of suicidal intent. The advocates of the dangerousness standard seem to be more comfortable with and pay more attention to the factor of dangerousness to others even though it is a much less frequent and much less significant consequence of mental illness than is danger to self.

3. The emphasis on dangerousness (again, especially to others) is a real obstacle to the right-to-treatment movement, since it prevents the hospitalization and therefore the treatment of the population most amenable to various kinds of therapy.

4. Emphasis on the criterion of dangerousness to others moves involuntary commitment from a civil to a criminal procedure, thus, as Stone put it, imposing the procedures of one terrible system on another.[22] Involuntary commitment on these grounds becomes a form of preventive detention and makes the psychiatrist a kind of glorified policeman.

5. Emphasis on dangerousness rather than mental disability and helplessness will hasten the process of deinstitutionalization. Recent reports (20, 21) have shown that these patients are not being rehabilitated and reintegrated into the community, but rather, that the burden of custodialism has been shifted from the hospital to the community.[23]

6. As previously mentioned, emphasis on the dangerousness criterion may be a tactic of some of the abolitionists among the civil liberties lawyers to end involuntary hospitalization by reducing it to an unworkable absurdity.[24]

## DISCUSSION

It is obvious that it is good to be at liberty and that it is good to be free from the consequences of disabling and dehumanizing illness. Sometimes these two values are incompatible, and in the heat of the passions that are often aroused by opposing views of right and wrong, the partisans of each view may tend to minimize the importance of the other. Both sides can present their horror stories—the psychiatrists, their dead victims of the failure of the involuntary hospitalization process, and the lawyers, their Donaldsons. There is a real danger that instead of acknowledging the difficulty of the problem, the two camps will become polarized, with a consequent rush toward extreme and untenable solutions rather than working toward reasonable ones.

The path taken by those whom I have labeled the abolitionists is an example of the barren results that ensue when an absolute solution is imposed on a complex problem. There are human beings who will suffer greatly if the abolitionists succeed in elevating an abstract principle into an unbreakable law with no exceptions. I find myself oppressed and repelled by their position, which seems to stem from an ideological rigidity which ignores that element of the contingent immanent in the structure of human existence. It is devoid of compassion.

The positions of those who espouse the medical model and the dangerousness approaches to commitment are, one hopes, not completely irreconcilable. To some extent these differences are a result of the vantage points from which lawyers and psychiatrists view mental illness and commitment. The lawyers see and are concerned with the failures and abuses of the process. Furthermore, as a result of their training, they tend to apply principles to classes of people rather than to take each instance as unique. The psychiatrists, on the other hand, are required to deal practically with the singular needs of individuals. They approach the problem from a clinical rather than a deductive stance. As physicians, they want to be in a position to take care of and to help suffering people whom they regard as sick patients. They sometimes become impatient with the rules that prevent them from doing this.

I believe we are now witnessing a pendular swing in which the rights of the mentally ill to be treated and protected are being set aside in the rush to give them their freedom at whatever cost. But is freedom defined only by the absence of external constraints? Internal physiological or psychological processes can contribute to a throttling of the spirit that is as painful as any applied from the outside. The "wild" manic individual without his lithium, the panicky hallucinator without his injection of fluphenazine hydrochloride and the understanding support of a concerned staff, the sodden alcoholic—are they free? Sometimes, as Woody Guthrie said, "Freedom means no place to go."

Today the civil liberties lawyers are in the ascendancy and the psychiatrists on the defensive to a degree that is harmful to individual needs and the public welfare. Redress and a more balanced position will not come from further extension of the dangerousness doctrine. I favor a return to the use of medical criteria by psychiatrists—psychiatrists, however, who have been chastened by the buffeting they have received and are quite willing to go along with even strict legal safeguards as long as they are constructive and not tyrannical.

## NOTES

1. D. A. Treffert, "The Practical Limits of Patients' Rights," *Psychiatric Annals* 5, no. 4 (1971), pp. 91–96.
2. T. Szasz, *Law, Liberty, and Psychiatry* (New York: Macmillan, 1963).
3. B. Ennis, *Prisoners of Psychiatry* (New York: Harcourt Brace Jovanovich, 1972).
4. T. Szasz, *The Myth of Mental Illness* (New York: Harper & Row, 1961).
5. R. Laing, *The Politics of Experience* (New York: Ballantine Books, 1967).
6. B. Ennis, "Ennis on 'Donaldson'," *Psychiatric News*, December 3, 1975, pp. 4, 19, 37.
7. T. Treffert, "Practical Limits of Patients' Rights"; R. Peele, P. Chodoff, and N. Taub, "Involuntary Hospitalization and Treatability: Observations from the DC Experience," *Catholic University Law Review* 23 (1974), pp. 744–53.
8. R. Michels, *The Right to Refuse Psychotropic Drugs*, Hastings Center Report (Hastings-on-Hudson, NY: Hastings Institute of Health and Human Values, 1973).
9. T. Parsons, *The Social System* (New York: Free Press, 1951).
10. R. M. Veatch, "The Medical Model: Its Nature and Problems," *Hastings Center Studies* 1, no. 3 (1973), pp. 59–76.
11. J. Katz, "The Right to Treatment—an Enchanting Legal Fiction?" *University of Chicago Law Review* 36 (1969), pp. 755–83.
12. M. S. Moore, "Some Myths about Mental Illness," *Archives of General Psychiatry* 32 (1975), p. 1483.

13. Peele, Chodoff, and Taub, "Involuntary Hospitalization and Treatability."
14. M. A. Peszke, "Is Dangerousness an Issue for Physicians in Emergency Commitment?" *American Journal of Psychiatry* 132 (1975), pp. 825–28; A. A. Stone, "Comment on Peszke MA: Is Dangerousness an Issue for Physicians in Emergency Commitment? ibid., pp. 829–31.
15. Peszke, "Is Dangerousness an Issue?" p. 825.
16. M. Siegler and H. Osmond, *Models of Madness, Models of Medicine* (New York: Macmillan, 1974).
17. A. Stone, lecture for course on "The Law, Litigation, and Mental Health Services," Adelphi, MD, Mental Health Study Center, September 1974.
18. *O'Connor v. Donaldson*, 43 U.S.L.W. 4929 (1975).
19. *Lessard v. Schmidt*, 349 F. Supp 1078, 1092 (E.D. Wis. 1972).
20. In re Johnnie Hargrove, Washington, DC, Superior Court Mental Health number 506–75, 1975.
21. Stone, "Comment on Peszke MA."
22. Ibid.
23. S. Rachlin, A. Pam, and J. Milton, "Civil Liberties versus Involuntary Hospitalization," *American Journal of Psychiatry* 132 (1975), pp. 189–91; S. A. Kirk and M. E. Therrien, "Community Mental Health Myths and the Fate of Former Hospitalized Patients," *Psychiatry* 38 (1975), pp. 209–17.
24. A. A. Dershowitz, "Dangerousness as a Criterion for Confinement," *Bulletin of the American Academy of Psychiatry and the Law"* 2 (1974), pp. 172–79.

# Involuntary Mental Hospitalization: A Crime against Humanity

## Thomas Szasz

*Thomas Szasz is the world's foremost critic of the tendency of his own profession, psychiatry, to incarcerate people forcibly in order to improve their mental health. In this selection, he defends a libertarian position, arguing that society commits people to mental institutions not to help them but as an exercise in power. He also makes an analogy between this practice and slavery.*

*Born in Hungary and a passionate libertarian, Thomas Szasz, MD, PhD, is a psychoanalyst and Professor Emeritus of Psychiatry at the State University of New York Health Sciences Center in Syracuse. His book* The Myth of Mental Illness *(1961) is a classic in both psychiatry and philosophy.*

### I

For some time now I have maintained that commitment—that is, the detention of persons in mental institutions against their will—is a form of imprisonment; that such deprivation of liberty is contrary to the moral principles embodied in the Declaration of Independence and the Constitution of the United States; and that it is a crass violation of contemporary concepts of fundamental human rights.[1] The practice of "sane" men incarcerating their "insane" fellow men in "mental hospitals" can be compared to that of white men enslaving black men. In short, I consider commitment a crime against humanity.

Existing social institutions and practices, especially if honored by prolonged usage, are generally experienced and accepted as good and valuable. For thousands of years slavery was considered a "natural" social arrangement

*Source: Ideology and Insanity* (Garden City, NY: Doubleday, 1970). Reprinted by permission of the author and publisher.

for the securing of human labor; it was sanctioned by public opinion, religious dogma, church, and state; it was abolished a mere one hundred years ago in the United States; and it is still a prevalent social practice in some parts of the world, notably in Africa.[2] Since its origin, approximately three centuries ago, commitment of the insane has enjoyed equally widespread support; physicians, lawyers, and the laity have asserted, as if with a single voice, the therapeutic desirability and social necessity of institutional psychiatry. My claim that commitment is a crime against humanity may thus be countered—as indeed it has been—by maintaining, first, that the practice is beneficial for the mentally ill, and second, that it is necessary for the protection of the mentally healthy members of society. . . .

## II

What is the evidence that commitment does not serve the purpose of helping or treating people whose behavior deviates from or threatens prevailing social norms or moral standards; and who, because they inconvenience their families, neighbors, or superiors, may be incriminated as "mentally ill"?

### 1. The Medical Evidence.

Mental illness is a metaphor. If by "disease" we mean a disorder of the physicochemical machinery of the human body, then we can assert that what we call functional mental diseases are not diseases at all.[3] Persons said to be suffering from such disorders are socially deviant or inept, or in conflict with individuals, groups, or institutions. Since they do not suffer from disease, it is impossible to "treat" them for any sickness.

Although the term "mentally ill" is usually applied to persons who do not suffer from bodily disease, it is sometimes applied also to persons who do (for example, to individuals intoxicated with alcohol or other drugs, or to elderly people suffering from degenerative disease of the brain). However, when patients with demonstrable diseases of the brain are involuntarily hospitalized, the primary purpose is to exercise social control over their behavior;[4] treatment of the disease is, at best, a secondary consideration. Frequently, therapy is nonexistent, and custodial care is dubbed "treatment."

In short, the commitment of persons suffering from "functional psychoses" serves moral and social, rather than medical and therapeutic, purposes. Hence, even if, as a result of future research, certain conditions now believed to be "functional" mental illnesses were to be shown to be "organic," my argument against involuntary mental hospitalization would remain unaffected.

### 2. The Moral Evidence.

In free societies, the relationship between physician and patient is predicated on the legal presumption that the individual "owns" his body and his personality.[5]

The physician can examine and treat a patient only with his consent; the latter is free to reject treatment (for example, an operation for cancer).[6] After death, "ownership" of the person's body is transferred to his heirs; the physician must obtain permission from the patient's relatives for a post-mortem examination. John Stuart Mill explicitly affirmed that "each person is the proper guardian of his own health, whether bodily, or mental and spiritual."[7] Commitment is incompatible with this moral principle.

## 3. The Historical Evidence.

Commitment practices flourished long before there were any mental or psychiatric "treatments" of "mental diseases." Indeed, madness or mental illness was not always a necessary condition for commitment. For example, in the seventeenth century, "children of artisans and other poor inhabitants of Paris up to the age of 25 . . . girls who were debauched or in evident danger of being debauched," and other "misérables" of the community, such as epileptics, people with venereal diseases, and poor people with chronic diseases of all sorts, were all considered fit subjects for confinement in the Hôpital Général.[8] And in 1860, when Mrs. Packard was incarcerated for disagreeing with her minister-husband, the commitment laws of the State of Illinois explicitly proclaimed that "married women . . . may be entered or detained in the hospital at the request of the husband of the woman or the guardian . . . without the evidence of insanity required in other cases."[9] It is surely no coincidence that this piece of legislation was enacted and enforced at about the same time that Mill published his essay *The Subjection of Women*.[10]

## 4. The Literary Evidence.

Involuntary mental hospitalization plays a significant part in numerous short stories and novels from many countries. In none that I have encountered is commitment portrayed as helpful to the hospitalized person; instead, it is always depicted as an arrangement serving interests antagonistic to those of the so-called patient.[11]

### III

The claim that commitment of the "mentally ill" is necessary for the protection of the "mentally healthy" is more difficult to refute, not because it is valid, but because the danger that "mental patients" supposedly pose is of such an extremely vague nature.

## 1. The Medical Evidence.

The same reasoning applies as earlier: If "mental illness" is not a disease, there is no medical justification for protection from disease. Hence, the analogy between mental illness and contagious disease falls to the ground: The justification for isolating or otherwise constraining patients with tuberculosis or typhoid fever cannot be extended to patients with "mental illness."

Moreover, because the accepted contemporary psychiatric view of mental illness fails to distinguish between illness as a biological condition and as a social role,[12] it is not only false, but also dangerously misleading, especially if used to justify social action. In this view, regardless of its "causes"—anatomical, genetic, chemical, psychological, or social—mental illness has "objective existence." A person either has or has not a mental illness; he is either mentally sick or mentally healthy. Even if a person is cast in the role of mental patient against his will, his "mental illness" exists "objectively"; and even if, as in the case of the Very Important Person, he is never treated as a mental patient, his "mental illness" still exists "objectively"—apart from the activities of the psychiatrist.[13]

The upshot is that the term "mental illness" is perfectly suited for mystification: It disregards the crucial question of whether the individual assumes the role of mental patient voluntarily, and hence wishes to engage in some sort of interaction with a psychiatrist; or whether he is cast in that role against his will, and hence is opposed to such a relationship. This obscurity is then usually employed strategically, either by the subject himself to advance *his* interests, *or* by the subject's adversaries to advance *their* interests.

In contrast to this view, I maintain, first, that the involuntarily hospitalized mental patient is, by definition, the occupant of an ascribed role; and, second, that the "mental disease" of such a person—unless the use of this term is restricted to demonstrable lesions or malfunctions of the brain—is always the product of interaction between psychiatrist and patient.

## 2. The Moral Evidence.

The crucial ingredient in involuntary mental hospitalization is coercion. Since coercion is the exercise of power, it is always a moral and political act. Accordingly, regardless of its medical justification, commitment is primarily a moral and political phenomenon—just as, regardless of its anthropological and economic justifications, slavery was primarily a moral and political phenomenon.

Although psychiatric methods of coercion are indisputably useful for those who employ them, they are clearly not indispensable for dealing with the problems that so-called mental patients pose for those about them. If an individual threatens others by virtue of his beliefs or actions, he could be dealt with by methods other than "medical": if his conduct is ethically offensive, moral sanctions against him might be appropriate; if forbidden by law, legal sanctions might be appropriate. In my opinion, both informal, moral sanctions, such as social ostracism or divorce, and formal, judicial sanctions, such as fine and imprisonment, are more dignified and less injurious to the human spirit than the quasi-medical psychiatric sanction of involuntary mental hospitalization.[14]

## 3. The Historical Evidence.

To be sure, confinement of so-called mentally ill persons does protect the community from certain problems. If it didn't, the arrangement would not have come into being and would not have persisted. However, the question we ought to ask is not *whether* commitment protects the community from "dangerous mental patients," but rather from precisely *what danger* it protects and by *what means?* In what way were prostitutes or vagrants dangerous in seventeenth century Paris? Or married women in nineteenth-century Illinois?

It is significant, moreover, that there is hardly a prominent person who, during the past fifty years or so, has not been diagnosed by a psychiatrist as suffering from some type of "mental illness." Barry Goldwater was called a "paranoid schizophrenic"; Whittaker Chambers, a "psychopathic personality"; Woodrow Wilson, a "neurotic" frequently "very close to psychosis";[15] and Jesus, "a born degenerate" with a "fixed delusional system," and a "paranoid" with a "clinical picture [so typical] that it is hardly conceivable that people can even question the accuracy of the diagnosis."[16] The list is endless.

Sometimes, psychiatrists declare the same person sane *and* insane, depending on the political dictates of their superiors and the social demand of the moment. Before his trial and execution, Adolph Eichmann was examined by several psychiatrists, all of whom declared him to be normal; after he was put to death, "medical evidence" of his insanity was released and widely circulated.

According to Hannah Arendt, "Half a dozen psychiatrists had certified him [Eichmann] as 'normal.' " One psychiatrist asserted: "his whole psychological outlook, his attitude toward his wife and children, mother and father, sisters and friends, was 'not only normal but most desirable'. . . And the minister who regularly visited him in prison declared that Eichmann was 'a man with very positive ideas.' " After Eichmann was executed, Gideon Hausner, the attorney general of Israel, who had prosecuted him, disclosed in an article in *The Saturday Evening Post* that psychiatrists diagnosed Eichmann as " 'a man obsessed with a dangerous and insatiable urge to kill,' 'a perverted, sadistic personality.' "[17]

Whether or not men like those mentioned above are considered "dangerous" depends on the observer's religious beliefs, political convictions, and social situation. Furthermore, the "dangerousness" of such persons—whatever we may think of them—is not analogous to that of a person with tuberculosis or typhoid fever; nor would rendering such a person "non-dangerous" be comparable to rendering a patient with a contagious disease non-infectious.

In short, I hold—and I submit that the historical evidence bears me out—that people are committed to mental hospitals neither because they are "dangerous" nor because they are "mentally ill," but rather because they are society's scapegoats, whose persecution is justified by psychiatric propaganda and rhetoric.[18]

## 4. The Literary Evidence.

No one contests that involuntary mental hospitalization of the so-called dangerously insane "protects" the community. Disagreement centers on the nature of the threat facing society, and on the methods and legitimacy of the protection it employs. In this connection, we may recall that slavery, too, "protected" the community: it freed the slaveowners from manual labor.

Commitment likewise shields the non-hospitalized members of society: first, from having to accommodate themselves to the annoying or idiosyncratic demands of certain members of the community who have not violated any criminal statutes; and, second, from having to prosecute, try, convict, and punish members of the community who have broken the law but who either might not be convicted in court, or, if they would be, might not be retrained as effectively or as long in prison as in a mental hospital. The literary evidence cited earlier fully supports this interpretation of the function of involuntary mental hospitalization.

## IV

I have suggested that commitment constitutes a social arrangement whereby one part of society secures certain advantages for itself at the expense of another part. To do so, the oppressors must possess an ideology to justify their aims and actions; and they must be able to enlist the police power of the state to impose their will on the oppressed members. What makes such an arrangement a "crime against humanity"? It may be argued that the use of state power is legitimate when law-abiding citizens punish lawbreakers. What is the difference between this use of state power and its use in commitment?

In the first place, the difference between committing the "insane" and imprisoning the "criminal" is the same as that between the rule of man and the rule of law:[19] whereas the "insane" are subjected to the coercive controls of the state because persons more powerful than they have labeled them as "psychotic," "criminals" are subjected to such controls because they have violated legal rules applicable equally to all.

The second difference between these two proceedings lies in their professed aims. The principal purpose of imprisoning criminals is to protect the liberties of the law-abiding members of society.[20] Since the individual subject to commitment is not considered a threat to liberty in the same way as the accused criminal is (if he were, he would be prosecuted), his removal from society cannot be justified on the same grounds. Justification for commitment must thus rest on its therapeutic promise and potential: it will help restore the "patient" to "mental health." But if this can be accomplished only at the cost of robbing the individual of liberty, "involuntary mental hospitalization" becomes only a verbal camouflage for what is, in effect, punishment. This "therapeutic" punishment differs, however, from traditional judicial punishment, in that the accused criminal enjoys a rich panoply of constitutional protections against false accusation and oppressive prosecution, whereas the accused mental patient is deprived of these protections.[21]

To support this view of involuntary mental hospitalization, and to cast it into historical perspective, I shall now briefly review the similarities between slavery and institutional psychiatry. (By the use of the term "institutional psychiatry" I refer generally to psychiatric interventions imposed on persons by others. Such interventions are characterized by the complete loss, on the part of the ostensible client or "patient," of control over his participation in his relationship with the expert. The paradigm "service" of institutional psychiatry is, of course, involuntary mental hospitalization.)[22]

## V

Suppose that a person wishes to study slavery. How would he go about doing so? First, he might study slaves. He would then find that such persons are generally brutish, poor, and uneducated, and he might accordingly conclude that slavery is their "natural" or appropriate social state. Such, indeed, have been the methods and conclusions of innumerable men throughout the ages. Even the great Aristotle held that slaves were "naturally" inferior and were hence justly subdued. "From the hour of their birth," he asserted, "some are marked for subjection, others for rule."[23] This view is similar to the modern concept of "psychopathic criminality" and "schizophrenia" as genetically caused diseases.[24]

Another student, "biased" by contempt for the institution of slavery, might proceed differently. He would maintain that there can be no slave without a master holding him in bondage; and he would accordingly consider slavery a type of human *relationship* and, more generally, a *social institution*, supported by custom, law, religion, and force. From this point of view, the study of masters is at least as relevant to the study of slavery as is the study of slaves.

The latter point of view is generally accepted today with regard to slavery, but not with regard to institutional psychiatry. "Mental illness" of the type found in psychiatric hospitals has been investigated for centuries, and continues to be investigated today, in much the same way as slaves had been studied in the ante-bellum South and before. Then, the "existence" of slaves was taken for granted; their biological and social characteristics were accordingly noted and classified. Today, the "existence" of "mental patients" is similarly taken for granted; indeed, it is widely believed that their number is steadily increasing.[25] The psychiatrist's task is therefore to observe and classify the biological, psychological, and social characteristics of such patients.[26] This perspective is a manifestation, in part, of what I have called "the myth of mental illness," that is, of the notion that mental illnesses are similar to diseases of the body;[27] and, in part, of the psychiatrist's intense need to deny the fundamental complementarity of his relationship to the involuntary mental patient. The same sort of complementarity obtains in all situations where one person or party assumes a superior or dominant role and ascribes an inferior or submissive role to another; for example, master and slave, accuser and accused, inquisitor and witch.

The fundamental parallel between master and slave on the one hand, and institutional psychiatrist and involuntarily hospitalized patient on the other, lies in this: in each instance, the former member of the pair *defines* the social role of the latter, and *casts* him in that role by force.

## VI

Wherever there is slavery, there must be criteria for who may and who may not be enslaved. In ancient times, any people could be enslaved. Bondage was the usual consequence of military defeat. After the advent of Christianity, although the people of Europe continued to make war upon each other, they ceased enslaving prisoners who were Christians. According to Dwight Dumond, "the theory that a Christian could not be enslaved soon gained such wide endorsement as to be considered a point of international law."[28] By the time of the colonization of America, the peoples of the Western world considered only black men appropriate subjects for slave trade.

The criteria for distinguishing between those who may be incarcerated in mental hospitals and those who may not be are similar: poor and socially unimportant persons may be, and Very Important Persons may not be.[29] This rule is manifested in two ways: first, through our mental-hospital statistics, which show that the majority of institutionalized patients belong in the lowest socioeconomic classes; second, through the rarity with which VIPs are committed.[30] Yet even sophisticated social scientists often misunderstand or misinterpret these correlations by attributing the low incidence of committed upperclass persons to a denial on their part, and on the part of those close to them, of the "medical fact" that "mental illness" can "strike" anyone.[31] To be sure, powerful people may feel anxious or depressed, or behave in an excited or paranoid manner; but that, of course, is not the point at all. This medical perspective, which defines all distressed and distressing behavior as mental illness—and which is now so widely accepted—only succeeds in confusing the observer's judgment of the quality of another person's behavior with the observer's power to cast that person in the role of involuntary patient. My argument here is limited to asserting that prominent and powerful persons are rarely cast into the role of involuntarily confined mental patient—and for obvious reasons: The degraded status of committed patient ill befits a powerful person. In fact, the two statuses are as mutually exclusive as those of master and slave. . .

## IX

The change in perspective—from seeing slavery occasioned by the "inferiority" of the Negro and commitment by the "insanity" of the patient, to seeing each occasioned by the interplay of, and especially the power relation between, the participants—has far-reaching practical implications. In the case of slavery, it meant not only that the slaves had an obligation to revolt and emancipate themselves, but also that the masters had an even greater obligation to renounce their roles as slaveholders. Naturally, a slaveholder with such ideas felt compelled to set his slaves free, at whatever cost to himself. This is precisely what some slaveowners did. Their action had profound consequences in a social system based on slavery.

For the individual slaveholder who set his slaves free, the act led invariably to his expulsion from the community—through economic pressure or personal harassment or both. Such persons usually emigrated to the North. For the nation as a whole, these acts and the abolitionist sentiments behind them symbolized a fundamental moral rift between those who regarded Negroes as objects or slaves, and those who regarded them as persons or citizens. The former could persist in regarding the slave as existing in nature; whereas the latter could not deny his own moral responsibility for creating man in the image, not of God, but of the slave-animal.

The implications of this perspective for institutional psychiatry are equally clear. A psychiatrist who accepts as his "patient" a person who does not wish to be his patient, defines him as a "mentally ill" person, then incarcerates him in an institution, bars his escape from the institution and from the role of mental patient, and proceeds to "treat" him against his will—such a psychiatrist, I maintain, creates "mental illness" and "mental patients." He does so in exactly the same way as the white man who sailed for Africa, captured the Negro, brought him to America in shackles, and then sold him as if he were an animal, created slavery and slaves.

The parallel between slavery and institutional psychiatry may be carried one step further: Denunciation of slavery and the renouncing of slaveholding by some slaveowners led to certain social problems, such as Negro unemployment, the importation of cheap European labor, and a gradual splitting of the country into pro- and anti-slavery factions. Similarly, criticisms of involuntary mental hospitalization and the renouncing by some psychiatrists of relationships with involuntary mental patients have led to professional problems in the past, and are likely to do so again in the future. Psychiatrists restricting their work to psychoanalysis and psychotherapy have been accused of not being "real doctors"—as if depriving a person of his liberty required medical skills; of "shirking their responsibilities" to their colleagues and to society by accepting only the "easier cases" and refusing to treat the "seriously mentally ill" patient—as if avoiding treating persons who do not want to be treated were itself a kind of malpractice; and of undermining the profession of psychiatry—as if practicing self-control and eschewing violence were newly discovered forms of immorality.[32]

# X

The psychiatric profession has, of course, a huge stake, both existential and economic, in being socially authorized to rule over mental patients, just as the slaveowning classes did in ruling over slaves. In contemporary psychiatry, indeed, the expert gains superiority not only over members of a specific class of victims, but over nearly the whole of the population, whom he may "psychiatrically evaluate."[33]

The economic similarities between chattel slavery and institutional psychiatry are equally evident: The economic strength of the slaveowner lay in the Negro slaves he owned. The economic strength of the institutional psychiatrist lies, similarly, in his involuntary mental patients, who are not free to move about, marry, divorce, or make contracts, but are, instead, under the control of the hospital director. As the plantation owner's income and power rose with the amount of land and number of slaves he owned, so the income and power of the psychiatric bureaucrat rise with the size of the institutional system he controls and the number of patients he commands. Moreover, just as the slaveholder could use the police power of the state to help him recruit and maintain his slave labor force, so can the institutional psychiatrist rely on the state to help him recruit and maintain a population of hospital inmates.

Finally, since the state and federal governments have a vast economic stake in the operation of psychiatric hospitals and clinics, the interests of the state and of institutional psychiatry tend to be the same. Formerly, the state and federal governments had a vast economic stake in the operation of plantations worked by slaves, and hence the interests of the state and of the slave-owning classes tended to be the same. The wholly predictable consequence of this kind of arrangement is that just as the coalition of chattel slavery and the state created a powerful vested interest, so does the coalition of institutional psychiatry and the state.[34] Moreover, as long as the oppressive institution has the unqualified support of the state, it is invincible. On the other hand, since there can be no oppression without power, once such an institution loses the support of the state, it rapidly disintegrates.

If this argument is valid, pressing the view that psychiatrists now create involuntary mental patients just as slaveholders used to create slaves is likely to lead to a cleavage in the psychiatric profession, and perhaps in society generally, between those who condone and support the relationship between psychiatrist and involuntary mental patient, and those who condemn and oppose it.

It is not clear whether, or on what terms, these two psychiatric factions could coexist. The practices of coercive psychiatry and of paternalistic psychiatrists do not, in themselves, threaten the practices of non-coercive psychiatry and of contracting psychiatrists. Economic relations based on slavery coexisted over long periods with relations based on contract. But the moral conflict poses a more difficult problem. For just as the abolitionists tended to undermine the social justifications of slavery and the psychological bonds of the slave, so the abolitionists of psychiatric slavery tend to undermine the justifications of commitment and the psychological bonds of the committed patient.

Ultimately, the forces of society will probably be enlisted on one side or the other. If so, we may, on the one hand, be ushering in the abolition of involuntary mental hospitalization and treatment; on the other, we may be witnessing the fruitless struggles of an individualism bereft of moral support against a collectivism proffered as medical treatment.[35]

# XI

We know that man's domination over his fellow man is as old as history; and we may safely assume that it is traceable to prehistoric times and to prehuman ancestors. Perennially, men have oppressed women; white men, colored men; Christians, Jews. However, in recent decades, traditional reasons and justifications for discrimination among men—on the grounds of national, racial, or religious criteria—have lost much of their plausibility and appeal. What justification is there now for man's age-old desire to dominate and control his fellow man? Modern liberalism—in reality, a type of statism—allied with scientism, has met the need for a fresh defense of oppression and has supplied a new battle cry: Health!

In this therapeutic-meliorist view of society, the ill form a special class of "victims" who must, both for their own good and for the interests of the community, be "helped"—coercively and against their will, if necessary—by the healthy, and especially by physicians who are "scientifically" qualified to be their masters. This perspective developed first and has advanced farthest in psychiatry, where the oppression of "insane patients" by "sane physicians" is by now a social custom hallowed by medical and legal tradition. At present, the medical profession as a whole seems to be emulating this model. In the Therapeutic State toward which we appear to be moving, the principal requirement for the position of Big Brother may be an M.D. degree.

## NOTES

1. T. S. Szasz, "Commitment of the Mentally Ill: Treatment or Social Restraint?" *Journal of Nervous and Mental Diseases* 125 (April–June 1957), pp. 293–307; idem, *Law, Liberty, and Psychiatry: An Inquiry into the Social Uses of Mental Health Practices* (New York: Macmillan, 1963), pp. 149–90, 223–55.

2. D. B. Davis, *The Problem of Slavery in Western Culture* (Ithaca: Cornell University Press, 1966); see R. Cohen, "Slavery in Africa," *Trans-Action* 4 (January–February 1967), pp. 44–56; R. L. Tobin, "Slavery Still Plagues the Earth," *Saturday Review,* May 6, 1967, pp. 24–25.

3. See T. S. Szasz, *The Myth of Mental Illness: Foundations of a Theory of Personal Conduct* (New York: Hoeber-Harper, 1961); idem, "Mental Illness Is a Myth," *New York Times Magazine,* June 12, 1966, pp. 30 and 90–92.

4. See, for example, A. P. Noyes, *Modern Clinical Psychiatry,* 4th ed. (Philadelphia: W. B. Saunders, 1956), p. 278.

5. T. S. Szasz, "The Ethics of Birth Control; or, Who Owns Your Body?" *The Humanist* 20 (November–December 1960), pp. 332–36.

6. B. D. Hirsch, "Informed Consent to Treatment," in *Tort and Medical Yearbook,* eds. A. Averbach and M. M. Belli (Indianapolis: Bobbs-Merrill, 1961), vol. 1, pp. 631–38.

7. J. S. Mill, *On Liberty* (1859) (Chicago: Regnery, 1955), p. 18.

8. G. Rosen, "Social Attitudes to Irrationality and Madness in 17th- and 18th-Century Europe," *Journal of the History of Medicine and Allied Sciences* 18 (1963), p. 223.

9. *Illinois Statute Book: Sessions Laws*, 15, sec. 10, 1851; quoted in E. W. P. Packard, *The Prisoner's Hidden Life* (Chicago: published by the author, 1868), p. 37.

10. J. S. Mill, *The Subjection of Women* (1869) (London: Dent, 1965).

11. See, for example, A. P. Chekhov, *Ward No. 6* (1892), in *Seven Short Novels by Chekhov* (New York: Bantam books, 1963), pp. 106–57; M. De Assis, "The Psychiatrist" (1881–82), in *The Psychiatrist and Other Stories* (Berkeley: University of California Press, 1963), pp. 1–45; J. London, *The Iron Heel* (1907) (New York: Sagamore Press, 1957); K. A. Porter, *Noon Wine* (1937), in *Pale Horse, Pale Rider: Three Short Novels* (New York: Signet, 1965), pp. 62–112; K. Kesey, *One Flew over the Cuckoo's Nest* (New York: Viking, 1962); V. Tarsis, *Ward 7: An Autobiographical Novel* (London: Collins and Harvill, 1965).

12. See T. S. Szasz, "Alcoholism: A Socio-Ethical Perspective," *Western Medicine* 7 (December 1966), pp. 15–21.

13. See, for example, A. A. Rogow, *James Forrestal: A Study of Personality, Politics, and Policy* (New York: Macmillan, 1964); for a detailed criticism of this view, see T. S. Szasz, "Psychiatric Classification as a Strategy of Personal Constraint," in *Ideology and Insanity* (Garden City, NY: Doubleday, 1970), pp. 190–217.

14. T. S. Szasz, *Psychiatric Justice* (New York: Macmillan, 1965).

15. "The Unconscious of a Conservative: A Special Issue on the Mind of Barry Goldwater," *Fact*, September–October 1964; M. A. Zeligs, *Friendship and Fratricide: An Analysis of Whittaker Chambers and Alger Hiss* (New York: Viking, 1967); S. Freud and W. C. Bullitt, *Thomas Woodrow Wilson: A Psychological Study* (Boston: Houghton Mifflin, 1967).

16. Quoted in A. Schweitzer, *The Psychiatric Study of Jesus* (1913), trans. Charles R. Joy (Boston: Beacon Press, 1956), pp. 37, 40–41.

17. H. Arendt, *Eichmann in Jerusalem: A Report on the Banality of Evil* (New York: Viking, 1963), pp. 22–23.

18. For a full articulation and documentation of this thesis, see T. S. Szasz, *The Manufacture of Madness: A Comparative Study of the Inquisition and the Mental Health Movement* (New York: Harper & Row, 1970).

19. F. A. Hayek, *The Constitution of Liberty* (Chicago: University of Chicago Press, 1960), especially pp. 162–92.

20. J. D. Mabbott, "Punishment" (1939), in *Justice and Social Policy: A Collection of Essays*, ed. F. A. Olafson (Englewood Cliffs, NJ: Prentice-Hall, 1961), pp. 39–54.

21. For documentation, see Szasz, *Law, Liberty, and Psychiatry* and *Psychiatric Justice.*

22. For further discussion, see Szasz, *The Manufacture of Madness*, especially the preface and chaps. 1–9.

23. Davis, *The Problem of Slavery*, p. 70.

24. R. W. Stock, "The XYY and the Criminal," *New York Times Magazine*, October 20, 1968, pp. 30–31, 90–104; F. J. Kallman, "The Genetics of Mental

Illness," in *American Handbook of Psychiatry*, ed. S. Arieti (New York: Basic Books, 1959), vol. 1, pp. 175–96.

25. G. Caplan, *Principles of Preventive Psychiatry* (New York: Basic Books, 1964); see, for example, L. Srole, T. S. Langer, S. T. Mitchell, M. K. Opler, and T. A. C. Rennie, *Mental Health in the Metropolis: The Midtown Manhattan Study* (New York: McGraw-Hill, 1962).

26. A. P. Noyes and L. C. Kolb, *Modern Clinical Psychiatry*, 5th ed. (Philadelphia: W. B. Saunders, 1958).

27. Szasz, *The Myth of Mental Illness.*

28. D. L. Dumond, *Antislavery: The Crusade for Freedom* (Ann Arbor: University of Michigan Press, 1961), p. 4.

29. D. Henderson and R. D. Gillespie, *A Textbook of Psychiatry*, 7th ed. (London: Oxford University Press, 1950), p. 684.

30. A. B. Hollingshead and F. C. Redlich, *Social Class and Mental Illness* (New York: Wiley, 1958).

31. Ibid., pp. xxi, 44, pp. 344–47.

32. See, for example, H. A. Davidson, "The Image of the Psychiatrist," *American Journal of Psychiatry* 121 (October 1964), pp. 329–33; F. G. Glaser, "The Dichotomy Game: A Further Consideration of the Writings of Dr. Thomas Szasz," ibid. (May), pp. 1069–74.

33. See W. Menninger, *A Psychiatrist for a Troubled World* (New York: Viking, 1967).

34. See Davis, *The Problem of Slavery*, p. 193.

35. T. S. Szasz, "Whither Psychiatry?" in *Ideology and Insanity*, pp. 218–45.

## PART TEN

# Genetic Information and Genetic Therapy

# Bad Axioms in Genetic Engineering

## C. Keith Boone

*In the following selection, C. Keith Boone analyzes a number of axioms, or assumptions, about the new genetics that prove wrongheaded. Included among these are "the Frankenstein factor," the notion of "playing God," the resistance to "interfering with nature," and some reductionistic assumptions.*

*Boone discusses the "slippery slope" or "wedge" argument in the context of application of new genetic knowledge, and his analysis should be compared to Leon Kass's in a very similar context in Selection 8. Boone also discusses an idea of Joseph Fletcher's on cloning human beings, mentioned in Selection 7.*

*Boone also considers whether science (genetics) is ethically neutral and whether science (genetics) can provide answers to man's quest for self-perfection. Finally, he argues against eugenics or human germ-line therapy.*

*C. Keith Boone is associate dean at the College of Arts and Sciences, Denison University, Granville, Ohio.*

The parade of wonders mounted by biological science marches by at an increasingly rapid pace. In a kind of mimicry of Genesis, we have synthesized a living, functioning gene from shelf chemicals in the laboratory. Through improved cloning techniques we are able to produce exact copies of lower life forms—genetic replicas down to the very shape and location of spots on the backs of leopard frogs. Even more significantly, recent techniques for gene mapping and recombination ("gene splicing") are throwing open doors to the treatment of diseases, ecological control, and the technological production of a wide range of goods from pharmaceuticals to peanuts.

In short, we are now able to control the destinies of ourselves, our offspring, and our environment in ways that are much more direct and trait-specific than previously imagined.

*Source: Hastings Center Report* 18 (August/September 1988), pp. 9–13. Reprinted by permission of the author and publisher.

**315**

Profound and fascinating moral dilemmas accompany the new biotechnical achievements, particularly those that involve manipulating the human genome, going to the very heart of who we are and how we think about ourselves. Many have argued that our technical advances have outpaced our ability to deal ethically with them. But they have not said why this is so, or what we ought to do about it. In fact, no ethical tradition seems sufficient to comprehend either the peculiarity of the genetic dilemma or the multiplicity of moral conundrums it presents.

## NEW MORAL CHALLENGES

The new methods of genetic engineering pose difficult ethical problems in part because they offer technological options that never before existed. Still, it is not the *fact* of options that is problematic, but rather their nature. What revisionist social philosophers and theologians of hope have described as the category of the *novum*, the generation of the qualitatively new, independent of any organic evolution from what already exists, has been its first genuine demonstration in the realm of the biological sciences. Inasmuch as many of the new genetic techniques allow scientists to bypass *development* in creating novel life forms, some scientific achievements can be appreciated only in these nonorganic, nonontologic terms. In the new biology, we confront in its most irreducible form the direct, minute, and purposeful design of life. That fact presents us with moral problems that are not just new in history, but new in kind.

As it applies specifically to human genetic manipulations, genetic engineering presents an unprecedented technological leap from merely designing the environment to "designing the designer."[1] These prospects threaten wholly to subvert traditional philosophical paradigms and undermine the standard ethical touchstones of "human nature," "humanity," and "rationality." These would become synthetic products rather than points of common reference. Of course, this scenario would result from proposed eugenic manipulations to alter human capacities in "positive" ways. It may be precisely such scenarios that give us a distinct basis for deciding where we would balk at further interventions.

An additional complicating feature is that genetic engineering is not a single problem at all, but rather a complex set of problems occurring in quite different domains of inquiry—epidemiological, ecological, evolutionary, human-genetic, and political. Many of the original concerns about recombinant DNA arose on the epidemiological level, involving fears about the accidental dissemination of altered, pathogenic bacteria for which there is no known antidote. And fear of the consequences of human germline alteration led fifty-six clergy and several scientists in 1983 to adopt a "Resolution," delivered to Congress, requesting a ban on all such interventions.

Finally, what Willard Gaylin has called the "Frankenstein factor" has influenced the tone of the genetic debate in negative ways. The specter of new life forms somehow "threatens our sense of identity, our sense of uniqueness, and our sense of primacy among the creatures of the earth."[2] Perhaps this is as it should be, that some nonrational element in our respect for extant genomes be maintained alongside our rational affirmations of them. But to the extent that these premonitions become exaggerated beyond what the facts can support, they tend to generate peremptory condemnations. The recombinant DNA controversy in this country was instantly polarized by disputants who charged that scientists were conspiring to create the master race and take control of our genetic futures. In response, many scientists joined battle and categorized their critics as anti-science ideologues.

## BAD AXIOMS

The combination of these characteristics of genetic engineering—its newness, its potential for manipulation of the "human," its complexity, and its capacity for arousing fear and recrimination—has proven fertile soil for the growth of an assortment of bad axioms whose distinguishing feature is that they are reductionistic. They substitute invocation of formula for careful analysis and in the process cut off precisely the kind of balanced scrutiny called for by this complex set of problems.

It is not the case that bad axioms contain no truth, however. Quite the contrary, it is their tendency to encapsulate a partial truth that makes them alluring. The problem with bad axioms is precisely their power to convince the hearer that a partial insight constitutes the whole truth, that looking through a single porthole provides panoramic vision. Thus the initial step in an appropriate ethical assessment of genetic prospects is to identify the axioms that have most obscured the issues. The second step is to consign them, as *axioms* to history. The final step is to discern what element of truth they may contain in their nonaxiomatic forms.

### Playing God

In the Jewish and Christian traditions "playing God" is characteristically associated with pride and arrogance, the aping of divine power, or the attempt to gain salvation without the help of the divinity. It is not the *use* of power and creativity that offends, but rather attributing power to one's own resources, denying its origin in what Jews and Christians believe is God's continuing creation. Those who object to any genetic medicine on religious grounds need to be clear that "playing God" is not, in this usage, an act against morality, but rather one against faith. Its verbal counterpart is blasphemy. However, it would not seem that individual genetic pursuits would be forbidden in any necessary sense, unless the motive were an attempt to stand in God's place. Therapeutic interventions are, in fact, consonant with the benevolent, other-regarding impulses of Judaism and Christianity.

Yet these traditions might well morally object to particular applications of genetic science, or point to problems with human conceits about our ability to predict or control the outcomes of our actions.

Such legitimate concerns are similar to those expressed in the secular usage of "playing God," in which the phrase is often used to remind us that it is only with caution that we should tamper with the most elemental organic forces in the universe. It intends to point to the great uncertainties we face as we consider how genetic science may eventually shape our physical being, our social structure, and our moral culture.

If these sorts of concerns lie beneath "playing God," then the concept has valid standing. Used in this sense, it ceases to be a bad axiom insofar as it rightly recommends a cautionary posture. The appropriate response, however, is not that we should not "play God," but that we must do so intelligently. That is the essence of making choices, and it undeniably is our destiny, whether we choose to accept genetic options or reject them.

## Interfering with Nature

There is nothing problematic in this axiom in its descriptive sense. *Homo faber* is, by definition, one who interacts with and reshapes the environment. But in the genetic context the phrase is often used as an indictment.

Behind such use of "interfering with nature" usually lies the notion that nature has a prescribed telos and a single program for reaching that telos. But it is not clear that the uncontrolled reign of nature produces the most humane world we can imagine. As molecular geneticist Stanley Cohen has noted, it is nature that gave us the genetic combinations for such afflictions as yellow fever, typhoid, and diabetes.[3] Humans have always danced a delicate ecological minuet with various other potent life forms, including bacteria and viruses. Deadly microorganisms have their own survivalistic ecology, and nowhere in nature's book is it written that human survival is the most preferred. The emergence of *Homo sapiens* in the evolutionary drama does not, according to biologists, represent a necessary, end-directed process. And we have always interfered with nature to protect the species and its likelihood, from the medical use of antibiotics to the draining of swamps that festered with malaria-bearing mosquitos.

The issue is not whether we interfere, but whether or not our incursions enhance or diminish the human prospect. Erwin Chargaff has put it eloquently: "This world is given to us on loan. We come and we go; and after a time we leave earth and air and water to others who come after us."[4] We have the ability to make genetic choices in symbiotic rhythm with nature, or to assault our contingent relationship with nature. We also have the ability to make intergenerationally sensitive choices or to take the short-term perspective.

This is not to underestimate the difficulty of deciding what is or is not an assault upon nature, particularly with regard to human genetic engineering. For example, whose definition of what is "natural" shall we accept? And as the President's Commission to study the question of gene splicing noted, the widely accepted belief that there is a fixed human genome is faulty, given that the "genetic basis of what is distinctively human continually changes through the interplay of random mutation and natural selection."[5] Our choices, then, should be based on some human conception of what is natural, not on a naturalistic definition of what is human. It is in the latter sense that the charge of "interfering with nature" becomes a bad axiom.

The truth in the axiom lies in its implicit invocation of the basic rule, *primum non nocere*, and in its explicit dual challenges for critical examination prior to action. First, it suggests an honest self-examination of motives for "intrusions" into the natural. Such motives can be venal and short-sighted, as has been frequently alleged against eugenics programs, or they can give relief to those who are or will be genetically crippled. Second, it suggests a careful examination of the external world for impacts and outcomes, not only on the physical, but on the social and cultural environments as well.

## Slippery Slopes

Those who use the "slippery slope" argument seem to imply two principles at work, one of momentum and one of logic. The principle of momentum states that, once you perform X, you will not be able to restrain yourself from doing Y, even though X does not necessarily imply Y. The principle of logic states that Y will inevitably follow from X, since doing X contains the *principle of permission* for doing Y. It is the latter that is more ethically relevant and seems to be operative in the following passage:

> Once we decide to begin the process of human genetic engineering, there is really no logical place to stop. If diabetes, sickle cell anemia, and cancer are to be cured by altering the genetic make-up of an individual, why not proceed to other "disorders": myopia, color blindness, left handedness. Indeed, what is to preclude a society from deciding that a certain skin color is a disorder? . . . What is the price we pay for embarking on a course whose final goal is the "perfection" of the human species?[6]

This line of reasoning mistakenly assumes that beginning the process of human genetic engineering means carrying it through to any conceivable application. It claims that if the principle of permission allows *some* kinds of interventions it will hold for all kinds of interventions. But morally to endorse positive eugenic measures would require justification by a very different, and certainly more disputable, principle. There is a seismic moral difference between treating leukemia and enhancing IQ, and to recognize that difference is one of the preeminent purposes of moral reasoning. The moral gulf between these two classes of action suggests that there is, in fact, a "logical place to stop"; it is just prior to the leap from therapeutic to eugenic measures. Once this boundary has been crossed, then there really is no logical place to stop. To be sure, in practice there are gray areas in what constitutes "eugenics." The better part of wisdom may tell us that we should not enter even that territory.

When used to refer to genetic enhancement of characteristics, the slope argument is no longer a bad axiom. It functions correctly in alerting us to the fact that permission for one eugenic measure inevitably establishes the principle of permission for other eugenic measures. Once the new moral rationale is in place, license would be the order of the day. It is not clear what could prevent us at that point from engaging in genetic wanderlust.

To assert that our final goal is the " 'perfection' of the human species" does not accurately report the motivation behind genetic research, except in the sense that all our endeavors aim at making the world a more hospitable place. Most of our genetic efforts are not even aimed at "final goals." They are more immediate attempts to find cures for diseases that disfigure, kill, or deny individuals the basic capacities to realize a minimally recognizable human existence. To deny afflicted individuals these therapies on the ground that we cannot make distinctions between remedial germline alterations and eugenic enhancements indicates a lack of trust in the human ability to act discriminately on the basis of distinctive ethical classifications.

## The Ethical Neutrality of Science

Taken in its most literal sense, the claim that science is ethically neutral is accurate. We would be hard put to defend the proposition that knowledge alone has a moral value or disvalue. But the claim is not usually made in this pure sense. It almost always conveys the notion that scientists do not have responsibility for the production of knowledge. As Jacob Bronowski has noted, however, this belief confuses the *findings* of science, which are ethically neutral, with the *activity* of science, which is not.[7]

Even so, the argument continues, it is not the activity of science to which notions of responsibility attach, but rather the applications of the products of that activity. Knowledge itself is value-neutral and "ambipotent"; for example, the same chemicals used to create nerve gases in the Great Wars turned out to be "elegant research weapons in the protein biochemistry revolution."[8] Therefore, the moral burden lies with those who choose to implement scientific information for ill purposes.

This argument combines a prima facie plausibility with some degree of disingenuity. The source of each is the attempt to form a cleavage between scientist *qua* scientist and scientist *qua* moral agent. But scientist *qua* scientist does not really exist except as a heuristic notion. The scientist in the laboratory is always moral agent at the same time that he or she is scientist. It is not possible for the scientist to hang the moral self on a coatrack on the way into the laboratory and then proceed indiscriminately with the scientific venture.

But in what precise sense is the scientist responsible for this production of knowledge? In his *Double Image of the Double Helix*, Clifford Grobstein distinguishes three kinds of research with recombinant DNA—basic, applied, and technological—and suggests that only the latter two be considered for any kind of external regulation, leaving the search for pure knowledge unfettered except for certain judicious forms of self-regulation.[9] Reasonable scientists may well agree with this recommendation, concurring that the connections between some kinds of applied or technological research and scientists' accountability can be readily established. For example, it is not hard to see the direct and predictable link between applied research on nerve gases and their use on human populations. But the same reasonable scientists may insist, along with Grobstein, that there is no such obvious connection between basic research and its unpredictable—perhaps even improbable—applications. Can the inventor of diesel engines be held responsible for Nazi submarines?

Still, the inability to predict the uses of pure knowledge does not relieve scientists of the responsibility for thinking in advance about how such knowledge might be used. The scientist, no less than other professionals, is required to exercise the "imagination principle" in projecting potential uses of scientific information."[10] I am speaking here of ordinary responsibility as a moral agent. In actual practice, scientists cannot be expected to think in terms of infinite causal chains into the future ("Only God can be a good utilitarian"). Since the eventual permutations of discovering pure knowledge are highly speculative, we would not expect to find frequent moral deterrence in the pursuit of basic knowledge. Nor is the moral responsibility to imagine uses the same as the moral responsibility to refrain from doing.

In its axiomatic form, then, the claim that scientific activity is ethically neutral is not accurate. Yet hidden within this bad axiom is often a more modest claim, that most knowledge may be used for good or ill, and that scientists should not shoulder the burden of responsibility for harmful applications. Corrupt persons, societies, and political regimes may misuse even the most innocent knowledge for deplorable ends, and therein lies considerable responsibility. If that is what is meant by the claim, then it ceases to be a bad axiom. Still, far from relieving scientists of all responsibility, it merely confirms that all share responsibility.

## Genetics Is the Answer

For many, the biological revolution has signaled the dawn of a bold new era of omnipotence. The euphoria of the 1970s, generated by rapid developments in genetic science, was for many a result of prospective applications in medicine, reproduction, agriculture, industry, and pharmacology. For others, it was the result of imagining these heady genetic technologies as the long-awaited solutions to perennial human problems and aspirations. Theoretical biologist James Danielli contended that "from the point of view of genetics, man is a barbarian," and it is only such radical interventions as genetic alteration that will allow civilization to "advance to a modestly stable state."[11] In a recent letter to the *New York Times*, Robert Davis spotted divine intentionality behind the new genetic powers: "God has put into our hands the possibility of what has so long been demanded by the great world religions, a change in man himself . . . To succeed will be to begin a new and glorious stage in the history of what has been so defective a humanity."[12]

Among others, Joshua Lederberg and Joseph Fletcher have argued for the direct, asexual copying of superior human traits, or of entire individuals, in the place of the genetic dice roll of ordinary reproduction.

In both their milder and more extreme expressions, these views share hope for instant genetic remedies that are themselves problematic. There are no single, discrete genes that code the complex arrangements of proteins that produce given human traits; and to manipulate one is to change the original, fragile configuration in unforeseeable ways. But even if such Promethean methods were developed in the distant future, who would decide what traits should be preferred? Who would decide what makes a person a more fit specimen, and under what idealized plan for human harmony and well-being? What would be the criteria for choosing alternatives that seem to some a social boon, to others a form of dehumanization?

Use of genetic methods for positive, eugenic purposes should give us sudden pause for another reason. It would involve us in the historic and shameful confession that we have not been able to resolve problems of social intercourse in ways that rely on human intelligence and character. Whatever problems we may have defining what is "human," it would be clear that use of these technological shortcuts would signal the repudiation of our current human abilities—in both material and immaterial senses. The legitimate desire to improve the human lot need not evolve into this sort of collective humiliation. Long before teleological thirst deteriorates into technological lust, it will need tempering by the acknowledgement of human finitude and by the willful determination to resolve problems by means that realize human integrity, not ones that undermine it.

Every such argument for "technological fix" merits counterargument from the fact of technological tragedy. The latter occurs in at least three senses. First, all inventions are two-edged swords. The obvious example is nuclear energy; on balance, it is not clear that the capability to split the atom nets human good. A second sense of technological tragedy is summarized in Chargaff's complaint about the microorganisms produced through the inexact and serendipitous methods of gene splicing: "You can stop splitting the atom; you can stop visiting the moon; you can stop using aerosols; you may even decide not to kill entire populations by the use of a few bombs. But you cannot recall a new form of life."[13]

It is not just new forms of life that are dubious in this respect, however. Once introduced, no unit of technological knowledge can be recalled, even if particular technologies can. In that sense, all technology is a new organism that insinuates itself into living cultures through altering them irrevocably.

Finally, the third meaning of technological tragedy is that technology's problem-solving innovations seem persistently to create new problems. What Reinhold Niebuhr articulated as a general social principle is equally true for genetic discovery: Every advance in the fulfillment of human aspirations creates problems at an entirely new level. An urgent example in the world of medical ethics is the host of moral dilemmas issuing from the new life-prolonging and resuscitative devices. We are still novices at resolving the legion of problems that accompany these otherwise beneficent technologies.

Of course, the fact that technology creates rich and challenging new problems is in no way determinative for the case against invention, either in genetics or in any other pursuit. But it does serve us notice to be perspicacious in the applications of science, and temperate in our expectations of it. Knowledge of tragic implications need not and should not paralyze action. To "know sin" is our ineluctable fate and fortune, and to lose nerve in the face of such knowledge would only enlarge the tragedy. On the other hand, that knowledge should take some of the color out of glib fantasies about what genetic science will do for us, as well as inform moral decisions about what we want to do with it.

## NOTES

1. Leon Kass notes that "engineering the engineer seems to differ in kind from engineering his engine"; "The New Biology: What Price Relieving Man's Estate?" *Science* 174 (November 19, 1971), p. 780.

2. Willard Gaylin, "The Frankenstein Factor," *New England Journal of Medicine* 97, no. 12 (September 22, 1977), pp. 665–66.

3. Stanley Cohen, "Recombinant DNA: Fact and Fiction," *Science* 195 (February 18, 1977), p. 655.

4. Erwin Chargaff, "On the Dangers of Genetic Meddling," *Science* 192 (June 14, 1976), p. 904.

5. President's Commission for the Study of Ethical Problems in Medicine and Biomedical and Behavioral Research, *Splicing Life: A Report on the Social and Ethical Issues of Genetic Engineering with Human Beings* (Washington, DC: U.S. Government Printing Office, 1982), p. 70.

6. Jeremy Rifkin, "Resolution" (June 8, 1983), Foundation on Economic Trends.

7. Jacob Bronowski, *The Identity of Man* (Garden City, NY: Doubleday, 1965), p. ix; quoted in William Lowrance, *Modern Science and Human Values* (New York: Oxford University Press, 1985), p. 5.

8. Lowrance, *Modern Science,* p. 5, uses this example to show the dual uses of scientific knowledge, not to argue that science is value-neutral, a position with which he does not identify.

9. Clifford Grobstein, *Double Image of the Double Helix* (San Francisco: W. H. Freeman, 1979).

10. Daniel Callahan, "The Social Responsibility of Science in the Face of Uncertain Consequences," *Annals of the New York Academy of Science* 265 (January 23, 1976), p. 4.

11. James Danielli, "Industry, Society, and Genetic Engineering," *Hastings Center Report* 2, no. 6 (December 1972), pp. 5–7.

12. Robert Davis, "What New Adam Lurks Inside the Gene Splice?" *New York Times,* March 15, 1987.

13. Chargaff, "On the Dangers of Genetic Meddling," p. 938.

# Moral Issues
# in Human Genetics:
# Counseling or Control?

## Ruth Macklin

*In this early classic, philosopher Ruth Macklin discusses a number of moral issues in genetics that have continued to be debated in the following two decades: presymptomatic screening for incurable hereditary diseases such as Huntington's, whether genetic counselors should be nondirective or directive, whether amniocentesis and abortion should be used to terminate fetuses with hereditary diseases, and whether genetic therapy should be used in "negative" ways to eliminate genetic defects in individuals and their offspring or also in "positive," eugenic ways to improve humans.*

*Ruth Macklin, PhD, is professor of bioethics at Albert Einstein College of Medicine in New York City. She was an early fellow at the Hastings Center. Her books include* Man, Mind, and Morality: The Ethics of Behavior Control, Moral Choices: Ethical Dilemmas in Modern Medicine, *and* Enemies of Patients.

> *[T]he question "valuable to what end?" is one of extraordinary complexity. For example, something obviously valuable in terms of the longest possible survival of a race (or of its best adaptation to a given climate, or of the preservation of its greatest numbers) would by no means have the same value if it were a question of developing a more powerful type. The welfare of the many and the welfare of the few are radically opposite ends.*
>
> —Friedrich Nietzche, *The Genealogy of Morals*

> *There is no question that genetic engineering in many forms . . . will come about. It is a general rule that whatever is scientifically feasible will be attempted. The application of these technics must, however, be examined from the point of view of ethics, individual freedom and coercion. Both the scientists directly involved and, perhaps more important, the political and social leaders of our civilization must exercise utmost caution in order to prevent genetic, evolutionary and social tragedies.*
>
> —Kurt Hirschhorn, July 1972

*Source: Dialogue* 16, no. 3 (1977), pp. 375–96. Reprinted by permission of the author and publisher.

**324**

# I

In the field of human genetics, the last several decades have witnessed a great increase in both theoretical knowledge and technological power.[1] Like so many other areas in biomedical ethics, the attainment of new knowledge and the development of new technology has given rise to moral problems that never had to be faced before. But while the biomedical contexts are new, the moral problems are ancient. Such problems arise at the level both of the individual and society, where decisions must be made about such matters as whether compulsory genetic screening programmes constitute a violation of individual privacy; whether enforced sterilization of genetically unhealthy individuals is ever justifiable in the interest of socially desirable outcomes; whether genetic counselors are obligated to tell the truth, and whole truth, and nothing but the truth to their clients even in cases where learning the truth is likely to be harmful. Ethical dilemmas about such matters as the rights of individuals when these conflict with anticipated social benefits, the morality of withholding the truth, the acceptability of paternalistic coercion of persons "for their own good"—these age-old moral problems are found in new settings created by advances in human genetics, as is the case in other biomedical areas.

A catalogue of representative moral issues in this domain would include at least the following concerns.

## 1. The Ethics of Screening for Incurable Heritable Disease.

Should tests such as the L-dopa test for presymptomatic Huntington's Chorea—a fatal, degenerative neurological disease—be made available to patients even in the absence of any treatment or cure? Should persons known to be at risk for such incurable hereditary conditions be informed of such tests? Urged to undergo them? Or should testing be withheld until there is something tangible to offer those who show a positive result? Ought information gained through genetic screening to be made available to others besides the patient, when such knowledge may affect the decision of other family members to bear children or undergo screening themselves?

## 2. Responsibilities of Genetic Counselors.

To whom is the genetic counselor responsible? The patient or married couple alone? Their unborn child? Other family members? Future generations who may suffer increasing numbers of persons with genetic defects? Should genetic counselors merely present "the facts" to those who come for counseling? Or does the greater theoretical knowledge and practical experience of the genetic counselor warrant his giving advice or urging a specific course of action? It is often noted that even in cases where a counselor believes himself to be simply imparting information, he nonetheless betrays his attitude in a way that is likely to influence a patient's decision. If this is so, does it suggest a reason for the counselor to render his own view explicit instead of trying (unsuccessfully) to remain neutral?

## 3. Moral Limits in the Use of Amniocentesis and Abortion.

Are there good reasons for remaining selective in the use of amniocentesis— the technique by which a small amount of amniotic fluid is taken from a woman early in pregnancy and fetal cells are cultured to ascertain the presence of genetic disorders? Do risks to the fetus—however slight—indicate that the procedure should be used selectively? Is the use of amniocentesis and subsequent abortion justifiable for reasons such as sex determination of the fetus? Should amniocentesis be ruled out in cases where the parents indicate that they are opposed to abortion in all circumstances?

## 4. The Morality of Positive and Negative Eugenics.

Do we have a moral obligation to refrain from "polluting" the human gene pool? How far into the future does our obligation to future generations lie? If there is such an obligation, ought it be mandated by government legislation and enforcement? What are the moral limits of developing and using radically new techniques such as high-precision surgery on genetic material, when there are significant risks in the form of accidental creation of hapless monsters, or abuse on the part of unethical investigators? Is some form of eugenics justifiable on the grounds that presently existing society must bear the enormous costs of maintaining defective infants and even adults who survive because of the capabilities of modern medicine?

In all of these questions and others we shall explore shortly, the moral categories include a number of alleged rights of the individual: the "right to know" (or *not* to know); the right to make autonomous decisions; the "right to bear children," even when a high probability exists that these children will either suffer from or be carriers of genetic disease. These moral issues need not be couched in the language of rights, but may instead (perhaps more profitably) be viewed as ethical dilemmas where cogent reasons can be offered for two or more alternative courses of action. It is the existence of just such alternatives that gives rise to the need for moral decision-making on the part of individual physicians, their patients, and the larger society.

Before we can begin to answer the question "who shall make the decisions?" we must first be clear about what decisions there are to be made. Since the issues in human genetics are so complex and multilayered, I shall spend a bit of time sorting them out and try to show how the practices of genetic screening, genetic counseling, and genetic engineering pose interconnected moral problems. In the course of this article, I shall argue for two separate but related theses. The first is that the individual (meaning also the individual couple, where appropriate) should have final decision-making authority in matters of his or her own reproductive acts and capacities, as well as continuation or termination of pregnancy, where the reasons for these decisions refer to genetic factors. The second thesis is that attempts at government-based or scientist-directed eugenic programmes—whether aimed at positive or negative eugenics—are bound to be misguided or dangerous or both. Having asserted these theses, let me now go back and lay the groundwork. I shall try, first, to identify the chief moral issues in human genetics, showing just where and in what ways the need for decision-making arises. Then I shall have the way paved for arguing the two theses just stated.

## II

As the terms imply, "genetic screening" denotes a process of detection and diagnosis of heritable conditions; "genetic counseling" refers to the activity of informing or advising those who are afflicted with such conditions or are carriers; and "genetic engineering" involves manipulation of either genetic material itself, or else the reproductive acts or capacities of persons. About each of these activities the following questions must be posed: What purposes is the practice designed to serve? Who stands to benefit from the practice? What individual rights or liberties stand to be abridged? What other values are involved in decision-making in these areas?

Beginning with genetic screening, let's look briefly at each of these activities to see where the need for decision-making arises and what sorts of decisions are involved. The range of diagnostic procedures known as genetic screening can be grouped roughly into the following five categories, of which I shall discuss the first four: (1) newborn metabolic screening; (2) chromosome screening; (3) carrier screening; (4) prenatal diagnosis; and (5) susceptibility screening.[2]

1. The most prevalent example of newborn metabolic screening is that of the relatively simple and inexpensive test for phenylketonuria (PKU), a rare autosomal recessive in which the afflicted infant has inherited one defective gene from each parent. Those suffering from phenylketonuria lack a critical enzyme for metabolizing phenylalanine, an essential amino acid. If left untreated, PKU leads to irreversible mental retardation; when treated by introducing a synthetic diet virtually free of phenylalanine and begun shortly after birth, children with PKU do not suffer the consequence of severe retardation; but there is now some evidence that the special diet does not restore intelligence totally.[3] While PKU screening is an example of genetic screening where some treatment or cure exists for afflicted individuals, its use is not free of difficulties. For one thing, there have been significant instances of false positives—a source of difficulty because the synthetic diet can be harmful to a normal child. Moreover, a serious reproduction problem has arisen, since PKU women give birth to children who are retarded, no matter what their genotype, because of a toxic uterine environment. A different sort of problem stems from the fact that most states in the U.S. have adopted a programme of mandatory PKU screening—a practice that some believe will serve as a model for increasing numbers of medical procedures compelled by law.[4] So while

PKU screening has the virtue of being a diagnostic procedure for a condition having a treatment or cure that now exists, it may, for that very reason, be an unwelcome paradigm of legally compelled medical procedures, which will make inroads into the privacy of individuals in our society.

2. The most notorious example of chromosome screening of newborns is that of the XYY chromosomal anomaly. The extra Y chromosome is thought by some to result in an unusual degree of antisocial, aggressive behaviour on the part of the so-called super-males who possess this abnormality. Unlike the case of PKU, there is no known "cure" or even a scientifically well-confirmed treatment programme for males who have this chromosomal abnormality, nor has it been fully ascertained that this special population is significantly different in behaviour patterns from "normal" XY males who come from similar backgrounds. But XYY screening has drawn sharp criticism for reasons other than those pertaining to theoretical and diagnostic uncertainties of this sort. Severe criticism has been leveled at a study in Boston, which has offered therapy to young boys found through screening to have the extra Y chromosome. One argument runs as follows:

> Either the researcher must withhold from the parents the information that the child being studied is XYY (which is probably immoral and perhaps also illegal), or that information must be disclosed, which will alter the way the parents feel about the child (probably for the worse). It will also render the study scientifically worthless, since for the study to demonstrate whether there are behavioral problems with the XYY male it is necessary that his upbringing be as "normal" as possible, so he can be compared with an XY boy.[5]

This argument is persuasive, especially given the circumstance that the therapy for aggressive or antisocial behaviour is, at best, uncertain, and at worst, coercive. But even if it is morally permissible or even desirable to seek to alter the deviant behaviour of XYY male children, the other points in the argument remain. The moral conflict surrounding how much and what specific information should be transmitted to whom arises directly in many cases of genetic counseling, as we shall see shortly. The problem of informing parents that they have an XYY child is wider than that raised by the Boston study. Even if no therapy were offered, there would remain the problem of adverse effects on the parents' expectations about and treatment of their sons whom they knew to possess an extra Y chromosome. While many screening programmes for XYY seem to have been dropped, controversy still rages over whether it is morally permissible to employ screening technics of this kind at all.

3. Carrier screening is different from the two varieties just discussed in that it is aimed not at those afflicted with a genetic disease, but rather, at a carrier—one "who is clinically well himself, but risks having a child with a disease. These programs do not involve case-finding and treatment in the conventional sense, but rather represent an attempt to identify the person at risk and to intervene in his or her reproductive life, an approach not taken by any previous screening program."[6] The two diseases for which carriers have been screened are Tay-Sachs disease, a rare metabolic disorder that leads to blindness,

paralysis and death usually before the age of four; and sickle-cell anemia, a painful and often life-shortening disease found largely among blacks. Tay-Sachs disease, found mostly among Jews of Eastern European descent, can be diagnosed *in utero* by means of amniocentesis, so afflicted fetuses can be aborted. While the condition itself has no cure, the purpose served by screening programmes is to supply information for those parents who would choose abortion rather than bear an afflicted child who will certainly suffer and die within a very few years after birth. The purpose served by screening for sickle-cell carriers is not so clear, however. The disease cannot be detected *in utero,* so screening for carriers does not present many options. Sickle-cell anemia is autosomal recessive, which means that both parents must be carriers before it is possible to give birth to a child with the disease, and there is a one-in-four chance with each pregnancy of having an afflicted child. So parents found to be carriers can either take their chances of bearing a child who will have the disease, or choose artificial insemination with a noncarrier donor, or else seek to adopt a child. Screening programmes for sickle-cell have come under fire on the grounds that they are potentially dangerous as weapons that might be used for racist purposes by whites against blacks. It is difficult to see what sorts of persuasive arguments could be offered for compulsory sickle-cell screening programmes, in the absence of intrauterine detection of diseased fetuses or else a cure for the disease. Optional screening programmes can be justified on the grounds that they enable couples to make a more informed choice about whether or not to have children; while some couples may well choose to take the one-in-four chance with each pregnancy, others will not. There seem to be no clear social benefits that accrue to mandatory programmes, and their disvalue lies largely in raising fear and suspicion about the possible repressive uses such programmes might serve.

4. Prenatal diagnosis as a form of genetic screening overlaps with the category of chromosomal screening discussed earlier. In one form of prenatal diagnosis, fetal cells from the amniotic fluid are cultured and subjected to chromosomal analysis. In this way, XYY males can be detected *in utero* and aborted; the moral permissibility of abortion on these grounds is another issue currently under debate. A more significant use of prenatal diagnosis is found in the case of Down's syndrome. Women over forty—or even over thirty-five—are known to be at greatly elevated risk for having a child with Down's syndrome—the type of retardation formerly known as mongolism. Again, controversy exists over whether prenatal diagnosis ought to be routinely offered to women of any age, or particularly to those over thirty-five. While there seem to be sound reasons for having such programmes available on a voluntary basis, there appear to be no good grounds for imposing prenatal diagnosis on women unwilling to undergo the slight physical risk or to receive genetic information about their child. There is, further, the consideration that a chromosomal analysis will turn up other genetic information, which even parents who are eager to learn about Down's syndrome may not wish to know. Here is where the moral dilemmas raised by genetic screening intersect with those of genetic counseling.

It is evident that the primary purpose for which genetic screening is now employed is for transmitting such information to prospective parents through genetic counseling, so that they can make as informed a choice as the circumstances allow. The primary and intended impact of transmitting the information obtained by screening is to reduce suffering of presently existing persons or their children. Thus the aim is to lessen the suffering of people in the present or next generation by preventing the birth of defective children, as in the case of Tay-Sachs and Down's syndrome, or by treating them at birth, like PKU children. But where there is no cure and no intrauterine detection programme, as in the case of sickle-cell anemia and Huntington's Chorea, there is some question about the purposes to which the information gained through screening may be put. We shall return to this issue later in connection with genetic engineering. But first, let us look at the overlapping yet distinct set of problems that arise in the area of genetic counseling.

## III

The moral issues that arise in the practice of genetic counseling are primarily those surrounding truth and information in medicine. As noted earlier, there is the overarching issue of whether the genetic counselor's role should be as neutral and objective as possible, or whether it is sometimes permissible or even desirable to offer advice or guide the patient or couple to a decision. This issue appears to be no different, in principle, in the area of genetic counseling from that of a wide range of therapeutic situations in medicine, such as elective surgery or treatment regimens for severely defective newborns. As usual in ethical contexts, it is probably unwise to adhere dogmatically to a rigid principle like "physicians or genetic counselors should never advise, but should always and only inform." While a general presumption in favour of fully autonomous decision-making by the patient or client is appropriate, sometimes the presumption may justifiably be overridden. There are cases in which a patient or couple asks directly for advice from the counselor, cases where it is evident to the counselor that the prospective parents fail to comprehend the enormity of caring for and raising a severely defective child, and still other instances where some measure of denial on the part of the parents stands in the way of their facing reality and making a rational decision. As with any other intermediate moral principle, the precept that genetic counselors should remain neutral and objective may justifiably be breached. Although some may argue that the genetic counselor's role includes some eugenic obligations, the purpose of counseling is to help the pregnant woman or prospective parents as much as possible in making an informed choice that is in accord with their own preferred values.[7] It has often been noted that many people suffer guilt, react unpredictably and often irrationally in the face of information about their role in transmitting defective genes to their offspring. A sensitive and compassionate genetic counselor, observing such situations, would be acting in accordance with a sound and widely held ethical precept in helping such parents come to a decision that is in accordance with their basic value scheme and that they can live with comfortably.

There are special circumstances, in addition to the more common problematic situations in counseling just noted, where the decisions to be made are straightforward medical decisions, requiring significant medical expertise. An example is the sex assignment for an intersex child, where the decision depends on knowledge and experience that the parents most likely do not have. As one physician argues:

> Sex assignment is basically a therapeutic problem because it requires surgery to correct the anatomical anomalies of intersex. Once you remove the phallus there's really not much choice any more—you have to raise that child as a female. And the basis for such a decision is medical experience regarding prospective adequacy of sexual performance. There are phalluses that will never be functional no matter how much surgery you do. Therefore, in such a situation it would be advisable to strongly suggest conversion to female gender . . . We still see many tragedies where the physician makes the wrong decision because of a lack of experience, or because the parents have their minds set on the sex of their child, and the physician allows his decision to be swayed by their attitude.[8]

These observations serve to remind us that although recent work in the field of medical ethics has uncovered a variety of contexts in which decisions formerly considered purely medical ones have been shown not to require special medical expertise, we must nevertheless be careful not to err in the opposite direction by relegating to patients decisions that properly require a knowledgeable medical judgment.

There are still other situations in genetic counseling, which pose different sorts of moral dilemmas from those just described. One such problem is whether or not it is ever permissible for a genetic counselor to withhold information from patients. In our discussion of the XYY chromosomal anomaly, we noted some difficulties that might arise if parents are apprised of the fact that their son's genetic endowment is one that has been found to correlate highly with overly aggressive behaviour and even with criminal tendencies. Other sorts of cases usually revolve around potential psychological harm to an individual or damage to a marriage likely to result from disclosure of genetic information. One physician cites the following two instances in which he believes that withholding information is justifiable.

> One example is where the genetic disorder of the child opens the possibility of nonpaternity—where the husband's genotype indicates he may not be the child's father. Disclosure of full information in this case could lead the father to question his acceptance of the child, as well as of his marital relationship.
>
> Another example would be the case of testicular feminization in which a genotype 46, XY male develops as a female because of the failure of tissues to respond to testosterone stimulation. One might withhold this information from some parents because they would have difficulty relating to the child or

would withhold it from the child herself when she is old enough to be counseled . . . In cases in which the information can do serious psychological
damage, I feel withholding it is justified.[9]

In these sorts of cases, it would seem that a rigid adherence to a moral principle that enjoins persons always to tell the truth, the whole truth, and nothing
but the truth is an instance of dogmatism in ethics. Other moral principles
sometimes override the precept that mandates truth-telling; or, to put it another way, the duty to tell the truth is sometimes superseded by another moral
duty, when the two come into conflict. The dilemma here seems to be more of
an epistemological one than an ethical one: How can we know in advance
when telling the truth or disclosing full information will yield greater harm
than good? How can we judge whether it is better, on the whole, for one member of a couple to be told about the infidelity of the other? Do we have an adequate basis for knowing how much and what sorts of psychological harm will
be done by informing parents about their child's sexual anomaly, as in the example cited earlier? The ethical principle here seems rather clear: perform that
act likely to produce least harm to everyone who stands to be affected. But one
can accept this consequentialist moral position and yet still not know how to
act because of the epistemological difficulties just noted. This should serve to
remind us that not all the problems in moral contexts arise out of uncertainty
about which ethical principle to adopt or what to do when two basic moral
precepts come into conflict. In the cases just noted, it is likely that general
agreement can be secured about the appropriateness of a utilitarian or consequentialist approach. Disagreement is more likely to arise over just which
course of action is, in fact, likely to produce more harm, on balance. Aside
from other kinds of disputes concerning what properly constitutes harm in
such cases, the difficulty does seem to be more of an epistemological one than
an ethical one.

The foregoing treatment of moral issues in genetic counseling has rested
on the presupposition that the genetic counselor's responsibility is to the patient or client. On the basis of this presupposition, I have supported the general presumption that favours decision-making autonomy on the part of those
being counseled. If, however, the genetic counselor were properly viewed as
having an obligation to society at large or to future generations, then the presumption about autonomy might have to be overridden in some cases. In answer to the question, "To whom is the genetic counselor responsible?" one geneticist replies:

> Basically, I think that genetic counselors may be misguided if they feel that
> their ethical obligation is in *any way* to future generations . . . All too often, I
> get the feeling that some genetic counselors are acting on the hidden assump-
> tion that they are somehow participating in that particularly Western
> predilection for attempting to create "ideal situations," in this instance, that of
> building a better gene pool through "negative eugenics" . . . The genetic
> counselor's obligation, I will maintain, never should extend beyond the family
> within his purview . . . Properly, a genetic counselor's job should not, in any
> way, be construed as eugenic in practice.[10]

Now, if we accept this view, that the genetic counselor has a responsibility to the family he is counseling and not to society at large or to future generations, then it is but a few small steps to the conclusion that individuals or couples should have final decision-making authority in matters of their own reproductive acts and capacities. But before such a conclusion can be reached, we must first explore the question of the feasibility or desirability of genetic engineering. Even if it is not the business of the genetic counselor to make recommendations to families on the basis of what is best for the human gene pool, it might still turn out that government-based or scientist-directed eugenic programmes could override personal decisions in these matters. So before concluding that ultimate decision-making authority ought to rest with individual persons or couples, we must first reject any presumptions to the contrary that stem from eugenic considerations. In the remaining time I shall explore some issues in genetic engineering, with the aim of showing that government-based or scientist-directed eugenic programmes are misguided or dangerous or both.

## IV

The notion of genetic engineering appears to have a narrower and a broader definition. The narrow conception refers to approaches involving laboratory manipulation of genes or cells: somatic cell alteration and germ cell alteration. When this meaning is assigned to genetic engineering, the term "eugenics" is used to refer to selection of parents or of their germ cells.[11] But sometimes the term "genetic engineering" is used in a fully general sense, to refer to any manipulation of the reproductive acts or capacities of persons or their parts. It is this latter sense that will be used in the remainder of this account.

At least the idea behind eugenics—if not the practice itself in some form—is ancient. Positive eugenics was promoted in Plato's *Republic,* long before the science of genetics provided the theoretical basis and systematic data that today's proponents of genetic engineering have to work with. The lack of personal freedoms allowed the citizens in the *Republic* is well known to those familiar with Plato's work, and is evident in the following passage discussing regulation of unions between the sexes:

> It is for you, then, as their lawgiver, who have already selected the men, to select for association with them women who are so far as possible of the same natural capacity . . . [A]nything like unregulated unions would be a profanation in a state whose citizens lead the good life. The Rulers will not allow such a thing . . . [I]f we are to keep our flock at the highest pitch of excellence, there should be as many unions of the best of both sexes, and as few of the inferior as possible, and . . . only the offspring of the better unions should be kept . . . Moreover, young men who acquit themselves well in war and other duties, should be given, among other rewards and privileges, more liberal opportunities to sleep with a wife, for the further purpose that, with good excuse, as many as possible of the children may be begotten of such fathers.[12]

But lest we conclude that a eugenics movement can only be promoted or gain adherents in a rigidly controlled society like Plato's *Republic* or a totalitarian regime such as Nazi Germany, let us consider the view of a 20th-century Nobel Prize–winning geneticist. The late Hermann Muller was an archpropo-nent of positive eugenics, the basis of his belief that the human gene pool is deteriorating. Muller argued for voluntary programmes of positive eugenics, rejecting any form of state-imposed regulations. He claimed that "democratic control . . . implies an upgrading of the people in general in both their intel-lectual and social faculties, together with a maintenance or, preferably, an im-provement in their bodily condition."[13] Muller was one of a number of con-temporary geneticists who have made gloomy prophecies about the increasing load of mutations in the human gene pool. The particular brand of positive eu-genics that he advocated was a voluntary artificial insemination programme using donor semen (AID). He envisaged preserving the semen of outstanding men for future use in artificial insemination, choosing such greats as Einstein, Pasteur, Descartes, Leonardo and Lincoln as men whose child no woman would refuse to bear.[14]

Muller's method of freezing the semen of intellectual and creative men is only one of several proposals favouring some form of *positive* eugenics—a programme for improving the species, breeding a better race, or trying to pre-vent further deterioration by taking active counter-measures. Greater atten-tion has been directed to the question of whether *negative* eugenics should be practiced on carriers or those afflicted with heritable diseases, in the form of enforced or encouraged abortions, sterilization, or less repressive but nonetheless coercive measures. The dilemma of choosing between preserving the individual freedom to marry and procreate as one chooses, and prevent-ing further pollution of the gene pool would, indeed, pose an agonizing moral choice if the facts were as clear-cut as the eugenicists take them to be. There seems, however, to be enough uncertainty about the possible and prob-able outcomes of any attempts at eugenics to warrant extreme caution in mounting such grandiose schemes for genetic improvement. Many scientists agree that trying to reduce the load of mutations in the human gene pool through negative eugenics would be ineffective, at best. And the arguments against positive eugenics point to a number of potentially infelicitous out-comes. There are at least five separate arguments against the feasibility or de-sirability of any large-scale attempt at genetic engineering for eugenic pur-poses—arguments which, if taken together, give strong support to my conclusion that genetic engineering with this aim is misguided or dangerous or both. A sixth argument is the religious one that creating or modifying the human species is a task not for man, but for God.[15] For those to whom this sort of argument is compelling, it may lend added strength to the other five. I shall confine my discussion to four of the five considerations that do not re-quire belief in a supernatural deity. Each of the following arguments against a systematic effort to mount any sort of eugenics programme will be dis-cussed in turn:

1. We're too ignorant to do it right.
2. In any case, we are likely to alter the gene pool for ill.
3. Negative eugenics can't possibly work unless carriers are eliminated, but this would soon eliminate the entire species.
4. Some methods of genetic engineering carry grave moral risks of mishap.

The fifth argument is essentially that most—if not all—methods of genetic engineering are dehumanizing in basic ways.[16] While I think this attack contains some interesting points and raises questions of value that generally deserve important consideration, it is a gratuitous argument in this context. If the first four arguments are sound, they obviate the necessity for the fifth, since the scientific and practical objections to eugenic programmes would rule them out before the value issues need be brought into consideration. So I shall treat only the first four arguments in what follows.

1. The claim that we are too ignorant to do the job right has several variants, each with significant implications. The first consideration points to our general ignorance about the value of a gene to a given race or to the species. As one prominent geneticist notes:

> We know only about its value to the individual carrying it and then only in instances where the effect is severe. In the light of such ignorance, it seems to me that the best procedure is to avoid all changes in the environment which are likely to change the mutation rate . . . The quality of a gene or genotype may be determined only by the reaction of the associated phenotype in the environment in which it exists. A phenotype may be disadvantageous in some environments, essentially neutral in others, and advantageous in others. In the face of a rapidly changing and entirely new environment (new in an evolutionary sense), I do not believe that we can determine the value of specific genotypes to the species.[17]

This brand of ignorance constitutes our lack of knowledge of what to select for—a form of ignorance that some may argue is confined to the present state of development of the science of genetics. But a second variant of the "we're too ignorant" argument notes that "if we alter the gene pool, independent of environment, we are acting on the basis of present environmental criteria to select a gene pool for the future. Since the environment is changing a thousandfold times faster than our gene pool, it would be a disastrous approach."[18] But the difficulty here is not simply one of our inability to predict accurately what the future will be like. Questions of value enter in—questions that invariably resurrect the memory of attempts at positive eugenics among the Nazis. One writer asks:

> Who will be the judges and where will be the separation between good and bad? The most difficult decisions will come in defining the borderline cases. Will we breed against tallness because space requirements become more critical? Will we breed against nearsightedness because people with glasses may not make good astronauts? Will we forbid intellectually inferior individuals from procreating despite their proved ability to produce a number of superior individuals?[19]

The last variant on the "we're too ignorant" theme that we shall consider here requires us to recall Hermann Muller's proposal for positive eugenics. Muller would not be alone in including Abraham Lincoln on a list of men whose child no woman would refuse to bear. Yet there is now considerable evidence that Lincoln was afflicted with Marfan's syndrome, a heritable disease of the connective tissue that is transmitted by a dominant gene. The evidence is based on a number of factors. Lincoln's bodily characteristics and facial features—the very qualities we term "Lincolnesque"—are typical features of bone deformities common to Marfan's syndrome. The disease was first named in 1896, some 30 years after Lincoln's death. It was believed for some time that Lincoln had Marfan's disease, on the basis of physical defects he was known to have had, as well as the early death of one of his children. One sign of the disease was Lincoln's abnormally long limbs. Also, casts made of Lincoln's body in the year of his inauguration reveal that his left hand was much longer than his right hand, and his left middle finger was elongated. He is also known to have suffered from severe farsightedness, in addition to having difficulty with his eyesight that stemmed from distortions in his facial bone structure. These bodily asymmetries are common to Marfan's syndrome, as is cardiac disease. It is believed that Lincoln inherited the disease from his father's side. His father was blind in one eye, his son Robert had difficulties with his eyes, and his son Tad had a speech defect and died at the age of eighteen, probably from cardiac trouble. The likelihood that Lincoln himself suffered from Marfan's syndrome was further confirmed in 1959, when a California physician named Harold Schwartz recognized the disease in a boy of seven who was known to share an ancestor with Lincoln.[20] Since the gene for Marfan's disease is dominant, those who have it and reach childbearing age stand a 50 percent chance of having an afflicted child.

Now consider the consequences for the gene pool if Lincoln's frozen sperm were to be disseminated widely in the population. At least until the facts became evident, the result would be exactly the opposite of what Muller intended by his proposal. And if the mistake went beyond the case of Lincoln and Marfan's syndrome, including other individuals who, despite their outstanding achievements, might be afflicted with or be carriers of other little-known or as yet undiagnosed genetic diseases, the results would be dysgenic in the extreme. This last consideration leads directly to the second argument against eugenics programmes, to which we turn next.

2. This argument holds that in any event, we are likely to alter the gene pool for ill. Leaving aside the less likely incidence of this occurrence as exemplified just now in the Abraham Lincoln story, we may look at another prominent consideration noted by some geneticists.

This consideration is often referred to as "heterozygote advantage." One geneticist explains the situation as follows:

> There is . . . good evidence that individuals who carry two different forms of the same gene, that is, are heterozygous, appear to have an advantage. This is true even if that gene in double dose, that is, in the homozygous state,

produces a severe disease. For example, individuals homozygous for the gene coding for sickle-cell hemoglobin invariably develop sickle-cell anemia, which is generally fatal before the reproductive years. Heterozygotes for the gene are, however, protected more than normals from the effects of the most malignant form of malaria. It has been shown that women who carry the gene in single dose have a higher fertility in malarial areas than do normals.[21]

Here again, it is not only in the cases where there is known heterozygote advantage that the likelihood exists of altering the gene pool for ill by trying to eliminate genes for heritable diseases. There are, in addition, all of the cases where heterozygote advantage may exist but is at present unknown. If one uses risk-benefit ratios or something like a utilitarian schema for deriding moral issues in biomedical contexts, the evidence seems clearly to indicate a greater risk of dysgenic consequences than a possibility of beneficial results from attempts to alter the human gene pool by means of negative eugenics. A successful effort to eliminate carriers for heritable diseases would result at the same time in eliminating heterozygote advantage, which is believed to be beneficial to the species or to sub-populations within the species. While little is known at the present stage of inquiry in genetics about all of the particular advantages that exist, it is an inference made by many experts in the field on the basis of present data and well-confirmed genetic theory. One biologist asks us to:

> Consider the gene leading to cystic fibrosis (C.F.). Until quite recently homozygotes for this gene died in infancy. Yet the gene causing C.F. is very common among all Caucasoid populations thus far studied . . . It is too widespread in the race to be accounted for by genetic drift. The gene is also too frequent for it to be likely to be maintained by mutation pressure. Hence, we are driven to assume heterozygote advantage.[22]

It would seem, then, that what is gained by the elimination of homozygotes may well be lost by the elimination of heterozygotes, resulting in no clear benefits and possibly some significant disadvantages in populations that suffer from genetic diseases. But the argument just given assumes that it would in fact be possible to eliminate genes for heritable diseases by preventing carriers from reproducing and thereby passing on such genes to future generations. The next argument against genetic engineering questions such a possibility.

3. This argument maintains, in sum, that negative eugenics can't possibly work unless carriers are eliminated as well as diseased individuals; but a successful attempt to prevent all carriers of potentially lethal genes from reproducing would effectively eliminate the entire species. The effects of negative eugenics on the general population are assessed by one geneticist as follows:

> With a few exceptions, dominant diseases are rare and interfere severely with reproductive ability. They are generally maintained in the population by new mutations. Therefore, there is either no need or essentially no need for discouraging these individuals from reproduction . . . The story is quite different for recessive conditions . . . [A]ny attempt to decrease the gene frequency of these common genetic disorders in the population by prevention of fertility of all carriers would be doomed to failure. First, we all carry between three and eight

of these genes in a single dose. Secondly, for many of these conditions, the frequency of carriers in the population is about 1 in 50 or even greater. Prevention of fertility for even one of these disorders would stop a sizable proportion of the population from reproducing.[23]

If this assessment is sound, it has significant implications for the prospects of favourably altering the human gene pool by negative eugenics. Such an argument is persuasive if the purpose of negative eugenics is viewed as that of improving the human gene pool for the sake of future generations. But if the purpose of negative eugenics is seen as improving the quality of life for those in the present and next generation, then the argument just given is beside the point. We should recall the dual purpose for which proposals for genetic engineering are put forth. The one we have been discussing here is the proposed improvement or prevention of deterioration of the gene pool for the sake of future generations of humans. The other purpose, tied to voluntary genetic screening programmes and the activity of genetic counseling, is to present options to individuals or couples that will help them avoid the birth of a defective child whose quality of life will be poor and who will most likely be a burden on both parents and society. For this latter purpose, the practice of negative eugenics through voluntary screening and sensitive genetic counseling can serve to improve the quality of life of persons in this and the next generation. But when transformed into a programme designed to control the reproductive acts or capacities of people for the sake of future generations, then the practice of negative eugenics seems to be scientifically and practically misguided. Indeed, taking this argument and the previous one together, the conclusion may be put succinctly in the words of one writer:

> Neither positive nor negative eugenics can ever significantly improve the gene pool of the population and simultaneously allow for adequate evolutionary improvement of the human race. The only useful aspect of negative eugenics is in individual counseling of specific families in order to prevent some of the births of abnormal individuals.[24]

4. The fourth argument against genetic engineering focuses specifically on those practices involving manipulation of genetic material itself. This argument raises questions about the grave risks involved in any such manipulation, especially since mishaps that may arise are likely to be far worse than what happens when nature takes its course. One geneticist sees the prospects as follows:

> The problem of altering an individual's genes by direct chemical change of his DNA presents technically an enormously difficult task. Even if it became possible to do this, the chance of error would be high. Such an error, of course, would have the diametrically opposite effect to that desired and would be irreversible; in other words, the individual would become even more abnormal.[25]

Some observers fear the creation of hapless monsters as a result of various manipulations on genetic material. Whether or not the laboratory techniques are sufficiently refined at present to enable researchers to develop procedures for widespread use, it is likely that these techniques will be available soon enough to deserve careful reflection now. We need to ask, once again, whether the purpose served by laboratory methods of genetic engineering is helping those who are at risk for bearing defective children to prevent such occurrences, or instead, breeding a genetically improved species for the future. If such techniques are perfected and become available for use in spite of the attendant risks of mishap, they would then be offered to couples on a voluntary basis in the same way that current methods of genetic intervention are employed. Where a practice is aimed at the genetic improvement of a couple's own progeny, there are no grounds for methods that involve coercion. What is needed in such cases is counseling and education, not coercion and control.

At the outset, I said I would argue for two separate but related theses. First, the individual or couple should have final decision-making authority in matters of his or her own reproductive acts and capacities, as well as continuation or termination of pregnancy where the reasons for these decisions refer to genetic factors. Second, attempts at government-based or scientist-directed eugenic programmes are bound to be misguided or dangerous or both. The four arguments at the end were offered in support of the second thesis. If those arguments are sound, they demonstrate that there is no warrant for those in power to take final decision-making authority away from the individual where the reasons for such actions refer to eugenic considerations. Recall also our earlier conclusion that final decision-making should be left to the individual or couple in the context of genetic counseling, except in cases where the decision requires medical expertise that a patient is unlikely to have. Now if genetic screening should be practiced on a voluntary basis; and if decisions arising out of counseling should be left to the individual; and if in addition, positive and negative eugenics aimed at future generations is basically misguided; then there seems to be only one consideration remaining that might argue in favour of limiting individual rights for the sake of social benefits. That consideration points to the burden placed on society for treating and maintaining defective infants and others who might have been aborted or never even conceived by dint of state policy. Time does not permit an examination of this last issue, but it is worth making a final observation in closing. If the notion of social benefit is understood largely in terms of increased financial resources that would otherwise be allocated to caring for those afflicted with heritable diseases, then something crucial is being left out of the balance between individual rights and social benefits. What is socially beneficial must be viewed not only in terms of increases in financial and other tangible resources, but also in terms of a range of freedom and autonomy that members of a society can reasonably expect to enjoy. It is important to preserve that freedom and autonomy through ensuring the individual's right to decide about his or her own reproductive acts and capacities. With increased availability of voluntary genetic screening programmes and widespread education of the public, it is hard to imagine that most people will choose to burden themselves and society with defective children when other options are open to them. Even if there are some who refuse screening or abortion, society as a whole would be better off to accommodate their freely chosen reproductive acts than to impose compulsory genetic screening, abortion, or sterilization on its members.

## NOTES

1. The second epigraph is from Kurt Hirschhorn, "Practical and Ethical Problems in Human Genetics," *Birth Defects,* 8, no. 4 (July 1972), pp. 29–30.
2. Tabitha Powledge, "Genetic Screening" in *Encyclopedia of Bioethics,* The Free Press, 1978, ed. W. Reich.
3. Ibid.
4. Ibid.
5. Tabitha Powledge, "The XYY Man: Do Criminals Really Have Abnormal Genes?" *Science Digest,* January 1976, p. 37.
6. Powledge, "Genetic Screening."
7. A view similar to this is argued by Marc Lappé. "The Genetic Counselor: Responsible to Whom?" *Hastings Center Report* 1 (September 1971).
8. Kurt Hirschhorn, "Symposium: Ethics of Genetics Counseling," *Contemporary OB/GYN* 2, no. 4, p. 117.
9. Robert F. Murray Jr., ibid., p. 120.
10. Lappé, "The Genetic Counselor," p. 6.
11. Bernard D. Davis. "Threat and Promise in Genetic Engineering," in *Ethical Issues in Biology and Medicine,* ed. Preston Williams (Cambridge, MA: Schenkman, 1973), pp. 17–24.
12. *The Republic of Plato,* trans. Francis MacDonald Cornford (New York: Oxford University Press), pp. 157–60.
13. Hermann J. Muller, "Genetic Progress by Voluntarily Conducted Germinal Choice," in *Man and His Future,* ed. Gordon Wolstenholme (Boston: Little, Brown, 1963), p. 256.
14. Theodosius Dobzhansky, *Mankind Evolving* (New Haven: Yale University Press, 1962), p. 328.
15. Such arguments are offered by Paul Ramsey in *Fabricated Man* (New Haven: Yale University Press, 1970).
16. This argument is given by Ramsey, *Fabricated Man,* by Leon R. Kass, "Making Babies—The New Biology and the 'Old' Morality," *Public Interest* 26 (Winter 1972).
17. Arthur Steinberg, "The Genetic Pool, Its Evolution and Significance—'Desirable' and 'Undesirable' Genetic Traits," in C.I.O.M.S., *Recent Progress in Biology and Medicine,* pp. 83–93.
18. Hirschhorn, "Symposium," p. 128.
19. Hirschhorn, "Practical and Ethical Problems in Human Genetics," p. 28.
20. Ibid., p. 23.
21. Steinberg, "The Genetic Pool."
22. René Dubos and Maya Pines, *Health and Disease* (New York: Time, 1965), pp. 123–24.
23. Hirschhorn, "Practical and Ethical Problems in Human Genetics," pp. 22–23.
24. Ibid., p. 25.
25. Ibid., p. 27.

# Resisting Reductionism from the Human Genome Project

## Robert N. Proctor

*Robert N. Proctor has devoted his career as a historian to studying the intersection of science and medicine. Proctor continues to argue that history has shown that people oversimplify new scientific results and then act incorrectly. Whether it is cancer or genetics, people usually fall into the trap of "reductionism," reducing complex facts to overly simplistic maxims, such as "It's all in the genes."*

*In this selection, Proctor predicts how results from the Human Genome Project and other genetic breakthroughs will be oversimplified and result in harm to people. He attacks the ideology behind many statements about genetics and urges us to resist biological (genetic) determinism.*

*Robert N. Proctor, PhD, is professor of history at Pennsylvania State University, Pennsylvania.*

Central to eugenics ideology was the view that biology is destiny—that human talents and institutions are largely the product of our anatomical, neurological, hormonal, genetic, or racial constitution. Eugenicists exaggerated the role of genetics predisposing one toward a life of alcoholism, crime, or other human defects or talent. At the root of the movement was a set of fears: that the poor were outbreeding the rich, that feminists were having too few babies, that the mentally ill and criminal were about to swamp the superior elements of the population with their high birth rates. Eugenics policies were designed to combat those fears.

Among all the potential dangers of human genomics, to my mind the most all-encompassing is the danger of its confluence with a growing trend toward biological determinism. Biological determinism is the view that the large part of human talents and disabilities—perhaps even our tastes and institutions—is

*Source: Genetic Mapping: A Guide to Law and Ethics*, ed. G. Annas and S. Elias (Oxford University Press, 1992). Reprinted by permission of the author and publisher.

anchored in our biology. The Human Genome Project has already been criticized by groups who fear that the ultimate rationale for the project is a biological determinist one. James Watson did little to dispel this concern, defending the Project as providing us with "the ultimate tool for understanding ourselves at the molecular level . . . We used to think our fate was in our stars. Now we know, in large measure, our fate is in our genes."[1] Critics point to the long, seamy tradition of eugenicists exaggerating the role of genes in human behavior; even without the impositions of a heavy-handed state, there are dangers of seeing biology as destiny. Genes have become a near-universal scapegoat for all that ails the human species. Even where genetic influence is well established, critics worry that aggressive promoting of genetic testing may generate fears out of proportion to actual risks. In the rush to identify genetic components to cancer or heart disease or mental illness, the substantial environmental origins of those afflictions may be slighted.

I want to emphasize this danger of exaggerating the role of genetics in the development of disease. Take the example of cancer. A number of rare cancers are known to be the result of heritable genetic defects. Highly heritable cancers include retinoblastoma (associated with a deletion in chromosome 13), certain leukemias, xeroderma pigmentosum (which predisposes one toward skin cancer), and a number of rare malignancies associated with a deletion in the recently discovered p53 gene (linked to the Li-Fraumeni syndrome). These are all germline defects—in other words, the genes causing these cancers can be passed from generation to generation.[2] A number of genes have also been found that predispose the carrier to more common kinds of cancers. In the spring of 1991 a research team headed by Bert Vogelstein at Johns Hopkins announced the discovery of a tumor suppressor gene on chromosome 5, the deletion of which seemed to be implicated in the onset of colon cancer.[3] A great deal of research has also gone into the search for predisposing genes for breast cancer.[4] E. B. Claus, N. Risch, and W. D. Thompson estimate that as many as 5 to 10 percent of all cases of breast cancer can be accounted for by inherited factors, and that the distribution of breast cancers is consistent with the existence of an autosomal (non-sex-linked) dominant gene affecting about one-third of 1 percent of all women.[5] Still other studies have tried to demonstrate differential susceptibilities to lung cancer. Smoking is clearly a cause of small-cell carcinoma of the lung, but only a fraction of those who smoke heavily do in fact develop lung cancer.[6] Predisposing genes may provide an answer to the question posed by *Science* magazine reporter Jean Marx, "Why doesn't everybody get cancer?"[7]

Genetic differences no doubt account for at least part of the differential susceptibility to cancer, though assertions about their frequency and what this implies for social policy are politically charged. Popularizers are fond of providing estimates for the frequency of susceptibility genes: a front-page *New York Times* article reporting on the March 1991 discovery of a tumor suppressor gene for colon cancer states that "at least 20 percent" of all colon cancers ("and possibly many more") begin through the action of the newly discovered gene.[8] Mark Skolnick, coauthor of a widely cited *New England Journal of Medicine* report on the genetics of colon cancer, speculates that genes predisposing to colon cancer are inherited "by as many as one-third of all Americans." Skolnick draws clear policy implications from the work: if suitable markers can be found, "we could use a simple blood test to screen the entire U.S. population. Those with the gene or genes would know they are carrying within them a potentially dangerous genetic defect. They would be warned to get regular checkups, and avoid the kinds of high-fat foods thought to trigger the cancer." Skolnick also states that "one-third of Americans stand some risk of developing colon cancer, while the other two-thirds probably aren't at risk at all."[9]

Quite apart from the logistical difficulties of screening "the entire U.S. population," a number of questions can be raised about such statements. For one thing, the figures commonly given for predisposing genes for cancer are somewhat speculative. The statistical models used to generate such figures (most recently for breast and lung cancers) are designed to measure the extent to which cancer runs in families,[10] but they also have notorious problems controlling for the fact that families often share common exposures to mutagens (through the "heritability" of occupation or household environment, for example). Furthermore, the genes discovered in the 1991 *Science* study headed by Vogelstein are genes in the DNA of tumor cells, not in germline DNA. The finding of damaged or deleted genetic loci in tumors does not mean that the same defects will be found in the remaining cells of the body and that the defects are therefore heritable. Finally, there is little evidence for the claim that two-thirds of Americans "probably aren't at risk at all" for a disease such as colon cancer. Such a claim presumes a small number of predisposing genes when the actual number might be quite large, producing a continuum of differential susceptibility rather than a simple yes or no, "susceptible or not." There is no evidence that a sizable fraction of the American population is invulnerable to cancer.

The most serious objection to predisposition studies, though, is that they can detract attention from the epidemiological fact that cancer is a disease whose incidence varies according to occupation, diet, socioeconomic status, and personal habits such as smoking. Genetics can do little to explain such patterns. Rates of lung and breast cancer, for example—two of the three deadliest cancers—have both risen dramatically in recent years; genetic propensities can have little to do with such increases. Lung cancer rates for U.S. males rose from 5 per 100,000 in 1930 to 75 per 100,000 in 1985—a fifteenfold increase.[11] Lung cancer rates for women rose some 420 percent over the last 30 years, and breast cancer rates have also grown. The American Cancer Society's 1991 *Cancer Facts and Figures* estimates that American women now face a one in nine chance of developing breast cancer—up some 10 percent from the risk calculated only 4 years earlier.[12] Such dramatic rises lead one to suspect environmental changes, rather than genetic propensities, as the primary culprit. Even Claus and his colleagues concede that "the great majority of breast cancers are nongenetic."[13]

A similar argument can be made for most of the systematic differences in cancer rates found between ethnic groups. Blacks, for example, have significantly higher cancer rates than do whites. But, as a National Cancer Institute study revealed in the spring of 1991, poverty—not race—is the primary cause of that difference.[14] And surely there are many other differences for which genetics will be irrelevant. Genetics is not going to explain the fact that asbestos miners have higher mesothelioma rates than people who work in air-conditioned offices, nor will it explain the fact that people who live in homes with radon seepage are more likely to contract cancer. Even if individuals vary in susceptibility to such agents, it may be wishful thinking to image that physicians will be able to assure people, from their genetic profiles alone, that they are or are not at risk for common diseases such as cancer. Nancy Wexler, president of the Hereditary Disease Foundation and chair of the ethics group of the Human Genome Project, has recently suggested that "[a]s geneticists learn more about diabetes or hypertension or cancer, at some point they will cross an important line. Instead of saying, as they do now, 'Lung cancer runs in your family and you should be careful,' physicians will be able to ask their patients, 'Would you like to take a blood test to see if you are going to get lung cancer?"[15] But if the majority of lung cancers are environmentally induced (and there is evidence that cigarette smoking alone accounts for as much as 90 percent of all lung cancers),[16] then physicians are unlikely ever to be able to predict cancers of this sort at an early age—except perhaps for the small percentage for whom a clear genetic defect can be discovered. It is misleading to suggest that physicians will ever have this power.[17]

Part of the confusion arises from the fact that cancers may be "genetic" in two very different senses. In one sense, all cancers are genetic. All cancer involves a runaway replication of cellular tissue; carcinogenesis invariably involves the switching on or off of genes that normally would not act in this fashion. Cellular replication involves genetic expression, and in this sense all cancers are genetic. Only a tiny proportion of cancers, however, are known to be heritable—that is, transmissible from generation to generation. There are thus two types of cancers, or rather two different ways cancers may originate: *somatic* cancers arise from genetic transformations in some particular bodily tissue (caused by exposure to mutagens or viruses, for example); *germline* or *heritable* cancers are passed from generation to generation through the genetic information in the germ cells (the sperm or eggs). The genetic defect is distributed differently in the two cases. In somatically induced cancers, the genetic malfunction lies only in the injured cells of the tumor. In heritable, germline cancers, the genetic defect will be found in every tissue of the body. The distinction is not always clear-cut: as already noted, some heritable genes confer an increased susceptibility to cancer, the ultimate trigger for which is some environmental mutagen. A given cancer (retinoblastoma, for example) may have both familial and sporadic (somatic) forms—the distinction being only in the timing and location of the mutation. The appropriate therapies for heritable and somatic cancers may be indistinguishable. Still, the root cause of cancer in the two extreme cases is quite different. Germline cancers may be expressed regardless of the environment to which one is exposed; somatic cancers are generally triggered by some postnatal environmental insult.

Knowledge of the genetic mechanisms involved in carcinogenesis has been growing rapidly in recent years. Since the late 1970s, several dozen different segments of the human genome have been discovered that, when mutated (sometimes by as little as one nucleotide, as in the case of human bladder cancer), produce cancer. "Oncogenes," as these segments are called, have been found associated with viruses that infect chickens, monkeys, and cats. Occurring naturally in certain animals, oncogenes may be picked up by these viruses and transmitted in the course of infection. Genes have also been discovered that, by contrast with oncogenes, allow cancer to flourish when the gene is absent. These "tumor suppressor genes" normally prevent the growth of cancer; when damaged or deleted, as seems to be required for the development of retinoblastoma, Wilms tumor (a kidney cancer), and certain forms of colon cancer, it is the absence or impairment of the gene that allows the malignancy to grow. How and why these growth-blocking genes are first activated or deactivated is not yet clear.[18]

The important question of policy interest, though, is: What causes a gene to mutate in the first place? Much has been made of the fact that carcinogenesis begins with genetic changes; Robert Weinberg of the Whitehead Institute (and one of the discoverers of oncogenes) states that "the roots of cancer lie in our genes."[19] Improved therapies may well emerge from investigating precisely what biochemical functions are curtailed by the loss of tumor suppressor genes. If, however, as most often appears to be the case, cancer begins through some kind of environmental insult—exposure to ionizing radiation, for example, or to one of the many chemical carcinogens in our air, food, or water—then the fact that oncogenes must be activated and suppressor genes turned off does not alter the fact that, from a long-run societal point of view, prevention is probably going to remain the best way to approach the problem of cancer.

One of the dangers of biological determinism, then, is that the root cause for the onset of disease is shifted from the environmental (toxic exposures) to the individual (genetic defects). The scientific search shifts from a search for mutagens in the environment to biological defects in the individual. Geneticists sometimes argue that identification of persons especially at risk will allow us to determine "who will benefit maximally from treatments designed to manipulate the environmental causes of those conditions."[20] Critics, however, point out that susceptibilities may be used for less benevolent purposes. *Consumer Reports,* in its July 1990 cover story on genetic screening, warned: "The danger is that industry may try to screen out the most vulnerable rather than clean up an environment that places all workers at increased risk."[21]

The threat screening poses to individual workers is well known;[22] less well known may be the fact that a number of industry spokesmen have sought to play the genetic card to defend a particular product as safe. The Council for Tobacco Research has spent more than $150 million on biomedical research since its founding in 1954; the overwhelming majority of its widely disseminated cancer studies have been devoted to genetic research.[23] Tobacco lobbyists have tried to argue that smoking causes cancer only in those persons for whom there is already a genetic predisposition.[24] The recent discovery of a gene triggering the onset of lung cancer (by converting hydrocarbons into carcinogens when exposed to cigarette smoke) prompted the discoverer to assert, "If we could identify those people in whom this gene is easily activated, then we could counsel them, not only not to smoke, but to avoid exposure to certain environmental pollutants."[25] Again, the danger in such arguments is that emphasis is placed on defects in the individual rather than defects in the industrial product or environment. The risk is what might be called an ideological one: if the (mis)conception grows that "nature" is more important than "nurture" in the onset of certain diseases, lawmakers may find themselves less willing to enact strong pollution prevention measures or consumer protection legislation.

It is not always easy, of course, to separate "nature" and "nurture" in such matters. Discoveries of genes for Alzheimer disease, manic depression, schizophrenia, Tourette syndrome, and lung cancer have all been announced with widespread media attention, only to be later found flawed.[26] Even for diseases that are clearly heritable, genes may vary widely in their manner of expression. Five percent of men who have heart attacks before the age of 60 carry a gene that prevents the liver from filtering out harmful cholesterol. Not all of those men with the gene, however, suffer early heart disease—only about half do. Diet or some other factor can apparently ameliorate the negative effects of the disease. Neil Holtzman, professor of pediatrics at Johns Hopkins, points out that genetic tests may have little predictive value in cases where genetic expression is highly variable: "For the vast majority of people affected by heart disease, cancer and the like, the origin is so complex that it's a gross oversimplification to think that screening for a predisposing gene will be predictive."[27]

## CONCLUSION

Popularizers and experts both often present the birth of genomics as heralding newfound technical and moral powers. The *Time* magazine cover story on the Human Genome Project of March 20, 1989, asserts that scientists are likely to be able eventually to predict an individual's vulnerability not just to diseases such as cystic fibrosis, but also to "more common disorders like heart disease and cancer, which at the very least have large genetic components."[28] Others imply sweeping moral transformations from the newfound knowledge of our nucleotides. An article in the *Hastings Center Report* envisions "a heightened societal attention to heritage, with DNA stored in banks becoming a new type of ancestral shrine"; the authors forecast a "renewed commitment to intergenerational relatedness." Daniel Koshland, in an editorial in *Science,* suggests that sequencing the human genome may result in "a great new technology to aid the poor, the infirm, and the underprivileged." George Bugliarello, of Brooklyn's Polytechnic University, states that human genome research may help us understand our "constitutional propensity to violence and aggression"; genome research is supposed to give us, for the first time, "a serious if distant hope of finding ways to change some of our dangerous ancestral traits."[29]

At the risk of dashing such fanciful hopes, it is important to keep in mind that there are not that many diseases that have a clear and simple genetic origin. Cystic fibrosis kills on the order of 500 Americans per year; death rates from Huntington disease are roughly comparable. These are not insignificant numbers, but they must be put into perspective. Cigarette smoking alone, for example, is estimated to cause the deaths of some 400,000 Americans per year—more, in other words, than all known genetic diseases combined.[30] Heart disease takes an even higher toll. If it is lives we want to save, where is the $3 billion antismoking initiative or the billion-dollar effort to reduce saturated fats or food additives? Where are the billions to reduce occupational exposures to toxins, or radon gas in homes? The U.S. infant mortality rate is among the worst for industrial nations; knowledge of genetics will do little to help change that. If improved health is our goal, then surely there is something wrong with the priorities of medical funding.

There is a great deal of concern about the "social control" likely to flow from the Human Genome Project. The argument I've made here is that there is an equal danger in the *illusion of control* that will flow from people's assuming that everything is genetic. We are in the midst of an upsurge in biological determinism, and not just in areas such as cancer theory. There is little danger today of the kinds of abuses that 1920s and 1930s eugenicists foisted on the world. The emphasis today is on treating or preventing genetic disease, not on elevation of the health of the race. Efforts are aimed at voluntary therapy, not forcible sterilization or marital bans. Counseling is supposed to be self-consciously "nondirective," meaning that it is left to individual patients to decide what kind of therapy they (or their offspring) will or will not have. Unlike in the eugenics movement, those who have genetic diseases are often those in the vanguard pushing for therapy. The champions of genomics are among those calling for research into the social and ethical implications on the project: the National Institutes of Health (NIH) working group formed to monitor the "Ethical, Legal, and Social Issues Related to Mapping and Sequencing the Human Genome" has already begun to fund research into most of the concerns outlined here, as well as several others.[31] The Department of Energy (DOE) has begrudgingly agreed to support ethics research.[32] Most important, perhaps, is the fact that American society as a whole has changed. Civil rights advocates have successfully pushed for laws protecting the status of minorities; disability movements have resulted in guarantees of access for the handicapped. The increasingly powerful voices of women and minorities have made it harder to stigmatize groups in the fashion of the 1920s and 1930s. Times have changed.

The biological determinism that underlay the 1930s eugenics movement, however, has by no means disappeared. Genetics remains very much a "science of human inequality" insofar as the more we look for differences, the more likely we are to find them. In the face of unequal powers and unequal access, there is a great danger of exaggerating the extent to which human behavior is rooted in the genes. Scientists still work to prove that intelligence, alcoholism, crime, depression, homosexuality, female intuition, and a wide range of other talents or disabilities are the inflexible outcomes of human genes, hormones, neural anatomy, or evolutionary history.[33] Endocrinologists still prescribe hormonal therapies to prevent homosexuality; psychologists still try to prove that average differences in black-white IQ scores are genetic. It is not so long since sociobiologists suggested that women were unlikely ever to achieve equality with men in the spheres of business and science.[34]

Biology is a common and convenient explanation for intractable social problems. In 1979, amid growing fears of international terrorism, *Science* magazine reported research claiming that "most terrorists probably suffer from faulty vestibular functions in the middle ear." In 1989, with violence growing in the schools, the physician Melvin Konner wrote in the *New York Times* that the tendency for people to do physical harm to others was "intrinsic, fundamental, natural."[35] Genetics has been blamed for nearly every conceivable vice and folly of human life; in 1991, scientists from Penn State and the University of Colorado's Institute for Behavioral Genetics announced that television viewing habits (including amount watched and even preferences for particular kinds of shows) were rooted in genes.[36] Scientific pronouncements on such issues are regularly picked up by the popular press: in 1978, at the height of the sociobiology controversy, *Playboy* magazine announced that scientists had found both rape and infidelity throughout the animal kingdom. The title of the article said it all: "Do Men *Need* to Cheat on Their Wives? A New Science Says YES: Darwin and the Double Standard."[37]

Critics worry that science in such cases is being used as a proxy for deeply held social values—that women cannot compete, that blacks are inferior, that war or crime or homosexuality or poverty is a disease that must be combated by medical means. Critics point out that there is little evidence that terrorism, or sexual preference, or personality traits such as "shyness" or "bullying" are genetically anchored, and that it is easy to mistake the intransigence of human cultural qualities (aggression or rape, for example) for biological anchoring.[38]

Of there is a disconcerting continuity between genomics and eugenics, it is the fact that both have taken root in a climate where many people believe that the large part of human talents and disabilities are heritable through the genes. The study of human biological differences is not an inherently malevolent endeavor,[39] but in late twentieth-century America, as in midcentury Germany, it is dangerous to assume that biology is destiny. Genetic disease is a reality, but the frequency of such disease should not be exaggerated. From the point of view of lives saved per dollar, monies would probably be better spent preventing exposures to mutagens, rather than producing ever more precise analyses of their origins and effects. Sequencing the human genome may be a technological marvel, but it will not give us the key to life. Pronouncements that "our fate is in our genes" may be good advertising for congressional support, but they may well exaggerate the benefit that will flow from knowledge of our nucleotides. The genome is not "the very essence" of what it means to be human, any more than sheet music is the essence of a concert performance.

But criticism must be concrete, not abstract. Critics sometimes warn about the "slippery slope" of technological development—that if you allow $x$, then what is to prevent you from doing $y$? The whole purpose of law, as ethics, is to draw lines through the continuum of social space—lines that limit what can or should be done, independent of nature's continuum. Criticism of technologies must be rooted in understanding how specific harms and benefits are distributed over particular social groups; it is as easy (and as mindless) to slide down the slippery slope of criticism, condemning any and all manipulations as "playing God," as it is to plunge headstrong across new technological frontiers.

Optimists might like to imagine that old-style abuses are a thing of the past, but a bit of perspective reveals otherwise. Singapore has launched a eugenics program that rivals those of the 1930s; China in 1989 began a systematic effort to sterilize its mentally retarded.[40] In the United States many safety nets are in place, but new forms of technological acrobatics create ever-new pits into which people are likely to fall. We should keep in mind that the potential for abuse of any technology is largely dependent on the social context within which that technology is used. This is the kernel of truth behind the claims that the Human Genome Project is not likely to raise any new ethical questions. The questions most commonly raised concerning discrimination, unequal access to resources, knowledge in the face of impotence, and rationalizations of social inequality are all old ones in medical ethics. Abuses stem from powers unequally distributed. The danger, to my mind, is therefore not that people will try to improve the genetic health of their offspring, or even that the health of groups as well as individuals will be the target of health planners. The danger is that in a society where power is still unequally distributed between haves and have-nots, the application of the new genetic technologies—as of any other—is as likely to reinforce as to ameliorate patterns of indignity and injustice.

## NOTES

1. James Watson, quoted in L. Jaroff, "The Gene Hunt," *Time*, March 20, 1989, pp. 62–67.
2. R. Weiss, "Genetic Propensity to Common Cancers Found," *Science News* 138 (1990), p. 342.
3. K. W. Kinzler et al. (including Bert Vogelstein), "Identification of a Gene Located at Chromosome 5q21 That Is Mutated in Colorectal Cancers," *Science* 251 (1991), pp. 1366–70; B. Vogelstein et al., "Genetic Alterations during Colorectal-Tumor Development," *New England Journal of Medicine* 319 (1988), pp. 525–32; L. A. Cannon-Albright et al., "Common Inheritance of Susceptibility to Colonic Adenomatous Polyps and Associated Colorectal Cancers," in ibid.

4. W. R. Williams and D. E. Anderson, "Genetic Epidemiology of Breast Cancer," *Genetic Epidemiology* 1 (1984), pp. 1–7; K. Wright, "Breast Cancer: Two Steps Closer to Understanding," *Science* 250 (1990), p. 1659.

5. E. B. Claus, N. Risch, and W. D. Thompson, "Genetic Analysis of Breast Cancer in the Cancer and Steroid Study," *American Journal of Human Genetics* 48 (1991), pp. 232–42. The authors estimate that 36 percent of all women with breast cancer aged twenty to twenty-nine are carriers of a gene predisposing them to the disease. Older women with the disease carry the gene with much lower frequency. Carriers' cumulative lifetime risk of developing the disease is estimated at 92 percent; noncarriers are estimated at 10 percent risk (the same as for the population as a whole).

6. N. Angier, "Cigarettes Trigger Lung Cancer Gene, Researchers Find," *New York Times*, August 21, 1990. Angier reports that only about 7 percent of those who smoke heavily develop lung cancer, but C. M. Pike and Richard Peto estimate that among men who smoke 25 or more cigarettes a day, 30 percent will develop lung cancer by age 75 in the absence of other causes of death; *Lancet*, 1965, pp. 665–68.

7. J. Marx, "A New Tumor Suppressor Gene?" *Science* 252 (1991), p. 1067.

8. N. Angier, "Crucial Gene Is Discovered in Detecting Colon Cancer," *New York Times*, March 15, 1991.

9. Mark Skolnick, quoted in J. E. Bishop and M. Waldoz, *Genome: The Story of the Most Astonishing Scientific Adventure of Our Time* (New York: Simon & Schuster, 1990), pp. 156, 163. Similar generalizations accompanied the November 30, 1990, publication in *Science* of evidence for predisposing genes for a rare form of breast cancer. Commenting on his discovery, David Malkin of Boston's Massachusetts General Hospital Cancer Center asserted, "We'll be able to say, 'Yes, you carry this mutation . . . and you are at risk' or 'No, you don't.' " See Weiss, "Genetic Propensity to Common Cancers Found."

10. Claus, Risch, and Thompson's "Genetic Analysis of Breast Cancer" is a recent example; compare also T. A. Sellers et al., "Evidence for Mendelian Inheritance in the Pathogenesis of Lung Cancer," *Journal of the National Cancer Institute* 82 (1990), pp. 1272–79.

11. E. Marshall, "Experts Clash over Cancer Data," *Science* 250 (1990), p. 902.

12. American Cancer Society, *Cancer Facts and Figures—1991* (Atlanta, 1991).

13. Claus, Risch, and Thompson, "Genetic Analysis of Breast Cancer," p. 241. In one sense, of course, breast cancer is overwhelmingly a genetic disease. More than 95 percent of all breast cancers occur in individuals with the XX rather than the XY karyotype—the disease strikes women far more often than men. Skin cancer is also genetic, insofar as populations with darker skin tend to suffer less from the disease. In both cases, however, genetic factors are incidental to the ultimate cause of the disease: males rarely get breast cancer because they don't have breasts; blacks suffer less from skin cancer because they are better protected from ultraviolet radiation. Predisposing genes for breast or skin cancer may well exist, but these are unlikely to have anything to do with either sex chromosomes or the genes controlling skin coloration.

14. "Poverty Blamed for Blacks' High Cancer Rate," *New York Times*, April 17, 1991. Adjusted for socioeconomic status, whites showed slightly higher rates than blacks for breast, rectal, and lung cancer; blacks showed greater risk for stomach, cervical, and prostate cancers.

15. Nancy Wexler, quoted in R. M. Henig, "High-Tech Fortune Telling," *New York Times Magazine*, December 24, 1989, p. 20.

16. R. Doll and R. Peto, *The Causes of Cancer* (Oxford: Oxford University Press, 1981). The authors estimate that in the United States smoking accounts for about one-third of *all* cancer deaths.

17. See E. S. Lander, "The New Human Genetics: Mapping Inherited Diseases," *Princeton Alumni Weekly,* March 25, 1987, pp. 10–16. Compare Natalie Angier's claim that "the study of oncogenes may not be the best hope of banishing cancer; it may be the only hope." More to the point may be the quip of Richard Rifkind, which Angier herself cites: "You want a cure for cancer? Tell the bastards to quit smoking." See her *Natural Obsessions* (New York: 1988), Warner Books, pp. 17, 141.

18. E. Fearon et al., "Clonal Analysis of Human Colorectal Tumors," *Science* 238 (1987), pp. 193–97; R. A. Weinberg, "Oncogenes and Tumor Suppressor Genes," in *Unnatural Causes: The Three Leading Killer Diseases in America*, ed. R. C. Maulitz (New Brunswick, NJ: Rutgers University Press, 1989).

19. R. A. Weinberg, "Finding the Oncogene," *Scientific American* 258 (1988), pp. 44–51.

20. A. Motulsky, *American Journal of Human Genetics* 48 (1991), p. 174.

21. "The Telltale Gene," *Consumer Reports,* July 1990, p. 485.

22. T. H. Murray, "Warning: Screening Workers for Genetic Risk," *Hastings Center Report*, February 1983, pp. 5–8.

23. *Report of the Council for Tobacco Research–U.S.A., Inc.* (New York, 1988).

24. M. Lappé, *Genetic Politics: The Limits of Biological Control* (New York: Simon & Schuster, 1979), p. 120.

25. N. Angier, "Cigarettes Trigger Lung Cancer Gene, Researchers Find, *New York Times*, August 21, 1990.

26. In the early 1970s, for example, a number of researchers postulated that individuals might differ genetically in their ability to metabolize certain lung carcinogens. Subsequent studies, however, showed that such differences were not heritable. For a review and criticism, see B. Paigen et al., "Questionable Relation of Aryl Hydrocarbon Hydroxylase to Lung-Cancer Risk," *New England Journal of Medicine* 297 (1977), pp. 346–50.

27. Neil Holtzman, quoted in R. Green, "Tinkering with the Secrets of Life," *Health* (January 1990), p. 84. See also N. Holtzman's extended discussion of these issues in *Proceed With Caution: Predicting Genetic Risks in the Recombinant DNA Era* (Baltimore: Johns Hopkins University Press, 1990).

28. L. Jaroff, "The Gene Hunt," *Time*, March 20, 1989, p. 62.

29. K. Nolan and S. Swenson, "New Tools, New Dilemmas: Genetic Frontiers," *Hastings Center Report*, October–November 1988, p. 42; D. E. Koshland, "Sequences and Consequences of the Human Genome," *Science* 246 (1989), p. 189; G. Bugliarello, "The Genetic and Psychological Basis of Warfare as a Challenge to Scientific Research," in C. Mitcham and P. Siekevitz, eds.

*Ethical Issues Associated with Scientific and Technological Research for the Military* (New York: New York Academy of Sciences, 1989). Compare also Marc Lappé's curious speculation that genomics may allow the establishment of files of persons "genetically at risk for acquiring AIDS following infection with the human immunodeficiency virus"; "The Limits of Genetic Inquiry," *Hastings Center Report,* August 1987, p. 6.

30. A recent article in *Circulation,* the official journal of the American Heart Association, estimates that more than 50,000 Americans may be killed each year by so-called "secondhand" or "environmental" smoke; S. A. Glantz and W. W. Parmley, "Passive Smoking and Heart Disease," *Circulation* 83 (1991), pp. 1–13.

31. The Working Group's report has been published as an appendix in the HHS and DOE's *Understanding Our Genetic Inheritance* (Washington, DC, 1990), pp. 65–73.

32. Benjamin Barnhart was reluctant to fund ethics as part of the DOE's Human Genome Project, despite the fact that Charles DeLisi had originally expressed an interest in this area. At a December 1989 meeting of the Joint DOE-NIH advisory committee for the project, James Watson cautioned Barnhart that if the DOE did not fund ethical analysis, "Congress will chop off your head" (quoted in R. Cook-Deegan, *Gene Wars: Science, Politics and the Human Genome Project* (New York: W. W. Norton, 1993).

33. R. C. Lewontin, S. Rose, and L. J. Kamin, *Not in Our Genes: Biology, Ideology, and Human Nature* (New York: Pantheon, 1983).

34. G. Dörner et al., "A Neuroendocrine Predisposition for Homosexuality in Men," *Archives of Sexual Behavior* 4 (1975), pp. 1–8; T. Bouchard et al., "Sources of Human Psychological Differences: The Minnesota Study of Twins Reared Apart," *Science* 250 (1990), pp. 223–28; E. O. Wilson, "Human Decency Is Animal," *New York Times Magazine,* October 12, 1975, p. 50. For a recent and unabashed effort to prove that the average economic underperformance of blacks (compared to whites) is traceable to differences in black-white genetic endowments, see the essays in the December 1986 *Journal of Vocational Behavior.*

35. C. Holden, "Study of Terrorism Emerging as an International Endeavor," *Science* 203 (1979), pp. 33–35; "Math Genius May Have Hormonal Basis," *Science* 222 (1983), p. 1312; M. Konner, "The Aggressors," *New York Times Magazine,* August 14, 1988, pp. 33–34.

36. M. Gooderham, "TV Viewing Habits Seen as Hereditary: 'Couch Potatoes' Born, Study Suggests," *Toronto Globe and Mail,* June 17, 1991.

37. S. Morris, "Do Men *Need* to Cheat on Their Wives? A New Science Says YES: Darwin and the Double Standard," *Playboy,* May 1978, pp. 109 ff.

38. Lewontin, Rose, and Kamin, *Not in Our Genes;* A. Fausto-Sterling, *Myths of Gender: Biological Theories about Women and Men* (New York: Basic Books, 1985).

39. The presumption of human biological equality can be as misleading as the presumption of inequality. Take, for example, the case of cystic fibrosis (CF). Discovery of "the" CF gene was announced amid great fanfare in

1989, but it soon became apparent that while a majority of cases in the U.S. population could be traced to a simple three-base-pair deletion, the disease could also be caused by some sixty other mutations. Early hopes for a simple, comprehensive test were further set back by the discovery that human populations differ substantially according to how common the three-base-pair deletion is relative to other mutations causing the disease. Among Eastern European Jews, for example, the simple three-base-pair deletion appears to account for only about 3 percent of all CF cases. In Denmark, by contrast, the simple deletion accounts for about 88 percent of all CF cases. The usefulness of the test is therefore likely to vary greatly according to the genetic background of the population in question.

40. N. D. Kristof, "Chinese Region Uses New Law to Sterilize Mentally Retarded," *New York Times,* November 21, 1989; idem, "Parts of China Forcibly Sterilizing the Retarded Who Wish to Marry," *New York Times,* August 8, 1991. For the case of India see Kaval Gulhati, "Compulsory Sterilization: The Change in India's Population Policy," *Science* 195 (1977), pp. 1300–5; for Latin America see Bonnie Mass, *Population Target, The Political Economy of Population Control in Latin America* (Toronto: Latin American Working Group, 1976); and for Singapore see C. K. Chan, "Eugenics on the Rise—Singapore," in *Ethics, Reproduction, and Genetic Control,* ed. R. Chadwick (New York: Routledge, 1987). The best recent U.S. review is Philip R. Reilly, *The Surgical Solution: A History of Involuntary Sterilization in the United States* (Baltimore: Johns Hopkins University Press, 1991).

In Britain, arguments have recently been put forward that DNA diagnostic laboratories should be judged in terms of how effectively they reduce the financial burden of caring for the handicapped. See, for example, J. C. Chapple, et al., "The New Genetics: Will It Pay Its Way?" *Lancet* 1 (1987), pp. 1189–92; Angus Clarke of the University of Wales's Institute of Medical Genetics has pointed to a danger in the more general use of audits to evaluate diagnostic departments, especially insofar as "efficiency" is measured in terms of aborted fetuses per unit of diagnosed defects. The danger, as he sees it, is that cost-benefit analyses of this sort will reintroduce eugenic criteria under the guise of "social responsibility in reproduction": "It is not at all far-fetched to imagine finance for the care of the handicapped being reduced on the grounds that there will be fewer handicapped children if the genetics services operated more 'efficiently.' To encourage such services to meet targets in terms of terminations, our funding might depend upon 'units of handicap prevented,' which would pressurise parents into screening programmes and then into unwanted terminations with the active collusion of clinical geneticists anxious about their budgets . . . There certainly is a role for public health genetics, but not for a system of eugenics by default, through the impersonal, amoral operation of a penny-pinching bureaucracy." See his "Genetics, Ethics, and Audit," *Lancet* 335 (1990), pp. 1145–47; and his remarks on "eugenics by accountancy" in *Lancet* 336 (1990), p. 120.

## PART ELEVEN

# Justice, Medical Finance, and Medical Care

# Saint Martin of Tours in a New World of Medical Ethics

## Richard D. Lamm

*For the last two decades, three-term governor of Colorado Richard D. Lamm has advo-
cated reform of the way America finances medicine. As an aspirant to be the Reform
Party's 1996 presidential candidate, he announced: "My platform would be to raise
your taxes and cut your services."*

*Such honesty has not won him election to national office, but has won him admir-
ers. Lamm urges that less money be spent on the last years of life and that adult children of those in nursing homes be made to pay more. Dubbed "Governor Gloom" for
such views, Lamm is widely known for his remark—taken out of context—that elderly
people have "a duty to die and get out of the way."*

*Writings on medical finance are usually boring, but not the following selection.
In it, Lamm argues that the Medicare system will collapse when the baby boomers re-
tire unless the system is soon reformed, and that the longer the solution is delayed, the
more painful the remedy will be. He maintains that it is profligate for half-empty hospitals to spend millions competing for decreasing numbers of well-insured customers,
while millions of under- or uninsured Americans lack basic services. Physicians, says
Lamm, must change their medical ethics to prevent a tragedy of the commons. If every
physician's ethics is to pursue the maximal good of each patient, there is an "unethical" result for the system. Consequently, changes in medical ethics may have to accompany financial reform.*

*Richard D. Lamm is professor and director, Center for Public Policy and Contem-
porary Issues, University of Denver.*

Source: *Cambridge Quarterly of Healthcare Ethics* 3 (1994), pp. 159–67. Reprinted by permission of the
author and Cambridge University Press.

In the Christian tradition, there is the story about Saint Martin of Tours who in the Middle Ages was riding his horse, alone and cold, through the deepening night toward the walled city that was his destination. Right outside the gate to the city, Saint Martin of Tours met a cold and starving beggar. In an act of charity that lives in Christian tradition, Saint Martin of Tours divided his cloak in half and gave that with half of his dinner to the cold and starving beggar. It was clearly the ethical and moral course to take. It has served as an example of Christian charity for centuries.

Yet Brecht, in his play *Mother Courage,* raises the issue of what if, instead of one cold and starving beggar, there were 40. Or, if you like, 100. What then is the duty of an ethical and moral person? It obviously does not make any sense to divide one's cloak into 40 or 100 painfully inadequate pieces. There is no reason to choose one among the many cold and starving beggars, and it is hard to solve this dilemma other than perhaps to say a prayer for them all as you ride past them into the city.

My passionate belief is that this parable applies to the dilemma we are faced with in healthcare. There is a new set of realities with which we are confronted, and we must develop a new set of values and a new way of looking at healthcare if we are to resolve the implications of this brave new world of healthcare. A whole new world has formed while we were busy inventing, developing, discovering, and innovating; a new world where our current and past values so agonizingly developed are no longer sustainable.

Ultimately our healthcare ethics are tethered to the economic life support system of our economy. We cannot deliver medically what we do not earn economically. The arm bone of healthcare is connected to the backbone of the economy.

The medical values developed by the world's largest creditor nation, with an economy that doubled every 30 years, with 9 percent of its citizens over 65, and modest biotechnology, cannot now be sustained by the world's largest debtor nation, that has already borrowed $4.3 trillion from its children and grandchildren, where the average worker has had no real growth in wages in 20 years, that has 12 percent of its population over the age of 65, and that has incredibly expansive biotechnology. No nation can long import more than it exports, borrow more than it earns, and spend medically what it does not produce economically.

Proust once observed that the real voyage of discovery lay not in discovering new worlds, but in seeing with new eyes. I see a healthcare world where nothing we have done for the past 40 years has even dented the volcanic upward thrust of healthcare costs—a world of medical innovation that has become a fiscal black hole that threatens to bankrupt our children—a world where our medical miracles are fiscal failures.

Medical technology does *not* save us money, as a genre. "Cured" is a marvelous word, but it also means "alive to die later of something else." We have reduced mortality but dramatically increased morbidity. Where we used to die inexpensively of the first or second disease, we now die expensively of the fifth or sixth disease, having consumed far more re-sources. A new world has formed.

## VALUE CHANGE NO. 1: STOP THE EGOISM ABOUT THE UNITED STATES HAVING "THE FINEST HEALTHCARE SYSTEM IN THE WORLD"

It is often said, almost as a mantra, that the United States has the best health-care system in the world. Whenever I hear this, I am reminded of the historian who said that the fourteenth century was a wonderful century, except for the Hundred Years' War.

America has much to be proud of in its healthcare system; but like the rooster that knew the sun came up just to hear him crow, it overstates its case. Clearly, the United States has the most sophisticated and the best medical tech-nology. I believe we have the best doctors. Yet, other industrialized countries have healthier people and lower healthcare costs. These countries deliver more healthcare services to more people more often with less administrative hassle and for substantially less money. Their doctors have more clinical freedom, and polls show both doctors and citizens in those countries are more satisfied.

As one of the most respected healthcare experts has found, "In compari-son with other major industrial countries, health care in the United States costs more per person and per unit of service, is less accessible to a large portion of its citizens, is provided at a more intensive level, and offers comparatively poor gross outcomes."[1]

The test of a system is not the quality of its individual parts but the effec-tiveness and efficiency of the total system. Like the man who knew seven lan-guages but had nothing to say in any of them, technical proficiency is not enough. You cannot have a good healthcare system without dedicated and brilliant doctors. Yet, dedicated and brilliant doctors are not enough to make a good healthcare system. A system can be flawed even if it is made up of indi-vidually spectacular parts. Clearly, the United States has a system that con-tains many spectacular parts. Yet, as society has come to recognize, the system contains two major flaws: (1) 35–37 million Americans are uninsured, and an equal number are underinsured; and (2) high cost.

The lack of access in America is well known but still worth repeating. We should take care we do not become hardened to these numbers. George Bernard Shaw once said, "The mark of a truly educated man [person] is to be moved deeply by statistics." In 1992, Louis Harris and Associates conducted a survey and found:

1. Approximately 23 million Americans needed medical care but did not get it in the last 12 months. Approximately 18 million could not get medical care for financial reasons.
2. Last year, for financial reasons 54 million people postponed care they thought they needed.

3. About 7 million Americans were denied health insurance because of a prior medical condition.

4. Nearly 22 million Americans said they themselves, someone in their family, or both had been refused healthcare during the last year because they did not have insurance or could not pay.[2]

These figures are a national disgrace. They show that for all our technical proficiency, our system contains major flaws. The largest flaw is lack of access, and the access problem is the ugly stepchild of the problems of out-of-control costs. We must start to understand that these two flaws are not blemishes of an otherwise ethical delivery system—but fatal flaws that go to the heart of the system.

## VALUE CHANGE NO. 2: HEALTHCARE MUST BE SEEN AS A SOCIAL GOOD

The first value issue involving access is to ascertain whether healthcare is a social good or a private commodity. It is important to first decide the context in which other decisions are made. Is healthcare a private commodity like a car or clothing or is it a social good like education or a police department? I believe this is actually a question of community values.

The hipbone of success is attached to the backbone of the values of our society. However imperfect, we have a democracy that eventually responds to public will. The problem is that we are schizophrenic about healthcare—we want everybody to have everything, but we do not want any more taxes or shifted costs. If we are to solve this problem of access, we shall have to form a new public consensus confirming that access is important. As Lawrence J. O'Connell, president and CEO of an ethics think tank, said, "All the talk from the campaign trail and the Oval Office is superficial. That is because it sidesteps the fact that before health care reform can succeed, we need to reexamine the fundamental societal values that gave birth to the health care system we have today."[3]

Our values must recognize that today uninsured Americans clearly have access to poorer medicine and poorer health. Blendon found that

> Despite considerable amounts of uncompensated care provided by hospitals and physicians, Americans without health insurance face major barriers to the receipt of needed health services. Although they suffer from higher rates of ill health than the insurance population, the uninsured report fewer hospitalizations and fewer visits to a physician, shorter hospital stays, and fewer discretionary in-patient hospital treatments and tests, at higher costs. The uninsured also experience higher mortality rates when hospitalized than persons with health insurance coverage who have similar diagnoses.[4]

The human toll was—and is—incredible though often unobserved. As John Kitzhaber said, "Legislatures never had to confront the victims of silent rationing or be accountable for the very human consequences. It was like high-level bombing where the crew never sees the faces of the people they are killing."[5]

In light of the foregoing, modern health reforms state that healthcare is not a private good for a social good—and should be available to all. As Charles Dougherty argued for universal access,

> The argument is simple but powerful. Respect for the incalculably great value of each person creates a duty not only to refrain from destroying health . . . but also a duty to take reasonable steps to preserve and restore health by ensuring access to basic health care. Failing to act on this duty, by allowing lives to be shortened or diminished in quality because of lack of access to basic health care, expresses callow disregard for the dignity of human life.[6]

## VALUE CHANGE NO. 3: ACCESS MUST GO FROM A SECONDARY VALUE TO A PRIMARY VALUE

Reinhard Priester, in a very thoughtful article, stated, "Since WWII, U.S. health policy has consistently subordinated access to other values, most notably to professional autonomy, patient autonomy, and consumer sovereignty." This stance is consistent, said Priester, with other American values, for in our past and present, "individualism and personal autonomy have superseded community values in American society."[7]

At least six values, focused on the individual, have had a major role in shaping our current healthcare system. These values have guided decisions of both individuals and policymakers in structuring our healthcare system.

1. Professional independence: The ability of health professionals, especially physicians, to regulate their own work and to determine what is medically appropriate.
2. Consumer freedom: The ability of individuals to choose their own insurance company, health organizations, and physicians.
3. Patient autonomy: The right of individuals to be informed about their medical and surgical options and to accept or refuse the advice given.
4. Patient advocacy: The duty of health professionals to act in the best interest of their patients, not the interest of the hospital, the insurance company, or the community.
5. High quality: The expectation that the services of health professionals meet the highest standards of competence and compassion.
6. Availability: The access to all (including the latest) that medicine and surgical technology has to offer.[8]

Priester suggested, given the new world of limited resources and unlimited demands, that we must add four new values, which put a priority on community good.

7. Resource scarcity: There is a limit to what can be spent on health and medical care if we wish not to undermine other important social needs.
8. Universal access: Society has a responsibility to provide access to all citizens regardless of income, job status, state of illness, and so forth.

9. Personal responsibility: Individual citizens have a responsibility to the community for staying well and keeping costs down.

10. Efficiency: The money spent on healthcare should help people stay well or get well. It should not be spent on needless administration or treatments that are not effective.[9]

Reforming the healthcare system will require that we consider these and other values that have given birth to the American healthcare system.

## VALUE CHANGE NO. 4: WE MUST START TO VALUE NOT ONLY THE INDIVIDUAL BUT THE WHOLE SOCIETY

The bottom line of modern healthcare is that there is no bottom line. "Modern men and women of medicine now have the capability to spend unlimited resources in heroic, and sometimes vain attempts to extend life . . . Theoretically, one could now spend all of his or her available time and money in the pursuit of health."[10]

Because healthcare is a public policy bottomless pit, we cannot build the new system looking only at the needs of the individual. We must never forget or abandon the individual, but we must look also at the needs of the entire population. There is an evolving new equation in this shift, and the shift will come only after considerable ethical debate: "Using resources for one patient necessarily means that fewer resources will be available to treat others."[11]

But the shift is coming. The Section on Health Care Systems of the American Hospital Association issued a report that found:

Health care in the U.S. should be redesigned around the needs of the population, not the needs of providers. "Population" is a broader term than patient, which has been our concern. We should all commit to a health population as one fundamental objective, then organize ourselves to support that objective. The measure of our success should be health status, not full hospitals; manageable costs per capita, not profitability for thousands of separate provider units; value, not just cost control.[12]

As Victor Fuchs said, "The difference between what is beneficial for the individual and what is beneficial to the society as a whole is the key element in the current health care debate."[13]

## VALUE CHANGE NO. 5: IN THE NEW WORLD OF HEALTHCARE REFORM, COMMUNITY HOSPITALS WILL OWE A DUTY TO THE COMMUNITY

The same analysis applies to hospitals. In the United States, hospitals focus almost entirely on the patients within the hospital. There seems to be little awareness of—let alone, a sense of responsibility for—the community. A community hospital should have geographical accountability. It should be considered unethical and wrong for community hospitals to make large profits while other people in the community are going without needed medical services.

Related to the sin of gluttony is the sin of excess. What if Saint Martin of Tours had come by in a camper stuffed with donated food and found six starving beggars and did nothing. Just passed on by.

America has a new sin—the sin of excess in the face of need. Half-empty hospitals hire marketing people and run expensive advertising campaigns—to win market share from a neighboring half-empty hospital which has hired a public relations firm and does expensive promotional spots on television—blocks away from women without prenatal care and children without vaccines. Half of the hospitals in Colorado are empty, filled with marketing people and advertising geniuses who are desperately trying to beat neighboring half-empty hospitals.

In the new world of healthcare, spending money to advertise your hospital would be like taking your neighborhood crime-protection money away to advertise your police department. A hospital is a community asset—like a fire department. If there are too many, they should be closed, not advertised.

Colorado has 2.8 hospital beds per 1,000 people—53 percent are empty. We have 21 hospitals that do open-heart surgery, many of them doing less than 50 each year (one per week), when 250 is the minimum number Medicare says is needed for proficiency.

Southern California also has 2.8 hospital beds per 1,000 people. HMOs operate at 1.5 hospital beds per 1,000 enrollees. California has 118 open heart units and 400 MRI machines.

The most health-producing ethical decision many Colorado hospitals could make is to close their doors or merge.

## VALUE CHANGE NO. 6: YOU CANNOT SAY "YES" TO NEW NEEDS IN HEALTHCARE UNLESS YOU ALSO SAY "NO"

There is a yin and yang to the issue of access; the issue is part expansion (people into the system) and part contraction (what is covered). We must expand the who and limit the what; we must give with one hand and take away with the other.

Access to healthcare could be a fiscal black hole into which we could pour unlimited societal resources. If we are going to grant universal access, we must put limits on what is covered. Healthcare is infinitely expandable.

It is estimated that in any given month,

> approximately three-fourths of the population have an acute or chronic illness that leads to some action, such as the restriction of activity or the taking of medication. Of these persons who report an illness during the month, approximately one-third seek medical consultation. Although, in general, illnesses that occur more dramatically or that cause greater discomfort or restriction of activity are more likely to lead to medical care, there is substantial overlap between the illnesses of treated and untreated persons.[14]

Although all politicians and many healthcare experts avoid the subject, society increasingly is recognizing a new world of limits: "Plainly, a positive right of access must be a limited right. Society is obliged only to provide basic care, not everything that medicine can offer. Defining basic care sets the moral limits of what government must provide or subsidize."[15] David Hadorn observed, "As costs continue to escalate out of control, nothing is more certain that an increasing number of patients will be forced to go without potentially life-extending or quality of life–enhancing treatments."[16] Priester further added, "While everyone ought to have access to health care, this does not require universal access to all potentially beneficial care. No society can afford to provide every service of potential benefit to everyone in need."[17]

Thus, the easy part of the access question is arranging access. The hard part is defining "access to what" and figuring out how to pay for the new access. A world of universal access is a world of choices and trade-offs: "Using resources for one patient necessarily means that fewer resources will be available to treat others."[18]

We are thus left, in this new and strange world, with the task of deciding not what is "beneficial" to a patient (which is a medical decision), but what is "appropriate" or "cost effective" (which is partly a social, economic, and a fairness decision). We shall have to balance quality of life with quantity of life, costs and benefits, preventive medicine versus curative medicine. We are, unfortunately but realistically, into prioritizing medicine. Medicine will never be the same.

Once we admit that we cannot pay for everything, we must ask ourselves not only what does a patient need, but how do we spend our resources to buy the maximum health for the largest number of citizens? This will inevitably impinge on a physician's judgment on what is the best medical treatment for an individual patient; when and where to admit patients to hospitals and when to discharge; under what conditions and symptoms are certain diagnostic or therapeutic procedures appropriate; and what prescriptions are appropriate under certain circumstances. It is the world of DRG (Diagnostically-Related Groups) writ large.

If the key to expansion is a matter of values, the key to defining the "appropriate" or "basic" healthcare also is largely a matter of values. The access question shifts the question from *who* is covered to *what* is covered.[19] This is an ethical earthquake to existing medical values. Providers in America have been trained to monomaniacally focus only on the patient. In the new world of access, "Providers should not do everything that may benefit an individual patient, since doing so may interfere with the ability of other patients to obtain basic services; rather, providers should treat each patient with a full range of resources as is compatible with treating patients yet to come."[20]

The illusion of unlimited resources has been very counterproductive for America. Once we admit that resources are limited, a whole new dialogue emerges. When we recognize that we cannot do everything, we start to ask: What do we do to maximize the health of the community? Both individuals and the community are important, but the emphasis shifts from individual centered to community centered.

## SUMMARY

I end with another parable, but it is also a true story. Harvey Cushing, the famous surgeon after whom the Cushing Lectures are named, made an international reputation in his allegiance to quality. He badgered his profession to a higher standard of self-effacement and railed against the debasement of clinical skills and overemphasis on research and pursuit of personal gain. We honor him to this day because those were, and remain, important points. Yet, Harvey Cushing served as a surgeon during World War I and at Ypres. Although the Allied mortality was as much as 50,000 soldiers a day, not counting the wounded. Cushing refused to operate on any more than two patients each day, arguing that to do so would have lowered his standard of care for his patients—a standard that made sense in one time but that became strikingly insensitive, and I suggest even unethical, in another when confronted with a different reality. "The ethical claims for professional autonomy based on such standards of professional ethics has had the effect of supporting widespread distributional inequities. These inequities are clearly a form of rationing that have been condoned implicitly by the professional ethics in the name of professional autonomy."[21]

Many of the condemnations we hear today of prospective payment systems and how they will "ration" medicine contain a similar sense of unreality. The high standards are laudatory, but they should not be used as an excuse to not meet other pressing needs. High standards should never be used to make a problem worse. At some point, all ethical doctors have to lift their eyes from the patient in front of them and survey the needs of the whole battlefield.

America is right now at the beginning of a debate about the entire battlefield. Our system needs challenging. We have built up a healthcare system that better serves the needs of the providers than the public. We must substantially revamp our values and goals in healthcare.

We must move part of our existing emphasis:[22]

### Emerging Changes

| | | |
|---|---|---|
| Individual Patient | TO | Population as a Whole |
| Acute Care | TO | Chronic Care |
| Specialized Care | TO | Primary Care |
| Institution Based | TO | Ambulatory Based |
| Technologically Oriented | TO | Humanistically Oriented |
| Individual Provider | TO | Team Provider |
| Cost Unaware | TO | Cost Aware |
| Governed Professionally | TO | Governed Managerially |

We are spending millions of dollars on esoteric improvements at the margin in American medicine while spending pennies on the access problem where we could buy far more health. We give some people too much healthcare and others too little. We have money for Ecmo machines but not prenatal care. We spend incredible amounts of money on kidney dialysis, but practically nothing on educating people to stop smoking and abusing alcohol. We have far too many MRI machines, but 30 percent of the women in America give birth without adequate prenatal care in their first trimester.

Our duty lies both to the individual and population, to the patient and to all citizens. In a world of unconstrained demands and limited resources, we must adapt ourselves to the new world of medical ethics.

## NOTES

1. G. Schieberg et al., "Health Care Systems in Twenty-four Countries," *Health Affairs* (Fall 1991), p. 23.
2. *Louis Harris Surveys, 1992* (Menlo Park: Henry J. Kaiser Foundation), April 8, 1992.
3. L. J. O'Connell, "Values and Health Care Reform," *Chicago Tribune,* June 18, 1992, p. 23.
4. R. Blendon, "Making the Critical Choices," *JAMA* 267 (1992), p. 2509.
5. J. Kitzhaber, "Oregon Blazes a Trail," *Washington Post,* June 9, 1992, p. 12.
6. C. Dougherty, "Ethical Values at Stake in Health Care Reform," *JAMA* 268 (1992), p. 2409.
7. R. Priester, "A Values Framework for Health System Reform," *Health Affairs* 11 (Spring 1992), pp. 89, 90.
8. Ibid., p. 92.
9. Ibid.
10. L. A. Graig, *Health of Nations: An International Perspective on U.S. Health Care Reform* (Washington, DC: Wyatt, 1991), p. xv.
11. Priester, "A Values Framework," p. 91.
12. "Reviewing the U.S. Health Care Systems," report of Ad Hoc Meeting, Section on Health Care Systems, American Hospital Association, Washington, DC, January 25–27, 1990.
13. V. Fuchs, "Poverty and Health," paper presented at the Cornell University Medical College Health Policy Conference, February 27–28, 1992.
14. C. Lewis, R. Fein, and D. Mechanic, *A Right to Health* (New York: John Wiley, 1976), p. 15.
15. Dougherty, "Ethical Values at Stake," p. 2409.
16. D. Hadorn, "The Problem of Discrimination in Health Care Priority Setting," *JAMA* 268 (1992), p. 1454.
17. Priester, "A Values Framework," p. 92.
18. Ibid., p. 91.
19. Ibid., p. 96.
20. Ibid.
21. G. J. Agich, "Rationing and Professional Autonomy," *Law, Medicine, and Health Care* 18 (1990), p. 81.
22. D. A. Shugars, E. H. O'Neil, and J. D. Bader, eds., *Healthy America: Practitioners for 2005. An Agenda for Action for U.S. Health Professional Schools* (Durham, NC: Pew Health Professions Commission, 1991).

# For and against Equal Access to Health Care

## Amy Gutmann

*In the following selection, Amy Gutmann discusses what the principle of equal access to medical care means, distinguishing it from equality of results. She explains how a "one-class," or one-tier, system would place restraints on individual patients and physicians in the medical marketplace. She argues that equal access to health care is a condition of maximizing self-respect of citizens in a democracy.*

*Gutmann defends her proposal against claims that a free market would work better; that a single-class, single-payer system is paternalistic to citizens; and that voluntary risks to health do not deserve the same, equal level of medical care as involuntary disease and accident. Gutmann does admit that restrictions will exist on the freedom of patients ("consumers") and physicians in a system of equal access.*

*Amy Gutmann, PhD, is a professor of political philosophy and dean of the faculty at Princeton University.*

There is a fairly widespread consensus among empirical analysts that access to health care in this country has become more equal in the last quarter century. Agreement tends to end here; debate follows as to whether this trend will or should persist. But before debating these questions, we ought to have a clear idea of what equal access to health care means. Since equality of access to health care cannot be defined in a morally neutral way, we must choose a definition that is morally loaded with a set of values.[1] The definition offered here is by no means the only possible one. It has, however, the advantage not only of clarity but also of having embedded within it strong and commonly accepted liberal egalitarian values. The debate is better focused upon arguments for and against a strong *principle* of equal access than [upon] disputes over

*Source: Milbank Memorial Fund Quarterly/Health and Society* 59, no. 4 (1981). Copyright Milbank Memorial Fund.

definitions, which tend to hide fundamental value disagreements instead of making them explicit.

An equal access principle, clearly stated and understood, can serve at best as an ideal toward which a society committed to equality of opportunity and equal respect for persons can strive. It does not provide a blueprint for social change, but only a moral standard by which to judge marginal changes in our present institutions of health care.

My purpose here is not only to evaluate the strongest criticisms that are addressed to the principle, ranging from libertarian arguments for more market freedom to arguments supporting a more egalitarian principle of health care. I also propose to examine the sorts of theoretical and practical problems that arise when one tries to defend an egalitarian principle directed at a particular set of institutions within an otherwise inegalitarian society. Since it is extremely unlikely that such a society will be transformed all at once into an egalitarian one, there ought to be room within political and philosophical argument for reasoned consideration and advocacy of "partial" distributive justice, i.e., of principles that are directed only to a particular set of social institutions and whose implementation is not likely to create complete justice even within those institutions.

## THE PRINCIPLE DEFINED

A principle of equal access to health care demands that every person who shares the same type and degree of health need must be given an equally effective chance of receiving appropriate treatment of equal quality so long as that treatment is available to anyone. Stated in this way, the equal access principle does not establish whether a society must provide any particular medical treatment or health care benefit to its needy members. I shall suggest later that the level and type of provision can vary within certain reasonable boundaries according to the priorities determined by legitimate democratic procedures. The principle requires that if anyone within a society has an opportunity to receive a service or good that satisfies a health need, then everyone who shares the same type and degree of health need must be given an equally effective chance of receiving that service or good.

Since this is a principle of equal *access*, it does not guarantee equal *results*, although it probably would move our society in that direction. Discriminations in health care are permitted if they are based upon type or degree of health need, willingness of informed adults to be treated, and choices of lifestyle among the population. The equal access principle constrains the distribution of opportunities to receive health care to an egalitarian standard, but it does not determine the total level of health care available or the effects of that care (provided the care is of equal quality) upon the health of the population. Of course, even if equality in health care were defined according to an "equal health" principle,[2] one would still have to admit that a just health care system could not come close to producing an equally healthy population, given the unequal distribution of illness among people and our present medical knowledge.

## PRACTICAL IMPLICATIONS

Since the equal access principle requires equality of effective opportunity to receive care, not merely equality of formal legal access, it does not permit discriminations based upon those characteristics of people that we can reasonably assume they did not freely choose. Such characteristics include sex, race, genetic endowment, wealth, and, often, place of residence. Even in an ideal society, equally needy persons will not use the same amount or quality of health care. Their preferences and their knowledge will differ, as will the skills of the providers who treat them.

### A One-Class System

The most striking result of applying the equal access principle in the United States would be the creation of a one-class system of health care. Services and goods that meet health care needs would be equally available to everyone who was equally needy. As a disincentive to overuse, . . . small fees for service could be charged for health care, provided that charges did not prove a barrier to entry to the poorest people who were needy. A one-class system need not, of course, be a uniform system. Diversity among medical and health care services would be permissible, indeed even desirable, so long as the diversity did not create differential access along nonconsensual lines such as wealth, race, sex, or geographical location.[3]

Equal access also places limits upon the market freedoms of some individuals, especially, but not exclusively, the richest members of society. The principle does not permit the purchase of health care to which other similarly needy people do not have effective access. The extent to which freedom of the rich must be restricted will depend upon the level of public provision for health care and the degree of income inequality. As the level of health care guaranteed to the poor decreases and the degree of income inequality increases, the equal access standard demands greater restrictions upon the market freedom of the rich. Where income and wealth are very unevenly distributed, and where the level of publicly guaranteed access is very low, the rich can use the market to buy access to health care goods unavailable to the poor, thereby undermining the effective equality of opportunity required by an equal access principle.

The restriction upon market freedoms to purchase health care under these circumstances creates a certain discomforting irony: the equal access principle permits (or is at least agnostic with respect to) the free market satisfaction of preferences for nonessential consumer goods. Thus, the rigorous implementation of equal access to health care would prevent rich people from spending their extra income for preferred medical services, if those services were not equally accessible to the poor. It would not prevent their using those same resources to purchase satisfaction in other areas—a Porsche or any other luxurious consumer good. In discussing additional problems created by an attempt to implement a principle of equal access to health care in an otherwise inegalitarian society, I return later to consider whether advocates of equal access can avoid this irony.

## Hard Cases

As with all principles, hard cases exist for the equal access principle. Without dwelling upon these cases, it is worth considering how the principle might deal with two hard but fairly common cases: therapeutic experimentation in medicine, and alternative treatments of different quality.

Each year in the United States, many potentially successful therapies are tested. Since their value has not been proved, there may be good reason to limit their use to an appropriate sample of sick experimental subjects. The equal access principle would insist that experimenters choose these subjects at random from a population of relevantly sick consenting adults. A randomized clinical trial could be advertised by public notice, and individuals who are interested might be registered and enrolled on a lottery basis. The only requirement for enrollment would be the health conditions and personal characteristics necessary for proper scientific testing.

How does one apply the principle of equal access when alternative treatments are each functionally adequate but aesthetically or socially quite disparate? Take the hypothetical case of a societal commitment to adequate dentition among adults. Replacement of carious or mobile teeth with dentures may preserve dental function at relatively minor cost. On the other hand, full mouth reconstruction, involving periodontal and endodontal treatment and capping of affected teeth, may be only marginally more effective but substantially more satisfying. The added costs for the preferred treatment are not inconsiderable. The principle would seem to demand that at equal states of dental need there be equal access to the preferred treatment. It is unclear, however, whether the satisfaction of subjective desire is equivalent to fulfillment of objective need.

In cases of alternative treatments, proponents of equal access could turn to another argument for providing access to the same treatments for all. A society that publicly provides the minimal acceptable treatment freely to all, and also permits a private market in more expensive treatments, may result in a two-class system of care. The best providers will service the richest clientele, at the risk of inadequate treatment for the poorest. Approval of a private market in alternative treatments would rest upon the empirical hypothesis that, if the publicly funded level of adequate treatment were high enough, few people would choose to short-circuit the public (i.e., equal access) sector; the small additional free market sector would not threaten to lower the quality of services universally available.

Most cases, like the one of dentistry, are difficult to decide merely on principle. Proponents of equal access must take into account the consequences of alternative policies. But empirical knowledge alone will not decide these issues, and arguments for or against a particular policy can be entertained in a more systematic way once one exposes the values that underlie support for an equal access principle. One can then judge to what extent alternative policies satisfy these values.

## SUPPORTING VALUES

Advocates of equal access to health care must demonstrate why health care is different from other consumer goods, unless they are willing to support the more radical principle of equal distribution of all goods. Norman Daniels provides one foundation for distinguishing between health care and other goods.[4] He establishes a category of health care needs whose satisfaction provides an important condition for future opportunity. Like police protection and education, some kinds of health care goods are necessary for pursuing most other goods in life. Any theory of justice committed to equalizing opportunity ought to treat health care as a good deserving of special distributive treatment. Equal access to health care provides a necessary, although certainly not a sufficient, condition for equal opportunity in general.

A precept of egalitarian justice that physical pains of a sufficient degree be treated similarly, regardless of who experiences them, establishes another reason for singling out certain kinds of health care as special goods.[5] Some health conditions cause great pain but are not linked to a serious curtailment of opportunity. The two values are, however, mutually compatible.

A theory of justice that gives priority to the value of equal respect among people might also be used to support a principle of equal access to health care. John Rawls, for example, argues that without self-respect "nothing may seem worth doing, or if some things have value for us, we lack the will to strive for them . . . Therefore the parties in the original position would wish to avoid at almost any cost the social conditions that undermine self-respect."[6]

### Conditions of Self-Respect

It is not easy to determine what social conditions support or undermine self-respect. One might plausibly assume that equalizing opportunity and treating similar pains similarly would be the most essential supports for equal respect within a health care system. And so, in most cases, the value of equal respect provides additional support for equal access to the same health care goods that are warranted by the values of equal opportunity and relief from pain. But at least some kinds of health care treatment not essential to equalizing opportunity or bringing equal relief from pain may be necessary to equalize respect within a society. It is conceivable that much longer waiting time, in physicians' offices or for admission to hospitals, may not affect the long-term health prospects of the poor or of blacks. But such discriminations in waiting times for an essential good probably do adversely affect the self-respect of those who systematically stand at the end of the queue.

Some of the conditions necessary for equal respect are socially relative; we must arrive at a standard of equal respect appropriate to our particular society. Universal suffrage has long been a condition for equal respect; the case for it is independent of the anticipated results of equalizing political power by granting every person one vote. More recently, equal access to health care has similarly become a condition for equal respect in our society. Most of us do not base our self-respect on the way we are treated on airplanes, even though the flight attendants regularly give preferential treatment to those traveling first class. This contrast with suffrage and health care treatment (and education and police protection) no doubt is related to the fact that these goods are much more essential to our society and opportunities in life than is airplane travel. But it is still worth considering that unequal treatment in health care, as in education, may be understood as a sign of unequal respect even where there are no discernible adverse effects on the health or education of those receiving less favored treatment. Even where a dual health care system will not produce inferior medical results for the less privileged, the value of equal respect militates against the perpetuation of such a system in our society.

## CHALLENGES

Equality of opportunity, equal efforts to relieve pain, and equal respect are the three central values providing the foundation of support for a principle of equal access to health care. Any theory of justice that gives primacy to these values (as do many liberal and egalitarian theories) will lend prima facie support to a health care system structured along equal access lines.

We are now in a position to consider alternative values and empirical claims that would lead someone to challenge, or reject, a principle of equal access to health care. These challenges also enable us to elaborate further the moral and political implications of the principle.

### Proponents of the Market

The most radical and vocal opposition comes from those who support a pure free market principle in health care. A foundation of support for the free market principle is the idea that the relative importance of satisfying different human desires is a purely subjective matter: we can distinguish between one person's desire for good medical care and another person's desire for a good Beaujolais only by the price they are willing to pay for each. If no goods are special because there is no way of ranking desires except by individual processes of choice, then what better way than the unconstrained market to allow us to decide among the smorgasbord of goods society has to offer?[7]

Health care goods and services are likely to be more equally allocated through the market if income and wealth are more equally distributed. Several defenders of the market as a means of allocating goods and services also support a moderate degree of income redistribution on grounds of its diminishing marginal utility, or because they believe that every person has a right to a "basic minimum."[8] Neither rationale for redistribution takes us very far toward a principle of equal access to health care. If one retains the basic assumption that human preferences are totally subjective, then the market remains the best way to order human priorities. Only the market appropriately decentralizes decision-making and eliminates all nonconsensual exchange of goods and services.[9]

Although a minimum income floor under all individuals increases *access* to most goods and services, even at a higher level than that supported by Friedman and others, a guaranteed income will be inadequate to sustain the costs of a catastrophic illness. An exceptionally high guaranteed minimum might result in almost universal insurance coverage at a fairly high level. Supporters of free market allocation do not, however, press for a very high minimum for at least two reasons. They fear its effects on incentives, and they cannot justify a high guaranteed income without admitting that there are many expensive goods that are essential to all persons, and are not just mere consumer preferences.

The first reason for opposing an exceptionally high minimum is probably a good one. A principle approaching equality of income and wealth is likely to have serious disincentive effects on productive work and investment. There are also better reasons for treating health care as a special good, a good that society has an obligation to provide equally to all its members, than there are for equally distributing most consumer goods.

A significant step beyond the pure free market principle is a position that preserves the role of the market in allocating different "packages" of health care according to consumer preferences, but concedes a role for government in supplying every adult with a "voucher" of a certain monetary value redeemable exclusively for health care goods and services. Proponents of health vouchers must assume that there is something special about health care to justify government in taxing its citizens to provide universally for these goods, and not all others. But if health care is a more important good, because it preserves life and expands opportunity, then what is the rationale for effectively limiting the demand a sick but poor person can make upon the health care system? Why should access to health care be dependent upon income or wealth at all?

Opponents of equal access generally imply that more than minimal access will unjustly curtail the freedom of citizens as taxpayers, as consumers, and as providers of health care. Let us consider separately the arguments with regard to the many citizens who are taxpayers and consumers, and the few citizens who are providers of health care.

## The Charge of Paternalism

Charles Fried has argued that equal access to health care is a particularly intrusive form of paternalism toward citizens. He claims further that "apart from a rather general commitment to equality and, indeed, to state control of the allocation and distribution of resources, to insist on the right to health care, where that right means a right to equal access, is an anomaly. For as long as our society considers that inequalities of wealth and income are morally acceptable . . . it is anomalous to carve out a sector like health care and say that *there* equality must reign."[10]

Would an equal access system necessarily be intrusive or paternalistic in its operation? A national health care system simply cannot be said to take away the income entitlement of citizens, since citizens are not entitled to their gross incomes. We can determine our income entitlements only after we deduct from our gross income the amount we owe the state to support the rights of others. To the extent that the rationale of an equal access principle is redistributive, those individuals who otherwise could not afford certain health care services will experience an expansion of their freedom (if we assume an adequate level of social provision). Of course, part of the justification of a national health care system is that it would also guarantee health care coverage to people who could afford adequate health care but who would not be prudent enough to save or to invest in insurance. Even if we accept the common definition of paternalistic actions as those that restrict an individual's liberty so as to further his or her interest, we still have to assess the assertion that this (partial) rationale for an equal access system entails a restriction of individual liberty. Unlike a law banning the sale of cigarettes or forcing people to wear seat belts, the institution of a national health care system forces no one to use it. If a majority of citizens decide that they want to be taxed in order to ensure health care for themselves, the resulting legislation could not be considered paternalistic: "Legislation requiring contributions to some cooperative scheme (such as medical care) . . . is not necessarily paternalistic, so long as its purpose is to give effect to the desires of a democratic majority, rather than simply to coerce a minority who do not want the benefits of the legislation."[11] It is significant in this regard that for the past twenty years the Michigan survey of registered voters has found a consistent and solid majority supporting government measures designed to ensure universal access to medical care.

The charge of paternalism levied against an equal access system is therefore dubious because it is extremely difficult, if not impossible, to isolate the self-protectionist rationale from the redistributive and the democratic rationales. Those who object to a national health care system on the grounds that it is coercing some people for their own good forget that such a system still could be justified as a means to avoid the threat to a one-class system that exempting the rich would create. To condemn such a system as paternalistic would commit us to criticizing all legislation in which a democratic majority decides to protect itself against the wishes of a minority when exemption from the resulting policy would undermine it. Other critics wrongly assume that people have an entitlement to the cash equivalent of the medical care to which society grants them a right. People do not have such an entitlement because taxpayers have a right to demand that their tax dollars are spent to satisfy health needs, not to buy luxuries. Indeed, our duty to pay taxes is dependent upon the fact that certain needs of other people must be given priority over our own desires for more commodious living.

## Other Restrictions

Nonetheless, two restrictions upon consumer freedom are entailed in an equal access system. One is the restriction imposed by the taxation necessary to provide all citizens, but especially the poorest, with access to health care goods. This restriction does not raise unique or particularly troublesome moral problems so long as one believes that the freedom to retain one's gross income is not an absolute right and that the resulting redistribution of income to the health care sector increases the life chances and thereby the effective freedom of many citizens.

But there is a second restriction of consumer market freedom sanctioned by the equal access principle: the limitation upon freedom to buy health care goods above the level publicly provided. Aside from reasserting the primary values of equality, there is at least one plausible argument for such a restriction. Without restricting the free market in extra health care goods, a society risks having its best medical practitioners drained into the private market sector, thereby decreasing the quality of medical care received by the majority of citizens confined to the publicly funded sector. The lower the level of public provision of health care and the less elastic the supply of physicians, the more problematic (from the perspective of the values underlying equal access) will be an additional market sector in health care.

Without an additional market sector, would the freedom of physicians and other providers to practice wherever and for whomever they choose be unduly restricted? The extent of such restrictions will also vary with the level of public provision and with the diversity of the health care system. Public funds already are crucial to providing many physicians with basic income (through Medicare and Medicaid fees), research opportunities through the National Institutes of Health (NIH), and many with hospitals and other institutions in which to practice (through the provisions of the Hill-Burton Act). In place of the time and resources now directed to privately purchased add-ons, an equal access system would redirect providers toward meeting previously unserved needs. These types of redirections of supply and redistribution of demand are commonly accepted in other professions that are oriented toward satisfying an important public interest. The legal and teaching professions are analogous in this regard. The equal access principle, strictly interpreted, however, adds another restriction, a limitation upon private practice that supplies health care goods not equally accessible to the entire population of relevantly needy persons. This restriction upon the freedom of providers does not have an analogue in the present practice of law or of education, although the arguments for equal access to the goods of these professions might be similar. And so, one's assessment of the strength of the case for such a restriction is likely to have implications beyond the health care system.

It is hard to see why one ought to prevent people, rich or poor, from spending money upon health care goods while permitting them to spend money on consumer goods that are clearly not essential, and perhaps even detrimental to health. One reason might be the possible systemic effect, mentioned above, that such additional expenditures would deprive the less advantaged of the best physicians. The freedom of providers as well as consumers would have to be restricted in order to curtail this effect. But beyond this empirically contingent argument for restricting any market in health care goods that are not equally accessible to all, the strict limitations upon market freedom in "extra" health care goods are hard to accept if one believes that medical services are at least as worthy items of expense as other consumer goods. One could argue that physicians ought to be free to meet the demand for additional medical goods, especially when that demand is a substitute for demand for less important goods.

This criticism illuminates a more general problem of attempting to equalize access to any good in an otherwise inegalitarian society. The more unequal the distribution of income and wealth within our society, the more likely that the freedom of consumers and providers to buy and sell health care outside the publicly funded sector will result in inequalities that cannot properly be regarded merely as the product of differences in consumer preferences. Therefore, in an inegalitarian society, we must live with a moral tension between granting providers the freedom to leave the publicly funded sector and achieving more equality in the satisfaction of health care needs.

A principle of equal access to health care applied within an otherwise egalitarian society might give little or no reason to restrict the freedom of providers or consumers. One argument often voiced against a publicly funded system that permits a marginal free market sector is that the government is a less efficient provider of goods than are private parties. But the equal access principle does not require that the government directly provide medical services through, for example, a national health service. Government need only be a regulator of the use and distribution of essential health care goods and services. This is a role that most people concede to government for many other purposes deemed essential to the welfare of all individuals.

Government regulation may, of course, be more expensive and hence less efficient than government provision of health care services of similar extent and quality. The tradeoff here would be between the additional market choice facilitated by government regulation or private providers and the decreased public cost of government provision. Despite utilitarian claims to the contrary, no simple moral calculus exists that would enable an impartial spectator to determine where the balance of advantage lies. Philosophers ought to cede to a fairly constituted democratic majority the right to decide this issue. What constitutes a fair process of democratic decision-making is an important question of procedural justice that lies beyond the scope of this paper.

## Liability for Voluntary Risks?

Another important criticism of the equal access principle cuts across advocacy of the free market and government regulation of health care. Supporters of both views might consistently ask whether it is fair to provide the same level of access for all people, including those who voluntarily adopt bad health habits, and who quite knowingly and willingly take greater-than-average risks with their lives and health. Even if it might be unjust not to provide health care for those people once the need arises, why would it not be fair to force those who choose to drink, smoke, rock climb, and skydive also to bear a greater burden of their ensuing medical costs than that borne by people who deliberately avoid these risky pursuits? An equal access principle seems to neglect the distinction between voluntary and nonvoluntary health risks in its eagerness to ensure that all people have an equal opportunity to receive appropriate health care.

Gerald Dworkin extensively and convincingly argues that it would not be unfair to force individuals to be financially liable for voluntarily undertaken health risks, but only under certain conditional assumptions. These include our ability (1) to determine the relative causal role of voluntary versus involuntary factors in the genesis of illness; (2) to differentiate between purely voluntary behavior and what is nonvoluntary or compulsive; and (3) to distinguish between genetic and nongenetic predispositions to illness.[12] For example, to satisfy the first condition one would have to determine the relative causal role of smoking and environmental pollution in the genesis of lung cancer; to fulfill the second, one must know when smoking (or drinking or obesity) is voluntary and when it is compulsive behavior; and to satisfy the third condition, one must distinguish among those who smoke and get cancer, and those who smoke and do not. In addition, so long as there are no good institutional mechanisms for monitoring certain risky activities or for differentiating between moderate and immoderate users of unhealthy substances, qualifying the equal access principle to take account of voluntary health risks is likely to create more unfairness rather than less. Finally, given great inequalities in income distribution, the poor will be less able to bear the consequences of their risky behavior than will the rich, creating a situation of unfairness at least as serious as the unfairness of equally distributing the burdens of health care costs between those who voluntarily impose risks upon themselves and those who do not. With respect to the health hazards of overeating and obesity, for example, the rich have recourse to expensive programs of weight control unavailable to the poor. Since we have such scanty knowledge of situations when sickness can be attributable to voluntary health risks, criticisms of the equal access principle from this perspective have more weight in principle than they do in practice.

## Equal Access to All Health Goods

All criticisms considered so far are directed at the equal access principle from a perspective suggesting that government involvement and public funding of health care would be too great and the role of the market too small in an equal access system. Now let us consider a powerful criticism of the principle for including too little, rather than too much, in the public sector. The criticism can be posed in the form of a challenge: if one crucial reason for supporting a principle of equal access is that health goods are much more essential than many other goods because they provide a basis for equalizing opportunity and relieving substantial pain, then why not require a government to provide equal access to *all* those health goods that would move a society further in the direction of equalizing opportunity and relieving pain for the physically and mentally ill? Without pretending that our society could ever arrive at a condition of absolute equality in health (or therefore strict equality of opportunity), proponents of this principle could still argue that we should move as far as possible in that direction.

In a society in which no tradeoffs had to be made between health care and other goods, equal access to *all* health goods might be the most acceptable principle of equity in health care.[13] Of course, we do not live in such a society. Given the advanced state of our medical and health care technology, and the prevalence of chronic degenerative diseases and mental disorders in our population, a requirement that society provide access to every known health care good would place an enormous drain upon social resources.[14]

Costliness per se is not the main issue. The problem with the principle of equal access to all health goods is that it demands an absolute tradeoff between satisfaction of health care needs and other needs and desires. The simplest argument against this principle is that other needs, such as education, police protection, and legal aid, will be sacrificed to health care, if the principle is enforced. But this argument is too simple. A proponent of equal access to all health goods could consistently establish some priority principle among these goods, all of which satisfy needs derived in large part from a principle of equal opportunity. The weightier counterargument is that, above some less-than-maximum level in the provision of opportunity goods, it seems reasonable for people to value what, for want of a better term, one might call "quality of life" goods: cultural, recreational, noninstrumental educational goods, and even consumer amenities. A society that maximized the satisfaction of needs before it even began to provide access to "quality of life" goods would be a dismal society indeed. Most people do not want to devote their entire lives to being maximally secure and healthy. Why, then, should a society devote all of its resources to satisfying human *needs?*

## Democracy and Equal Access

We need to find some principle or procedure by which to draw a line at an appropriate level of access to health care short of what is socially and technologically possible, but greater than what an unconstrained market would afford to most people, particularly to the least advantaged. I suspect that no philosophical argument can provide us with a cogent principle by which we can draw a line within the enormous group of goods that can improve health or extend the life prospects of individuals.

This problem of determining a proper level of guaranteed social satisfaction of need is not unique to health care. Something similar can be said about police protection or education in our society. Philosophers can provide reasons why police protection and education are rightly considered basic collective needs and why they should be given priority over individual consumer preferences. But no plausible philosophical principle can tell us what level of police protection or how much education a society ought to provide on an egalitarian basis.

The principle of equal access to health care establishes a criterion of distribution for whatever level of health care a society provides for any of its members. And further philosophical argument might establish some criteria by which to judge when the publicly funded level of health care was so low as to be unfair to the least advantaged, or so high as to create undue restrictions upon the ability of most people to live interesting and fulfilling lives. The remaining question of establishing a precise level of priorities among health care and other goods (at the "margin") is appropriately left to democratic decision-making. The advantage of the democratic process in determining the precise level of health care provision is that citizens have an equal and collective voice in determining a decision that, according to the equal access principle, ought to be mutually binding. Citizens not only reap the benefits; they also share the burdens of the decision to expand or limit access to health care.

There is yet another advantage to this procedural method of establishing a fair level of health care provision. If the democratic decision will be binding upon all citizens, as the equal access principle assumes it must be, then one might expect the most advantaged citizens to exercise more political pressure to increase access to health care and hence increase the opportunity of the least advantaged above the level that they could afford in a free market system, or in a system where the rich were not included within the publicly funded health care sector. One finds some evidence to support this hypothesis in comparing the relative immunity from budget cutbacks of the program under universal entitlement of Medicare compared with the income-related Medicaid program. Of course, if costliness to the taxpayer is one's only concern, this added political pressure for health care expenditures is a liability rather than a strength of a one-class system. But from the perspective of equal access, the cost of a two-class system, one privately and one publicly funded, is an inequitable distribution of quantity and quality of care according to wealth, not need. The added nonproductive costs required merely to keep the two classes apart are seldom taken into account. And from the perspective of those supporters of an equal access principle who also want to increase the total level of health care provision, the two-class system threatens to work in the opposite direction, siphoning off the pressure of citizens who have a disproportionate share of political influence. A democratic decision, the results of which are constrained by the principle of equal access, will give a relatively accurate reading of what most people believe to be an adequate level of health care protection. The major disadvantage of the equal access constraint is that the decision of the majority or its representatives binds everyone, even those people who want more than the socially mandated level of health care.

Given the great economic inequalities of our society, it is politically impossible for advocates of equal access to fulfill their task. No democratic legislator could possibly succeed in winning support for a proposal that restricted market freedom as extensively as a strict interpretation of the equal access principle requires. And it probably would be a mistake to insist upon strict philosophical standards: one thereby risks throwing the possibility of greater access to health care for the poor out with the insistence upon curtailing access for the rich.

## CONCLUSION

I began by arguing that a principle of equal access to health care was at best an ideal toward which our society might strive. I shall end by qualifying that statement. A sufficiently high level of public provision of health care for all citizens and a sufficiently elastic supply of health care would significantly reduce the threat to universal provision of quality health care of a private market in extra health care goods, just as a very high level of police protection and education reduces the inequalities of opportunity resulting from purchase of private bodyguards or of private school education by the rich.

In the best of all imaginable worlds of egalitarian justice, the equal access principle would be sufficiently supported by other egalitarian social and economic institutions that a market in health care would complement rather than undercut the goals of equal respect and opportunity. But philosophers ought to resist basing their political recommendations solely upon a model of the best of all imaginable worlds.

## NOTES

1. N. Daniels, "Equity of Access to Health Care: Some Conceptual and Ethical Issues," paper delivered to the President's Commission for the Study of Ethical Issues in Medicine and Biomedical and Behavioral Research, Washington, DC, March 13, 1981.
2. R. Veatch, "What Is a Just Health Care Delivery," from *Ethics and Health Policy,* eds. R. Veatch and R. Bransen (Cambridge, MA: Ballinger Publishing Group, 1976).
3. P. Starr, "A National Health Program: Organizing Diversity." *Hasting Center Report* 5:11–13, 1975.
4. N. Daniels, "Health-Care Needs and Distributive Justice," *Philosophy and Public Affairs* 10 (1981), pp. 146–79.

5. A. Gutmann, *Liberal Equality* (New York: Cambridge University Press, 1980).
6. J. Rawls, *A Theory of Justice* (Cambridge, MA: Harvard University Press, 1971).
7. C. Fried, "Health Care, Cost Containment, Liberty," paper presented to the Institute of Society, Ethics, and the Life Sciences, Hastings-on-Hudson, NY, October 1979; R. Nozick, *Anarchy, State, and Utopia* (New York: Basic Books, 1974); R. N. Sade, "Medical Care as a Right: A Refutation," *New England Journal of Medicine* 285 (1971), pp. 1288–92.
8. M. Friedman, *Capitalism and Freedom* (Chicago: University of Chicago Press, 1962); C. Fried, *Right and Wrong* (Cambridge, MA: Harvard University Press, 1978).
9. Fried, *Right and Wrong*, pp. 124–26.
10. C. Fried, "Equality and Rights in Medical Care," *Hastings Center Report* 6 (1976), p. 31.
11. D. F. Thompson, "Paternalism in Medicine, Law, and Public Policy,"; D. Callahan and S. Boll (eds.), *Ethics Teaching in Higher Education* (New York; Plenum, 1980), pp. 245–75.
12. G. Dworkin, "Responsibility and Health Risks," paper presented to the Institute of Society, Ethics, and the Life Sciences, Hastings-on-Hudson, NY, October 1979.
13. R. Veatch, pp. 127–53.
14. A. R. Somers, Health Care in Transition: Directions for the Future (Chicago, IL: Hospital Research and Educational Trust, 1971).

## PART TWELVE

# AIDS

# How Society Should Respond to AIDS

## Richard Mohr

*Richard Mohr is the foremost American philosopher writing about the rights of gay males and lesbians. In this selection he discusses how serious the dangers or indirect harms of HIV infection might have to be before state coercion is justified.*

*Richard Mohr, PhD, writes monthly columns for* The Advocate. *His landmark pieces on gays and lesbians have been published in* The Right Thing to Do, *edited by James Rachels. He is the author of* Gays' Justice: A Study of Ethics, Society, and Law, Gay Ideas: Outing and Other Controversies, *and* A More Perfect Union: Why Straight America Must Stand Up for Gay Rights. *He is a professor of philosophy at the University of Illinois, Urbana. Professor Mohr also writes about Plato and ancient Greek philosophy.*

*Source: Bioethics* 1, no. 1 (1987). Copyright 1986, Richard Mohr. For Robert W. Switzer. This essay partially overlaps "AIDS, Gay Life, State Coercion," *Raritan: A Quarterly Review* 6, no. 1 (Summer 1986), pp. 38–62. It was widely circulated in draft form. The author thanks the following people for offering comments that prompted revisions or amplifications: the editors and referees of *Bioethics;* Jennifer Bremer (Robert Nathan Associates, D.C.); Sandra Panem (the Brookings Institution); Ronald Bayer (Hastings Center); Doug Mitchell (University of Chicago Press); Thomas Edwards (Rutgers University); James Rachels (University of Alabama); Michael Slote and Fred Suppe (University of Maryland); Joyce Trebilcot (Washington University); Christopher Morris (Bowling Green State University); Timothy Murphy (Boston University); Larry Thomas (Oberlin College); Mark Chekola (Moorhead State University); Larry Klein (San Francisco City College); Ferdinand Schoeman (University of South Carolina); Mary Mahowald (Case Western Reserve University); Donald Levy (Brooklyn College–CUNY); and David Luban, Bob Fullinwider, Claudia Mills, Judy Lichtenberg, Henry Shue, and Doug MacLean of the University of Maryland's Center for Philosophy and Public Policy, where the paper was written while the author was the Rockefeller Foundation Fellow in the Humanities for 1985–86; and my husband, the dedicatee.

## ALARUMS AND EXCURSIONS

Of those dead and dying from AIDS three-quarters are gay men. Government funding for AIDS research was at best sluggish till the disease appeared to the dominant non-gay culture as a threat. That perceived threat has spawned state-mandated discrimination against groups at risk for AIDS in employment and access to services, allegedly on medical grounds but in pointed contradiction to the judgments of the very medical institutions to which society has entrusted the determination of such grounds (the U.S. Department of Health and Human Services, the Centers for Disease Control, and the National Institutes of Health).[1]

Government's disregard for medical opinion and for the lives of gays strongly suggests that prejudicial forces are at work. There is of course nothing new in this, but the stakes here are high. The armed forces have already established quarantines of those at risk for AIDS on some bases.[2] With state-mandated discriminations installed and calls for civilian quarantines circulating, it is clear that the AIDS crisis is going to test the country's mettle. Not since the Supreme Court affirmed the internments of Japanese-Americans in World War II has so live a danger existed to America's traditional commitment to civil liberties. And again the danger is created by hysteria and not a reasoned necessity.

The hysteria, when not simply an expression of old anti-gay prejudices, is based on the presumption that the disease is spread indiscriminately. This presumption permitted Jeane Kirkpatrick to begin a syndicated column by using AIDS as a metaphor for international terrorism—"it can affect anyone"—in the serene belief that her audience, educated America, already thought this about AIDS and might even be ready for extreme measures.[3]

## ALLEGED HARMS TO OTHERS

For public policy purposes, the most important fact about AIDS is not that it is deadly but that it, like hepatitis B, is caused by a blood-transmitted virus. For the disease to spread, bodily fluids of someone with the virus must *directly enter the bloodstream of another:* "It appears that, in order to infect, this virus must be virtually injected into the bloodstream."[4] But not just any bodily fluid will do. Only blood and semen have been implicated in the transmission of the virus.[5]

That the virus is blood transmitted means first and foremost that, in countries with reasonable sanitation, groups at risk for the disease are clearly definable—more so than for virtually any other disease known—with 96 percent of cases having clearly demarcated modes of transmission and cause.[6] And now that blood supplies are screened with a test for antibodies to the AIDS virus, the number of these groups is indeed dropping. Hemophiliacs not already exposed and blood transfusion recipients are now no longer groups at risk.

Admittedly, in countries without adequate sanitation, blood-transmitted viruses like hepatitis B are rampant. If a population prone to cuts and abrasions bathes in the same water in which it bleeds and urinates, it will have blood-transmitted viruses dispersed widely through its membership. Perhaps a quarter of the Third World suffers from hepatitis B, which in the U.S. infects the same groups that are at risk for AIDS. Though hepatitis B has always been around, it has not been a threat to the general U.S. population and has never caused much social or government concern, even though for high-risk groups—basically gays and intravenous drug users—it is occasionally fatal. At the very least it causes weeks or months of debilitating pain and exhaustion, and threatens chronic recurrence and a greatly increased risk of liver cancer. Indeed, the very close epidemiological modeling of AIDS to hepatitis B was what first led medical investigators to hypothesize that AIDS was caused by a blood-transmitted virus, long before the virus itself was discovered.[7] Those who take Zaire as their model of AIDS contagion for the U.S. conveniently fail to weigh these facts or even mention them.[8] Fear of general, indiscriminate contagion by AIDS is unwarranted—though it makes for terrific press.

The July 1985 cover of *Life* informed the nation in three-inch red letters that "NOW NO ONE IS SAFE FROM AIDS." The magazine used as its allegedly compelling example a seemingly typical Pennsylvania family all but one of whose members has the disease. But it turns out that all those members with the disease were indeed in high-risk groups. The father was a hemophiliac, his wife had sex with him, and she conveyed the virus to a child in the process of giving birth. No one got the disease either mysteriously or through casual contact. The family example in fact was evidence *against* the article's generic contagion thesis. Equally irresponsible journalists, lobbyists, and elected officials have compared AIDS to air-borne viral diseases like influenza and the common cold.[9]

The case for general contagion cannot be made. In consequence government policy which is based on that fear is unwarranted. The extraordinary measures—including the suspension of civil liberties—which government might justifiably take, as in war, to prevent wholesale slaughter simply do not apply here. In particular, quarantining the class of AIDS-exposed persons in order to protect society from indiscriminate harm is unwarranted.

## HARM TO SELF

The disease's mode of contagion assures that those at risk are those whose actions contribute to their risk of infection, chiefly through intimate sexual contact and shared hypodermic needles.[10] In the transmission of AIDS, it is the general feature of self-exposure to contagion that makes direct coercive acts by government—like bathhouse closings—particularly inappropriate as efforts to abate the disease.

If independence—the ability to guide one's life by one's own lights to an extent compatible with a like ability on the part of others—is, as it is, a major value, one cannot respect that value while preventing people from putting themselves at risk through voluntary associations. Voluntary associations are star cases of people's acting in accordance with the principle of independence, for mutual consent guarantees that the "compatible extent" proviso of the principle is fulfilled. But the state and even the courts have not been very sensitive to the distinction between one's harming oneself and one's harming another—nor has the medical establishment.[11] It appears to all of them that a harm is a harm, a disease a disease, however caused or described. The moral difference, however, is enormous. Preventing a person from harming another is required by the principle of independence, but preventing someone from harming himself is incompatible with it. While no further justification is needed for the state to protect a person from others, a rather powerful justification is needed if the state is to be warranted in protecting a person from himself.

In the absence of such a justification, the state sometimes tries to split the moral difference and argues that state coercion *may* be used when the harm to others is remote and indirect. Such an argument from indirect harms runs to the effect that state-coerced use of, say, seatbelts and motorcycle helmets is warranted, for helmetless motorcycle crashes and seatbeltless car accidents harm even those not involved in the accidents, by raising everyone's insurance costs and burdening the public purse when victims end up in county hospitals. Here state coercion comes in through the backdoor.

This line of argument has been used with increasing frequency even by self-described liberals like New York's Governor Cuomo, and it is beginning to be heard in AIDS discussions. This is not surprising, for the cost of AIDS patient care from diagnosis to death is somewhere between $35,000 and $150,000. Private funds are often quickly exhausted, and the patient ends up on the dole—harming everyone, and so allegedly warranting state coercion of the means of possible AIDS transmission.

J. S. Mill's rule of thumb for appraising such appeals to indirect harms is exactly on target: an indirect harm counts toward justifying state coercion only when the harm grows large enough to be considered a violation of another person's right. This understanding of harm to others is necessary so that independence is not rendered nugatory and, *as a right,* is only outweighed by something comparable to it. Now, while it is nice if products (like insurance) are cheap and taxes low, the considered opinion of our society is not that one's rights have been violated when taxes or the price of milk goes up. Indeed, in the case of taxes, the considered opinion is cast as a constitutional provision. So arguments that smuggle coercion in through the backdoor of indirect harms are not successful.[12]

In general, heed should be given to Douglas' warning in his dissent to *Wyman* that the welfare state is gradually being allowed to buy up rights. In *Wyman* the Court ruled, among other horribles, that an indigent woman in accepting welfare for her child had simply waived her Fourth Amendment rights.[13] Actions infringing upon rights are most likely to go unnoticed or be misperceived, and so be most insidious when they are performed for an end that is good. Many addressing the AIDS crisis seem to be operating with bad motives. They generally can be easily spotted; appeals to consistency are usually enough to trip them up. But those with good motives yet anxious to do something quickly are those most likely to effect policies which destroy rights. The problem identified by Justice Douglas is part of a wider problem detected in Justice Brandeis' vindicated dissent in *Olmstead:* "Experience should teach us to be most on our guard to protect liberty when the Government's purposes are beneficent. Men born to freedom are naturally alert to repel invasion of their liberty by evil-minded rulers. The greatest dangers to liberty lurk in insidious encroachment by men of zeal, well-meaning but without understanding."[14]

## STATE PATERNALISM CONSIDERED

The important question remains whether AIDS warrants paternalistic state coercion to prevent those not exposed from harming themselves, through banning or highly regulating the means of possible viral transmission. Usually paternalistic arguments cannot be made sensible and consistent. For example: federal AIDS funding for FY 1986 in the House came with a paternalistic rider giving the surgeon general a power he already has—to close bathhouses, gay social institutions, if they are determined to facilitate the transmission or spread of the disease, which indeed they do. (So do parks and bedrooms.)[15] The sponsor of the rider argued that it was "a small step to help those who are unable or unwilling to help themselves."[16] Cast *so* baldly, the argument simply denies independence as a value. For it is consistent with the presumption that the majority gets both to determine what the good life is and to enforce it coercively. The argument could as well be used to justify compulsory religious conversion—those who are unable or unwilling to see the light are helped to see it.

## REASON ASSURED

Occasionally, to be sure, the case for paternalism can be made to work. One legitimate way to justify paternalistic coercion is to claim as warrant a lack of rationality on the part of an agent (say, a child). By "rationality" here I mean having relevant information and certain mental capacities, including the ability to reason from ends to means, but I do not presume that making the best possible assessment of means to an end is a requirement for rationality—error is compatible with rationality.

A presumption of an agent's rationality is a necessary condition for the very respect which is owed to his making his own decisions and guiding his life by them. Thus, paternalistic interference is warranted when a person is operating at risks which he is unable to assess as a result of diminished mental skills or lack of information. But education, not coercion, is the solution which is tailored to, and so appropriate for, such incapacities. Coercion in such cases is warranted only temporarily, to permit a check of whether a person indeed knows the risks he is taking. Thus (to borrow an example from Mill) it is justified to forcibly detain someone about to cross a structurally compromised bridge just long enough to inform him of its condition. Dilated to an extreme, this line of argument permits paternalistic labelling of possibly dangerous products and other means of placing a decision-maker in a reasonable position to make decisions for himself.

But far from justifying major paternalistic coercion of gay institutions, say, closing gay baths, the argument from rationality here indeed suggests that paternalistic arguments surrounding AIDS are not even being advanced in good faith. For though education is one of government's highest spending priorities, governments have made no serious attempt to educate people about medically informed risk of AIDS and of safe alternatives to high-risk sexual practices. It took the federal government five years even to put out bids for studies of ways in which programs of AIDS education might be effected.[17] The government then stalled in releasing the funds and finally barred their use for sexual messages that would be explicit enough to be effective. James Mason, the director of the CDC, which administered the grants, claimed, "We don't think that citizens care to be funding material that encourages gay sex lifestyles."[18]

Local governments in many cases have positively hampered private attempts at such education. In Los Angeles and Philadelphia, for instance, government sponsorship of private-sector distribution of safe-sex literature was denied or withdrawn when some officials branded the literature as pornography—neo-feminists take note. Thus one is probably justified in seeing as disingenuous any governmental argument for the coercion of gay institutions on paternalistic grounds. At most the argument from rationality warrants placing warning labels on baths as they are placed on cigarettes, the use of which also threatens death.[19]

## SELF-INDENTURED GAYS?

The other legitimate argument for paternalistic coercion is that one should be protected from ceding away the very conditions that enable one to be an independent agent. Thus one cannot legitimately contract to become a slave or to sign away rights to the fair administration of the enforcement of contracts or more generally the equitable administration of justice.

When dilated to the extreme, this line of justifying paternalistic coercion is used to support legislation mandating seat belt use: it's good for you, since it preserves you as an independent agent (though usually politicians cast the argument in terms of indirect harm to others). How does putting oneself at risk for AIDS weigh into this conceptual scheme? Does AIDS, invariably fatal in full-blown cases, rise to a level of seriousness to warrant on these paternalistic grounds a state-imposed bar to putting oneself at risk for it?

Admittedly, minimally good health is a central personal concern and its possession a necessary condition for being viewed seriously as an independent agent. So at first blush the AIDS case may seem relevantly similar to the contracting-to-slavery case. It differs, however, in two significant, severally decisive ways.

First, slavery *by definition* is a condition of lost independence. However, as with other venereal diseases, not every sexual encounter with a virus-exposed person exposes one to the AIDS virus, and even exposure to it is nowhere near a guarantee of actually contracting AIDS, since only some portion of those exposed actually get the disease.[20] Because the risk is high but the results not invariably catastrophic, putting oneself at risk for AIDS becomes less like contracting into slavery and more like being a race-car driver, mountain climber, or astronaut. In the absence of inevitability, the assessment of risk should be left to the individual, and indeed, as the examples of space flight, mountaineering, and race-car driving show, this is the considered standard of society as well. Deviations from the standard in other similar cases are likely to be motivated by something other than honest paternalistic concerns.

Second, it is hard to imagine even dispassionately and impartially that the momentary gain—say, some psychological thrill—from submitting to slavery could be reasonably balanced against the value *to the individual* of independence permanently lost. This differs significantly from "slavery" in sex play, where the thrill to the "slave" lies in continuous voluntary submission. To imagine the pure case, however, is as hard as trying to imagine (Mishima aside) someone seeing suicide as the culmination and chief organizing principle of his life rather than as an exit from a life that has become incapable of significance.

## SEX AND LIFE

However, an impartial examination of the role of sex in an individual's life would show that, far from having any imaginable value or at most a trifling one, sex, like health, is in general a central personal concern, and that for those people with a sex drive, addressing sex as central and appropriating it to oneself in some way or another is probably necessary to meaningful life. Or at least the lives of those like priests and nuns who renounce it altogether would support a belief that one's sexual choices are as central as any aspect of one's life. For vows of chastity are as central to their religious life—their most meaningful life—as any vows they take.

The centrality of sex as a value is indicated by the very vocabulary, or *lack* of it, that surrounds sex. Sex used to seem so central and yet seemingly frightening that for centuries, as Murray S. Davis has noted, only theologians and pornographers could discuss it.[21] Only the power of considerable and complex institutions was strong enough to preserve this gap in discourse and thought, a power so pervasive as to appear invisible. Thus when one looks at a newspaper's cavalcade of engagement and wedding photos, it never even crosses one's mind to think "gosh, what a slew of heterosexuals." When discourse about sex simply could not be avoided, the institutions were strong enough to fill the void with euphemisms so automatic and arcane as not to suggest a present presence—the language of "to have and to hold" and "blessed events". Even so some "things" were so powerful and frightening that they had to remain unnamed and unmentionable, to be dealt with not by appeal to and through institutional arrangements but only by extraordinary direct appeal to some allegedly preinstitutional fundament.

When now sex is discussed forthrightly, the terms are not merely those of desire but also those of need, and correctly so for two reasons. First, though sexual activity is not necessary to the continued biological existence of the individual as are some things that are called natural needs, it is a desire (unlike addictions) that is recurrent independently of its satisfaction—a natural object, not a product. Second, (like addictions and desires for the prerequisites of continued biological existence) its frustration tends to sponsor aggression. The pleasures of sex are not mere forgoable pleasures like the quest for sugar. To forgo them would itself have to be a major life commitment.

The centrality of sex to life means that it may have to be balanced with the value of continued independence—all the more so if independence is chiefly, like health, a generalized means to individuals' ends rather than an end in itself. Independence is not the only value of life, nor one prior to all other values. Further, central values are not equally central for all—some people indeed do not find sex very important and yet do not seem repressed. These people seem to be missing something, not to be morally lesser beings but somehow, like Gertrude Stein's Oakland, to have less there there. It would be silly for them to take high sexual risks, for the balance for them is so clearly tilted in one direction, and little would be lost if the state nudged them that way. But this tilt will in general not be so clear. The balancing in cases of conflicting personally affecting values is not a decision that the state could reasonably make across the board for all. The state is not capable of the probings of the soul that would be necessary for such a decision. Individuals, not the state, must make the difficult choices where values centrally affecting the self come in conflict.

That such choice falls to the individual is generally recognized where religious commitment and health come in conflict. The state cannot legitimately make the trade-offs that an informed adult will make between religious values and health by, say, coercing a person—for the sake of preserving his own independence—to have a blood transfusion against his belief that a transfusion, even a coerced one, will damn him for all eternity. Sexual attitudes and acts in accord with them are at least as central to a person as religious beliefs and acts, and so they too are not fit subjects of state coercion for the individual's own good, even when that good is the continued ability to make choices.

Governments that have written off the value of gay sex altogether by having made it illegal, largely on religious or other grounds that do not appeal to the causing of harms to others, should be viewed as especially suspect when they make paternalistic arguments on behalf of gays. For they have already clearly shown that they do not respect gays as independent beings.

## PUBLIC HEALTH AND TOTALITARIANISM

Arguments offered so far by the medical community against quarantines and bathhouse closings have largely adopted the terms of mere practicality, appealing to such facts as the large number of people involved, the permanence of the virus in those exposed, and the possibility that the sexual arena may simply shift away from bathhouses where some educational efforts may be possible.[22] I have suggested to the contrary that quarantines and closings should be opposed, not because they are impractical (though they may be), but because they are immoral.

Doctors tend to hold their unrefined view that health policy is merely a matter of strategy because they, not surprisingly, tend to see health itself as a trumping good, second to none in importance. This is a dangerous view, especially when coupled with their idea that health is an undifferentiated good. They fail to distinguish between my harming my health and my harming your health. Behind this oversight lies the further (sometimes unarticulated) presumption that you and I both are absorbed into and subordinated under something called the public health—a concept that tends to be analyzed in inverse proportion to the frequency with which it is used when trying to justify coercive acts.[23]

No literal sense exists in which there could be such a thing as a public health. To say the public has a health is like saying the number seven has a color: such a thing cannot have such a property. You have health or you lack it and I have health or lack it, because we each have a body with organs that function or do not function. But the public, an aggregate of persons similarly disposed as persons, has no such body of organs with functions which work or fail. There are, however, two frequently used metaphoric senses of public health that do have a reference: one is a legitimate use but largely inapplicable to the AIDS crisis; the other, when used normatively, is the pathway to totalitarianism.

The legitimate sense places public health in the same conceptual scheme as national defense and water purification. These are types of public goods in a technical sense—not what most people want and thus what democratic governments give them nor what tend to maximize by state means some type of good (pleasure, happiness, beauty), but what everyone wants but cannot get or get efficiently through voluntary arrangements and which thus require coercive coordinations from the state, so that *each* person gets what he wants. Thus, the private or voluntary arrangements of the market system do not seem likely to provide adequate national security, because a defense system that protects those who pay for it will also protect those who do not; everyone (reasonably enough) will tend to wait for someone else to pay for it, so that national security ends up not being purchased at all, or at least far less of it is purchased than everyone would agree to pay for if there were some means to manifest that agreement. The coercive actions of the state through taxation are then required to achieve the public good of national defense.

For exactly the same reason, the state is warranted in using coercive measures to drain swamps and provide vaccines against air-borne viruses. But the state is not warranted by appeal to the public good in coercing people to take the vaccine once it is freely available, for then *each* person is capable on his own—without further state coercion—of getting the protection from the disease he wants.[24] The mode of AIDS contagion makes it relevantly like this latter case. Each person on his own—without state coercion—can get the protection from the disease that he wants through his own actions, and indeed can get it by doing himself what he might be tempted to try to get the state to force upon others, say, avoiding bathhouses. As far as the good of protection is concerned, it can be achieved with no state coercion.

Is there a public good involved simply in reducing the size of the pool of AIDS-exposed people? I see just one, the one I argued for—the ability to have a robust sex life, without fear of death. But this good does not permit every form of state coercion. Not every public good motivates every form of coercion. The public goods mentioned so far could all be achieved by *equitable* coercion (e.g., universal conscription, taxation, compensated taking a property). When equitable coercion is the means, the public good can be quite slight and still be justified (as in government support for the arts). But when the coercion is inequitably dispersed, the public good served must be considerably more compelling than the means are intrusive. Thus, dispersed coercion against select individuals that involves restricted motion and physical suffering is warranted only by unqualifiedly necessary ends: when the individuals coerced have harmed others (as in punishment) or when it is necessary to the very existence of the country (as a partial military draft may be for a nation at defensive war). And thus too, the substantial good of civil rights protections is advanced only through the considerably weak intrusion of barring the desire of employers to indulge in whimsical and arbitrary hiring practices. The public good of an unencumbered sex life, however, fails this weighted ends-to-means test if the means are a dispersedly coerced sex life. For the intrusion and the good are on a par—on the one hand encumbered sex, on the other unencumbered sex. And so it appears that only equitably coercive means are available to achieve the end of reducing the pool of AIDS-exposures—taxation for preventive measures like vaccine development, but not coercive measures that affect some but not others, like closing bathhouses or banning or regulating sex practices selectively.

Those who do not find the possibility of carefree sex a public good—probably the bulk of those actually calling for state coercion—will find no legitimate help in the notion of public health for state coercion here. Those who do will find it justifies only equitable measures.

The other metaphoric sense of public health takes the medical model of the healthy body and unwittingly transfers it to society—the body politic. But this transfer (when it has any content at all) bears hidden and extremely dangerous assumptions. Plato in the *Republic* was the first thinker systematically to press the analogy of the good society to the healthy body. The state stands to the citizenry and its good, as a doctor stands to the body and its health.

Society, so it is claimed, is an organism in which people are mere functional parts, ones that are morally good and emotionally well-off only insofar as they act for the sake of the organism. The analogy is alive and well today and calling out for extreme measures now: "Much as a physician treating one organ must consider the effects on the entire organism, a public official has the community as the patient and must attend to all factors in seeking the greatest overall good."[25] On this view, the individual, however harmed, cannot fulfill his role. A damaged organ, the spleen for example, can be, to continue the analogy, simply cut out. By comparison, quarantines and coerced sex lives might appear as mild remedies on this analogy. But something has been lost here—persons.

The medical model of society is the conceptual engine of totalitarianism. It presumes not that the goods of individuals are final goods but that individuals are good only as they serve some good beyond themselves, that of the state or body politic. The state exists not for the sake of individuals—to protect and enhance their prospects as rational agents—but rather individuals exist for the state and are subordinated to society as a whole, the worth of which is to be determined only from the perspective of the whole. The individual, thus, is not an end in himself but exists for some social good—whether that good be some hoped-for overall happiness or some social idea—like purity, wholesomeness, decency, or "traditional values." Unconscious obedient servicing is dressed up as virtue.

The worst political consequence of the AIDS crisis would not be simply the further degradation of gays. Gay internments would not be anything new to this century. In the European internment camps of World War II, gypsies wore brown triangle identifying badges, Jehovah's Witnesses purple, political prisoners red, race defilers black, and gays pink triangles. Worse than the further degradation of gays in America would be a general, and not easily reversed, shift in the nation's center of gravity toward the medical model and away from the position, acknowledged in America's constitutional tradition, that individuals have broad yet determinate claims against both general welfare and social ideals. The consequence of such a shift would be that people would come to be treated essentially as resources, sometimes expendable—a determination no less frightening when made by a combined father, colonel, and doctor than by a fearful mob.

## NOTES

1. See particularly the CDC's guidelines for preventing transmission in the workplace, "Recommendations for Preventing Transmission of Infection with Human T-Lymphotrophic Virus Type III/Lymphadenopathy-Associated Virus in the Workplace," *Morbidity and Mortality Weekly Report (MMWR)*, 34, no. 45 (November 15, 1985), pp. 682–95.
2. *Washington Post*, October 19, 1985, p. A12; *The Advocate*, no. 442 (March 18, 1996), p. 14.

3. *Washington Post,* October 13, 1985, p. B8. If a *Los Angeles Times* poll of 2,300 Americans is to be believed, the country indeed is ready for extreme measures: 51 percent favored quarantines of people with AIDS, 48 percent closing gay bathhouses, 42 percent closing gay bars, and 14 percent tattooing people with AIDS. Twenty-eight percent thought AIDS was God's punishment for homosexuals, and 23 percent thought AIDS victims were "getting what they deserve" (December 19, 1985, p. I1). For discussions of civil liberties issues raised by the AIDS crisis, see, for example, "AIDS and Individual Rights," *New York Times,* December 15, 1985, p. E6; and "Quarantines Considered to Combat AIDS," *Washington Post,* December 16, 1985, pp. A1, 26–27.
4. Mathilde Krim, "AIDS: The Challenge to Science and Medicine," *AIDS: The Emerging Ethical Dilemmas, A Hastings Center Report Special Supplement,* 1985, p. 4.
5. "Recommendations for Preventing Transmission," p. 682.
6. "Strictly heterosexual adult men and women who cannot be classified as belonging to any high-risk group" constitute only 1 percent of AIDS cases, and this figure has been constant; Krim, "AIDS," p. 6. See also Colin Norman, "AIDS Trends," *Science* 230 (November 29, 1985), p. 1021.
7. For a comparison of AIDS virus transmission with that of the hepatitis B virus, see "Recommendations for Preventing Transmission," pp. 682–83. The close modeling of the two viruses continues to be the chief basis of the CDC's guidelines for AIDS prevention.
8. For example, Krim, "AIDS," p. 6. The much-reported finding that AIDS occurs in Zaire in equal numbers between men and women weighs no more in favor of the thesis that heterosexual transmission is the chief cause of African AIDS cases than that lack of sanitation is the chief cause.

    Alternatively, the widespread practices in central Africa of female circumcision, excision, and infibulation and attendent consequences for sexual behavior may account for the high incidence of AIDS in central African women (see "AIDS in Africa," *Science* 231 [January 17, 1986], 203). If so, again the circumstances of blood-borne contagion in Africa are strongly disanalogous to those in America.
9. For an irresponsible analogy of AIDS to air-borne disease, see Dr. Richard Restak's widely reprinted op-ed piece "Worry about Survival of Society First; Then AIDS Victims' Rights," *Washington Post,* September 8, 1986, p. C1. For claims of casual transmission, see Tom Johnson, 1986, "Congressman AIDS," *Los Angeles* 1986, pp. 125 ff., especially 199. For a history of irresponsible and hysteria-pandering reportage in the mass media, see William Check, "Public Education on AIDS: Not Only the Media's Responsibility," *AIDS: The Emerging Ethical Dilemmas,* pp. 27–31. For a readable social history of the disease, see Dennis Altman, *AIDS in the Mind of America* (New York: Doubleday, 1986).
10. A small exception is those whose well-being and life chances are already substantially at the mercy of the person who infects them—newborns of

infected mothers. For this set of cases social policy should be whatever it already is for cases of parents who pass fatal congenital disease to their children.

11. For instance, Mervyn F. Silverman, former Director of Health for San Francisco, shows no cognizance of the distinction in his argument for his unsuccessful 1984 attempt to close that city's bathhouses: Mervyn F. Silverman and Deborah B. Silverman, "AIDS and the Threat to Public Health," *AIDS: The Emerging Ethical Dilemmas*, pp. 21–22.

12. Whether it is legitimate for the state to condition, for instance, motorcyclists' access to county hospitals upon the wearing of helmets cannot be determined independently of an assessment of the arguments for such free health care in the first place. The arguments advanced in R. Mohr, "AIDS, Gay Life, State Coercion," *Raritan: A Quarterly Review* 6, no. 1 (Summer 1986), pp. 50–58, for AIDS patient funding bar any such conditioning of relief upon cost-reducing conformity.

    A wife who contracts AIDS from a bisexual husband does not have a right that has been violated by the bathhouse where he may have been AIDS-exposed. Rather if she has a legitimate plaint, it is against the direct harm caused by the husband or against the institution of marriage itself if it has kept her in a position of enforced ignorance. But it should be remembered that traditional marriage vows pledge the participants to joint risk taking and place commercial and medical risks on a par. The institution of marriage itself, then, acknowledges what is independently true: it is as little a good reason to shut down bathhouses to protect "innocent" wives as it is to shut down stock markets to spare them lost spousal income.

    Further, it is wholly unfair to coerce one institution because of the patent immoralities of another. The immoralities which occur within marriage (lying, cheating, promise-breaking, willful ignorance) or which are endemic to it (enforced ignorance, indenture) cannot ground the coercion of gay bathhouses. For an excellent discussion of the procedural and substantive abuses inherent in traditional marriage contracts, see Sara Ann Ketchum, "Liberalism and Marriage Law," in *Feminism and Philosophy*, ed. Mary Vetterling-Braggin (Totowa, NJ: Littlefield, Adams, 1977), pp. 247–76.

13. Wyman v. James, 400 U.S. 309, 328 (1971), J. Douglas, dissenting: "The central question is whether the government by force of its largesse has the power to 'buy up' rights guaranteed by the Constitution. But for the assertion of her constitutional right, Barbara James in this case would have received the welfare benefit."

14. Olmstead v. U.S., 277 U.S. 438, 479 (1969).

15. A directive from New York's Governor Cuomo mandated in late 1985 the closing of public accommodations where oral or anal sex occur. But the distinction between a public accommodation and a private dwelling, given the nature of the disease, is medically irrelevant. So is the distinction between providing for profit a location for sex and providing one for free.

Public accommodations, private clubs, parks, and bedrooms—even marital ones—are medically all equally suspect. The line of thought that has led to bathhouse closings, if carried out consistently, would require shutting down realtor's offices that make a profit from selling homes to gays.

Further, the directive curiously enough omits banning vaginal sex. Though there is some reason to believe that anal sex is extremely risky, there is no evidence that vaginal penetrations are any less likely a mode of transmitting the virus than oral sex. Cuomo's directive disingenuously re-criminalizes sodomy in New York (*Washington Post,* October 31, 1985, p. A1). New York City's corporation counsel has argued that restrictions on oral and anal sex do not discriminate against gays because they also apply to non-gays (*New York Times,* December 15, 1985, sec. 4, p. 6). One could as well argue that a law against sleeping under bridges does not discriminate against the poor because it also bars the wealthy from sleeping there.

In applying the directive both the governor and New York City's Mayor Koch claimed that their acts were not to be construed in any way as assaulting the gay community. But instead of showing good faith in this regard by doing something that would be politically unpopular (like first shutting down, say, a marriage with an AIDS-exposed hemophiliac member), they chose instead to shut down as their very first target a central part of gay male mythology, the notorious private membership sex club The Mineshaft (*Washington Post,* November 8, 1985, p. A7). Subsequently, New York state's health commissioner reported that his "investigators will enter hotel rooms if necessary to stop sexual activities linked to the spread of AIDS" (*Washington Post,* November 18, 1985, p. A4). His office has assured gays that the free enterprise system will preclude discrimination against gays in hotel accommodations (*Washington Blade,* November 22, 1985, p. 12). New York, like forty-eight other states, has no legislation that would bar such discrimination against gays.

16. *Washington Blade,* October 4, 1985, p. 1.
17. *Federal Register* 50, no. 143 (July 25, 1985), p. 30298.
18. James Mason, *The Advocate,* no. 437 (January 7, 1986), p. 20.
19. Whether warning labels *should* be placed on bathhouses turns on considerations of consistency: some dangerous products are labelled, others not. What gets labelled should not depend on ideology, prejudice, or politics. Getting right on this point is particularly important in the case of bathhouses, since such labelling, even when carried out in good faith, will have the side effect of saying to most people that gay sex is bad. The relevant question, one for which I do not have an answer, is whether bathhouses present the same degree of risk to the user as other products that are already so labelled.
20. Krim, "AIDS," pp. 4, 5.
21. Murray S. Davis, 1983, *Smut: Erotic Reality/Obscene Ideology* (Chicago: University of Chicago Press, 1983). Davis' book offers an excellent phenomenology of sex acts and an intriguing account of the conservative mind on matters sexual.

22. For examples, see Kenneth H. Mayer, "The Epidemiological Investigation of AIDS," *AIDS: The Emerging Ethical Dilemmas*, p. 15 (against both quarantines and bath closings); and Silverman and Silverman, "AIDS and the Threat to Public Health," p. 21 (against quarantines).

23. For a signal example, see "Additional Recommendations to Reduce Sexual and Drug Abuse-Related Transmission of HTLV-III/LAV," *MMWR* 35, no. 10 (March 14, 1986), p. 154, recommending the closing of bathhouses "on public health grounds." No definition, elaboration, or analysis is offered of the notion "public health." The recommendation stands in marked contrast to the CDC's employment recommendations ("Recommendations for Preventing Transmission"), for which elaborate analysis and argumentation are offered.

24. The Supreme Court's leading medical case, Jacobson v. Massachusetts, 197 U.S. 11 (1905) (upholding criminal penalties—a five-dollar fine—for refusing a free vaccination), because it leaves the notion public health wholly unanalyzed, contradicts its own declaration that the principle of independence is overridden only by public goods on a par with national defense. The upheld law's resort to criminal penalties for a person refusing the vaccine rather than to coercing directly the taking of the vaccine shows that the law is incoherent as a measure aimed to protect against indiscriminate harms.

25. Silverman and Silverman, "AIDS and the Threat to Public Health," p. 22.